ADOLESCENT MEDICINE: STATE OF THE ART REVIEWS

Sports Medicine and Sports Injuries

GUEST EDITORS

Albert C. Hergenroeder, MD

Rebecca A. Demorest, MD

April 2015 • Volume 26 • Number 1

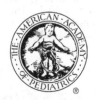

ADOLESCENT MEDICINE:
STATE OF THE ART REVIEWS
April 2015
Editor: Carrie Peters
Marketing Manager: Marirose Russo
Production Manager: Shannan Martin
eBook Developer: Houston Adams

Volume 26, Number 1
ISBN 978-1-58110-886-6
ISSN 1934-4287
MA0729
SUB1006

The recommendations in this publication do not indicate an exclusive course of treatment or serve as a standard of medical care. Variations, taking into account individual circumstances, may be appropriate.

Statements and opinions expressed are those of the author and not necessarily those of the American Academy of Pediatrics.

Products and Web sites are mentioned for informational purposes only. Inclusion in this publication does not imply endorsement by the American Academy of Pediatrics. The American Academy of Pediatrics is not responsible for the content of the resources mentioned in this publication. Web site addresses are as current as possible but may change at any time.

Every effort has been made to ensure that the drug selection and dosage set forth in this text are in accordance with the current recommendations and practice at the time of publication. It is the responsibility of the health care provider to check the package insert of each drug for any change in indications and dosage and for added warnings and precautions.

Adolescent Medicine: State of the Art Reviews is published three times per year by the American Academy of Pediatrics, 141 Northwest Point Blvd, Elk Grove Village, IL 60007-1019. Periodicals postage paid at Arlington Heights, IL.

POSTMASTER: Send address changes to American Academy of Pediatrics, Department of Marketing and Publications, Attn: AM:STARs, 141 Northwest Point Blvd, Elk Grove Village, IL 60007-1019.

Subscriptions: Subscriptions to Adolescent Medicine: State of the Art Reviews (AM:STARs) are provided to members of the American Academy of Pediatrics' Section on Adolescent Health as part of annual section membership dues. All others, please contact the AAP Customer Service Center at 866/843-2271 (7:00 am–5:30 pm Central Time, Monday–Friday) for pricing and information.

Adolescent Medicine: State of the Art Reviews

Official Journal of the American Academy of Pediatrics
Section on Adolescent Health

EDITORS-IN-CHIEF

VICTOR C. STRASBURGER, MD, Distinguished Professor Emeritus of Pediatrics, Founding Chief, Division of Adolescent Medicine, University of New Mexico, School of Medicine, Albuquerque, New Mexico

DONALD E. GREYDANUS, MD, Dr HC (ATHENS), Professor & Founding Chair, Department of Pediatric & Adolescent Medicine, Western Michigan University Homer Stryker M.D. School of Medicine, Kalamazoo, Michigan

GUEST EDITORS

ALBERT C. HERGENROEDER, MD, Baylor College of Medicine, Texas Children's Hospital, Department of Pediatrics, Section of Adolescent Medicine and Sports Medicine, Houston, Texas

REBECCA A. DEMOREST, MD, Pediatric and Young Adult Sports Medicine, Webster Orthopedics, Dublin and San Ramon, California

CONTRIBUTORS

JON ALMQUIST, ATC, VATL, ITAT, Fairfax Family Practice Comprehensive Concussion Center, Fairfax, Virginia

ROBERTA H. ANDING, MS, RD/LD, CDE, CSSD, Baylor College of Medicine, Texas Children's Hospital, Department of Pediatrics, Section of Adolescent Medicine and Sports Medicine, Houston, Texas

HOLLY J. BENJAMIN, MD, Associate Professor of Pediatrics and Orthopedic Surgery, Director of Primary Care Sports Medicine, University of Chicago, Chicago, Illinois

DAVID BERNHARDT, MD, University of Wisconsin School of Medicine and Public Health, Madison, Wisconsin

NICOLE T. BONIQUIT, MD, Resident Physician, Department of Pediatrics, University of Chicago, Chicago, Illinois

JOEL S. BRENNER, MD, MPH, Medical Director, Children's Hospital of The King's Daughters' Sports Medicine Program, Director, Division of Sports Medicine and Adolescent Medicine, Associate Professor of Pediatrics, Eastern Virginia Medical School, Children's Specialty Group, PLLC, Norfolk, Virginia

SUSANNAH M. BRISKIN, MD, Assistant Professor of Pediatrics, Division of Pediatric Sports Medicine, Rainbow Babies and Children's Hospital, Cleveland, Ohio

ALISON BROOKS, MD, MPH, Assistant Professor, Departments of Orthopedics and Pediatrics, Division of Sports Medicine, University of Wisconsin–Madison, Madison, Wisconsin

GABRIEL BROOKS, PT, DPT, MTC, SCS, Baylor College of Medicine, Texas Children's Hospital, Department of Pediatrics, Section of Adolescent Medicine and Sports Medicine, Houston, Texas

JOSEPH N. CHORLEY, MD, Baylor College of Medicine, Texas Children's Hospital, Department of Pediatrics, Section of Adolescent Medicine and Sports Medicine, Houston, Texas

MARY JANE DE SOUZA, PhD, The Pennsylvania State University, University Park, Pennsylvania

LEDA A. GHANNAD, MD, Pediatric Sports Medicine Fellow, Division of Orthopaedic Surgery and Sports Medicine, Ann & Robert H. Lurie Children's Hospital of Chicago, Chicago, Illinois

JORGE E. GOMÉZ, MD, MS, Baylor College of Medicine, Texas Children's Hospital, Section of Adolescent Medicine and Sports Medicine, Houston, Texas

ANDREW J. GREGORY, MD, Associate Professor of Orthopedics, Pediatrics and Neurosurgery, Vanderbilt University School of Medicine, Nashville, Tennessee

MARK E. HALSTEAD, MD, Washington University School of Medicine, St. Louis Children's Hospital, St. Louis, Missouri

ELISABETH S. HASTINGS, MPH, RD, CSSD, LD, Instructor, Baylor College of Medicine, Department of Pediatrics, Section of Adolescent Medicine and Sports Medicine, Houston, Texas

ALBERT C. HERGENROEDER, MD, Baylor College of Medicine, Texas Children's Hospital, Department of Pediatrics, Section of Adolescent Medicine and Sports Medicine, Houston, Texas

AMANDA WEISS KELLY, MD, Division Chief, Pediatric Sports Medicine, UH Case Medical Center and Rainbow Babies and Children's Hospital, Program Director, Pediatric Sports Medicine, UH Case Medical Center, Associate Professor, Pediatrics, CWRU School of Medicine, Cleveland, Ohio

CHRIS G. KOUTURES, MD, Pediatric and Sports Medicine Specialist, Private Practice, Anaheim Hills, California

CYNTHIA R. LABELLA, MD, Associate Professor of Pediatrics, Division of Orthopaedic Surgery and Sports Medicine, Ann & Robert H. Lurie Children's Hospital of Chicago, Chicago, Illinois

MICHELE LABOTZ, MD, InterMed Sports Medicine, South Portland, Maine

GREGORY L. LANDRY, MD, University of Wisconsin–Madison School of Medicine and Public Health, Madison, Wisconsin

KATHLEEN A. LINZMEIER, MD, Pediatric Resident, University of California–Irvine, Children's Hospital of Orange County Pediatric Residency Program, Orange, California

KELSEY LOGAN, MD, MPH, Associate Professor of Pediatrics and Internal Medicine, University of Cincinnati College of Medicine, Director, Division of Sports Medicine, Cincinnati Children's Hospital Medical Center, Cincinnati, Ohio

ANDREW R. PETERSON, MD, MSPH, Assistant Professor, University of Iowa Carver College of Medicine, Stead Family Department of Pediatrics, Iowa City, Iowa

KEVIN D. WALTER, MD, Medical College of Wisconsin, Children's Hospital of Wisconsin, Milwaukee, Wisconsin

ANDREW M. WATSON, MD, MS, Clinical Instructor, Departments of Orthopedics and Pediatrics, Division of Sports Medicine, University of Wisconsin–Madison, Madison, Wisconsin

CONTENTS

Most team physicians at the youth and high school levels and even some team physicians at the collegiate level do not have formal training in sports medicine, but they all share a keen interest in the health and well-being of athletes. This article summarizes the duties and responsibilities of the team physician, game preparation and handling of on-the-field emergencies, and duties of the team physician related to drug testing. It reviews the legal guidelines for communication of protected health information and for medical practice outside the physician's home state when the physician travels with the team.

The preparticipation physical evaluation (PPE) is a required component of sports participation for many young athletes and often is their only nonacute contact with the health care system. Unfortunately, recent evidence indicates that many physicians are not comfortable with the PPE and are not aware of resources that will assist in the quality and efficiency of these examinations. This article reviews the most pertinent issues to address during the PPE and examines topics of current interest, including cardiac evaluation, concussion, and screening for sickle cell trait. The current recommended history and physical forms are included.

Sport-related concussion is a common injury in the adolescent athlete. Despite increasing awareness in both the lay public and medical communities, it still is too often unreported or missed, and management strategies remain quite varied among medical practitioners. Understanding how to diagnose and manage concussions is an important component for any physician who cares for pediatric and adolescent patients. If diagnosed and treated appropriately, concussions generally completely resolve; however, delayed diagnosis and improper management can result in prolonged recovery and life-altering complications. Concussions cannot be prevented, but there are many strategies that may decrease the incidence.

Adolescence is a period of rapid musculoskeletal growth, and with this growth comes increased susceptibility to injuries unique to this age group. The purpose of this article is to focus on those musculoskeletal conditions that necessitate early diagnosis and management to improve outcomes and decrease morbidity. Topics discussed include the diagnosis and management of upper and lower extremity ligamentous injuries, neurovascular injuries, traumatic fractures, stress fractures, and other high-risk bone lesions.

Youth sports provide many benefits, including learning lifelong physical activity skills, peer socialization, teamwork, leadership, improving self-esteem, and allowing young athletes to have fun. Unfortunately, sports for teenagers have changed from adolescent-driven games and activities to adult-driven activities. Now a group of teenagers is less likely to congregate after school or on a weekend to play in a "pick-up" game, as was common practice in the 1970s and 1980s. Along with the paradigm shift of adults becoming the driving force came increased pressure to participate at a high level, specialize in a single sport early, and play year-round, sometimes on multiple teams. This has led to an increase in overuse injuries and overtraining. This article reviews the scope of the problem of overuse and overtraining injuries, discusses common overuse injuries using a case-based format, presents a few overtraining issues, and offers general prevention recommendations.

Musculoskeletal disorders and diseases are the leading causes of pain, physical disability, and physician visits throughout the world. Yet there is a well-documented disparity between the frequency of medical visits for musculoskeletal injuries and the preparedness of many physicians to adequately care for these injuries in office practice. This article reviews the key principles of primary and secondary care for musculoskeletal injuries and provides recommendations to assist the physician in the management of the young athlete.

Exercise has demonstrated benefits for young women. However, a subgroup of young women exercises to the extent that the high-energy expenditure of their exercise is not balanced with adequate calories, thereby resulting in an energy deficit. This energy deficit, when chronic, can have adverse health consequences. When the chronic energy deficit involves menstrual dysfunction and low bone mass, it is referred to as the *female athlete triad*. This article discusses the pathophysiology of the female athlete triad, its clinical presentations, and a treatment approach to address it.

The significant time commitments and physical requirements of dance during the adolescent growth and development period can place unique stressors for injury and disability. Adolescent medicine specialists who combine an understanding of dance demands with particular anticipatory guidance recommendations can become outstanding resources for adolescent dancers and their families. Appreciation of different dance disciplines, popular movements or positions, and types of dance classes and performances while addressing common nutritional issues, development concerns, and particular anatomic predispositions to both overuse and acute injury will enable the adolescent specialist to directly and effectively communicate dance-specific recommendations and injury management information.

equipment, specialty food, and a routine physical examination that includes immunizations, infection prophylaxis, and updated prescriptions are necessary. Adequate time for acclimatization, jet lag, and training as well as handling unanticipated delays must be accounted for in the travel schedule. Above all, the general health and readiness of an adolescent athlete to compete is highly dependent on proper hydration and balanced nutrition. Maintenance of a proper balance requires discipline and lifestyle alterations tailored to each athlete's individual needs based on the athlete's general health, performance goals, and type of sport. The traveling athlete faces additional challenges in order to maintain adequate hydration and nutrition necessary to support peak performance.

Preface

Sports Medicine and Sports Injuries

Welcome to a whirlwind of up-to-date, practical, evidence-based information on teens and sports for the adolescent physician.

With more than 30 million US children and teenagers participating in both recreational and team sports, the adolescent physician is faced with many medical, parental, and community questions and concerns regarding the diagnosis, treatment, and prevention of youth sports injuries. Whether a teenager is a competitive travel soccer player, recreational rock climber, or outdoor explorer, or simply hangs out with friends at the skate park, salient advice on physical activity, nutrition, injury, and prevention of injury is important for all adolescents.

This issue of *AM:STARs* tackles many pertinent concerns about today's young athletes. Starting with the preseason preparticipation physical evaluation (PPE), this issue discerns the most important topics to address regarding healthy sports participation. It attends to the ECG debate, discusses concerns regarding sickle cell trait, and outlines potential issues for the special needs athlete. With chronic overuse sports injuries taking center stage over many acute sports injuries, this issue details both the acute and chronic injuries seen in active teenagers and provides advice on how to best diagnose and manage them. The newest findings regarding sports concussions, their management, and return to play guidelines will supply physicians with up-to-date information on this current and evolving field. Issues regarding performance and dance medicine are expertly discussed along with the signs of overtraining and burnout in young athletes.

The safety, availability, and efficacy of popular performance-enhancing supplements (PES), including nutritional supplements, anabolic steroids, human growth hormone (HGH), and creatine, are addressed. We discuss the recognition and treatment of psychological stresses and provide an overview of mental health in today's young athletes. Bone health and the female athlete triad, along with nutritional, safety, and health recommendations for traveling athletes, are reviewed and practical current guidelines are provided.

For those taking an active role in managing teen athletes, this issue addresses the role of the team physician, including the physician's duties and responsibilities, game preparation and handling of on-the-field emergencies, and duties related to drug testing. It reviews legal guidelines for communication of protected health information and for medical practice outside of the physician's home state when the physician travels with the team. Ongoing challenges related to the popular "extreme" teen sports and the principles of rehabilitation when returning athletes to sports after injury are explored in detail.

We generously thank all of the authors for their tireless efforts in adhering to tight timelines and providing such excellent detailed manuscripts. We thank the American Academy of Pediatrics (AAP) Council on Sports Medicine and Fitness (COSMF) and the Section on Adolescent Health (SOAH) for supporting our efforts. We also thank Carrie Peters and the AAP for giving us the opportunity to share our passion with the adolescent community.

We hope that this issue gives you as much academic information as it does practical advice for you to use in your office on a daily basis. Our goal was to make this issue readable, worthwhile, and transferrable to everyday life for you—the physician, your adolescent athlete patients, and their parents. We want to supply you with pertinent information so all teens have the ability to safely engage in any sort of physical activity, whether it be competitive play or pure recreational adventure, so sports and physical activity become a doable reality for them for the rest of their lives. Let's keep them safe, healthy, strong, and knowledgeable so they can keep on playing!

Rebecca A. Demorest, MD, FAAP
Pediatric and Young Adult Sports Medicine
Webster Orthopedics
Dublin and San Ramon, California

Albert C. Hergenroeder, MD, FAAP
Baylor College of Medicine
Texas Children's Hospital
Department of Pediatrics
Section of Adolescent Medicine and Sports
Medicine
Houston, Texas

Adolesc Med 026 (2015) 1–17

Being a Team Doctor

Jorge E. Goméz, MD, MS[a]*; Gregory L. Landry, MD[b]

[a]Baylor College of Medicine, Texas Children's Hospital, Section of Adolescent Medicine and Sports Medicine, Houston, Texas; [b]University of Wisconsin–Madison School of Medicine and Public Health, Madison, Wisconsin

THE TEAM PHYSICIAN

Qualifications

The team physician ideally should have formal training in sports medicine and have completed either a primary care or orthopedic sports medicine fellowship. However, most team physicians are primary care physicians or orthopedic surgeons who have not completed a sports medicine fellowship; they simply have a strong interest in caring for athletes. Many of these team physicians regularly participate in sports medicine continuing education. The team physician should be board certified in a specialty (eg, pediatrics, family medicine) and should maintain cardiopulmonary resuscitation (CPR) certification.

Duties and Responsibilities

The duties and responsibilities of the team physician will vary depending on the practice setting (Table 1).

Liability

Under most circumstances the team physician, even one who does not receive payment, is not protected by the particular state's Good Samaritan laws. Therefore, it is the physician's responsibility to contact his[†] insurance carrier and obtain liability coverage for any activities he will perform as the team physician.

---

*Corresponding author
E-mail address: jxgomez@texaschildrens.org

[†]The information and advice in this article apply equally to physicians of both sexes. To indicate this, we have chosen to alternate between masculine and feminine pronouns throughout the article.

Table 1
Duties and responsibilities of the team physician

Familiarity with medical policies set forth by a governing body (league, organization, federation)
Familiarity with policies and clinical guidelines set forth by expert panels and organizations regarding
    issues in sports medicine
Responsibility for ensuring that members of the team (coaches, trainers, other physicians, players)
    adhere to recommended guidelines
Game and event medical preparation
Diagnosis and treatment of injuries and sport-related conditions

---

THE SPORTS MEDICINE TEAM

Care of an athlete, both for prevention and treatment, involves the coordinated efforts of several partners, each with unique skills and interests. The team physician is primarily responsible for coordinating this care between the athlete, the athlete's parents and coaches, the team's athletic trainers, and other health care professionals involved in the athlete's care.

The keys to coordinating care are good communication and having protocols in place not only for how injuries should be managed but also how information will be provided to coaches, parents, and the media.[1] Communication of information regarding injured athletes is governed by laws applicable to all confidential health information, and the team physician not only needs to be aware of these laws but also is responsible for ensuring that appropriate safeguards are in place, including signed *consent to treat* forms and authorizations to release medical information to essential parties (parents, coaches, and other medical staff).

The team physician should be clear about her responsibilities with regard to making *return to play* decisions. In situations in which a formal or written contractual agreement exists between the school or team and the physician, the team physician may be primarily responsible for return to play decisions, whereas in less formal arrangements, these decisions may be made by the physician directly treating the athlete, whether it is the team physician or the athlete's treating physician.

Parents

The team physician should introduce himself as early as possible to the parents of the group being cared for, particularly in school and youth team settings. This introduction is ideally done in a setting, such as a booster club meeting for a high school, where most of the involved parents are present. It also can be achieved via handouts given to parents, such as the information packet parents must read and sign before the student participates in athletics. If possible the team physician should convey the following points to parents: (1) his primary responsibility is to ensure the health and safety of the athlete; (2) he will adhere to the highest standards of athletic care; and (3) he will not allow his judgment to be clouded by team metrics, such as how many players are available to play, what the team's win/loss record is, how important the next game is, or how valuable the player is to the team.

The team physician should remain in close contact with parents during a player's injury and recovery.

Athletic Trainers

Athletic trainers are the team physician's direct extension in providing ongoing athlete care. The team physician should be able to rely on the athletic trainer for support in daily surveillance and treatment activities. Any concerns regarding adherence to standards of care or differences in approach to injury management should be immediately and explicitly addressed by the team physician, with an attitude of respect for the athletic trainer's expertise and experience. For schools that do not have athletic trainers, the coaches usually act as the medical liaisons between the player, parent, and physician. In these settings the team physician can define her role, such as covering live events, and the follow-up of injuries can be made on a case-by-case basis.

Coaches

Coaches are an integral part of the athlete's health care team.[2] Most coaches willingly and gladly leave medical decisions to the team's athletic trainer and team physician. When coaches seem to be making medical decisions on behalf of the athlete that, to the team physician, are counterproductive to the athlete's treatment and recovery, the best approach is to respectfully discuss the rationale of the treatment plan with the coaching staff, to answer any questions they may have, and to try to better incorporate the coaches into the treatment plan. Situations in which such factual discussions have no effect on a coach's inclination to subvert or ignore the treatment plan call for involvement of administrative personnel.

Other members of the health care team may include sports dietitians, sports psychologists, strength and conditioning specialists, and other physician specialists. It is important for the team physician to be familiar with the expertise of each of these physician in order to properly and fully utilize their talents in caring for injured athletes and keeping athletes healthy. The team physician should insist on timely communication with these specialists regarding an athlete's illness or injury.

PREPAREDNESS

Game Day Planning

Duties of the team physician, whether preparing for a single game, tournament, or mass participation event, are listed in Table 2. Details of preparation will vary depending on whether the team physician is responsible for a mass participation event, a tournament involving many teams, or a single contest. This is especially important for teams that do not have trainers.

As part of the team physician's preparation for a game or tournament, getting to know the names of the individual members of the team or teams covered, especially key players or injured players, is of great benefit not only for enhancing reporting of injuries but also for promoting communication regarding treatment effectiveness and recovery from injuries.

The Field Bag

Table 3 lists the supplies and equipment recommended for the team physician covering athletic events. Each physician will have a personal preference and thus may stock the bag slightly differently according to that preference as well as to the demands of the particular event.[3]

The medications stocked in the field bag will also depend on the group of athletes being cared for (eg, master's athletes, Special Olympics athletes).[4] The contents of the field bag should be reviewed on a weekly basis to ensure adequate supplies and to keep the bag organized. A disorganized bag will only add to confusion, hesitation, and delay in treatment in emergency situations. A recent survey indicated that 68% of team physicians did not carry an inventory list in their bag.[5]

Table 2
Athletic event preparation

Be familiar with the types of injuries and emergency situations that may arise in a particular athletic setting.
Have all equipment and supplies on hand to deal with common and emergency conditions.
Have proper training in recognizing and managing sport-specific acute injuries and illnesses.
Be aware of rules and laws governing specific events and event-related conditions.
Ensure that all necessary personnel will be available (athletic trainers, therapists, nurses, emergency medical personnel, physicians, record-keepers, equipment managers, personnel to manage and direct athletes, emergency medical personnel, security personnel) before, during, and after the event.
Predetermine lines of communication and responsibilities to be used in emergency situations.
Make whatever preparations are necessary in advance of an athletic event to ensure that personnel are well informed of event-specific rules, conditions, security warnings, and deadlines, through direct communication (e-mail) and pre-event meetings.

Table 3
Team physician's field bag

Administrative
  Cell phone
  Emergency contact numbers
  Prescription pad and pen
  Business cards
First-Aid Supplies and Wound Dressings
  Examination gloves (4-8 pair)
  Gauze sponges: 2×2, 4×4 (½ dozen each)
  Roll gauze: 2 inch, 4 inch (2 of each)
  Elastic bandages: 2 inch, 4 inch, 6 inch
  Nonadherent (Telfa) dressing pads (4-6)
  Dental rolls (8-10)
  Cotton-tipped applicators (6-12)
  Micropore tape (1 roll)
  Benzoin swab sticks (6-8)
  Betadine swab sticks (6-8)
  Alcohol pads (1 dozen)
  Antibiotic ointment
  Antiseptic towelettes
Eye Kit
  Pocket vision card
  Sterile saline eye wash
  Fluorescein strips (½ dozen)
  Cotton eye patches (½ dozen)
  Rigid eye shield
  Cobalt light
  Ophthalmic antibiotic
Wound Closure Supplies
  Sterile saline (½ liter)
  Syringes: 40-60 cc (1), 20 cc (1), 10 cc (2),
    3 cc (4-6)
  Needles: 21-gauge (6), 23-gauge (6), 25-gauge
    (4), 27-gauge (4)
  Sharps container
  Minor laceration kit (1-2)
  Sterile gloves (3-4 pair)
  Towel clip (1)
  Sutures: Nylon: 3-0 (4), 4-0 (6), 5-0 (4);
  Vicryl, Dexon, or PDS: 4-0 (4)
  Drapes, disposable (2-3)
  Adhesive wound closures: ¼ inch (1 package),
    ⅛ inch (1 package)
  Suture removal kit
Training Supplies
  Elastic bandages: 2 inch (1), 3 inch (2),
    4 inch (2), 6 inch (1)

Cloth tape: 1 inch (2 rolls), 2 inch (2 rolls)
Elastic tape: 2 inch
Pre-wrap (1 roll)
Bandage scissors or tape cutter
Foam adhesive padding: ⅛ inch (1 sheet),
  ¼ inch (1 sheet)
Finger splints
Aluminum splint
Sam splint
Arm sling
Tongue depressors
Bags for ice
Skin lubricant
Mouth guard (1)
Horseshoe pads (4)
Medications
  Antibiotic ointment (1 tube)
  Acetaminophen (1 bottle)
  Afrin nasal spray
  Albuterol MDI (1)
  Antacid/Pepto-Bismol
  Benadryl 25-mg caplets
  Carmex ointment
  Dextrose 50% (30-mL vial)
  Decadron
  Epi-Pen (1) or epinephrine 1:1000 (1 vial)
  Glucose tablets, liquid, or paste
  Ibuprofen (1 bottle)
  Lidocaine: 1% without, 1% with epinephrine
  Nitrostat (1 bottle)
  Sodium bicarbonate 8.4%
  Styptic powder
  Thera-Gesic
Medical Equipment
  Stethoscope
  Pen light
  Diagnostic kit (otoscope)
  Glucometer
  Thermometer, digital, oral (1)
  Pocket mask
  Reflex hammer
  Tuning fork
  23-gauge butterfly needle

ON-THE-FIELD EMERGENCIES

Many of the on-the-field emergencies described here occur infrequently. There-fore, the team physician should seek to gain as much experience as possible covering athletic events of various types. This nearly always requires the team physician to devote many hours of uncompensated time to the team(s). How-ever, there is no substitute for experience.

Cervical Spine Injury

Cervical spine injury is one of the most frightening and dire situations encoun-tered in sports. The highest level of suspicion should be used in evaluating every athlete who has sustained an injury to the neck. Any athlete who is rendered unconscious should be assumed to have a cervical spine injury.

The team physician should be thoroughly familiar with procedures for stabiliza-tion of the cervical spine, particularly in athletes wearing protective equipment (helmet, shoulder pads), and for transferring athletes from the field, court, or ice to a spine board.[6] The team physician's familiarity with these procedures should be based not only on review of written protocols but also on careful and regular practice, ideally before the start of each season. Viewing videos of proper tech-nique (eg, www.youtube.com/watch?v=tR4O9pvnFuw) can be helpful.

The team physician or athletic trainer typically will be in charge of immobilizing the head and neck, if necessary, and will direct all personnel who are assisting in stabilizing and transferring the injured athlete. When both a team physician and athletic trainer are present, duties should be assigned before an emergency situa-tion arises to prevent any delay in treatment. Evaluation of a possible cervical spine injury should be performed in all athletes with head injuries and in all athletes who are down or unconscious in the field of play. The team physician should first assess airway, breathing, and circulation. Next, assess consciousness. If the athlete remains unconscious, the physician must assume that a cervical spine injury is present, activate emergency medical services (EMS), and main-tain control of the head and neck. If the athlete is conscious and responsive, palpate for midline cervical tenderness. If cervical spine pain or tenderness is present, immobilize the spine by keeping the head and neck in anatomic align-ment. It is important to remember that passively or actively returning the head and neck to anatomic position is unlikely to cause or worsen any neurologic compromise. If the athlete is prone or lying on 1 side, the athlete should, with assistance, be carefully repositioned to the supine position, following recom-mended guidelines.[6] Instruct the athlete to lie still. Occasionally an athlete with a neck injury will panic and begin thrashing. In this situation, the team physi-cian should instruct others assisting to gently restrain the athlete's limbs until the athlete is calm and the physician can complete assessment of the spine. Assess neurologic functioning (active movement of limbs). If bony cervical spine injury is suspected because of significant reported pain, abnormal neurologic function, or the presence of concomitant head injury, the team physician should continue to maintain control of the head and neck until EMS arrives.

If the athlete does not have significant pain, does not have midline cervical tenderness, and has intact neurologic function, the team physician may ask the athlete to actively flex, extend, rotate, and bend the neck. If the athlete demonstrates full active range of motion, cervical spine injury is unlikely, and the athlete may gently be helped to his feet for further evaluation on the sideline. Range of motion of the neck in an athlete with possible cervical spine injury should *never* be checked passively.

Concussions

Concussions are the most common head injury in athletics. It is important for the team physician to be knowledgeable about the diagnosis and management of concussions.

Collapse

Collapse of an athlete on the field may constitute a true medical emergency. The differential diagnosis of collapse includes cardiac arrest, closed head injury, seizure, heat illness, vasovagal syncope, hypoglycemia, syncopal migraine, postrace collapse from venous pooling, and drug effect. The first priority is to ensure an adequate airway and to confirm breathing and a pulse. If a pulse is absent, CPR should be started immediately and an automated external defibrillator (AED) applied, if available. When an athlete has collapsed and is unconscious, regardless of what is known about the collapse, a cervical spine injury must be assumed to be present and appropriate actions taken until proven otherwise.

Fractures

Fracture should be suspected after trauma when significant bony tenderness or deformity is present. Angulated or displaced fractures should not be reduced in the field but should be immobilized and the athlete sent or transported to an emergency facility for definitive care. Table 4 lists fractures that require and those that do not require immediate transport.

Suspected fractures should be immobilized with any available splinting materials before the athlete is moved or transported. Ready-made splints are expensive but convenient and should be used if available. If a ready-made splint is not available, a splint should be improvised using available materials (Table 5). Soft materials should be applied for padding, then the rigid materials applied and secured with tape or bandage. The neurovascular examination should be repeated after the splint has been applied.

Table 4
Fracture requiring and not requiring immediate transport

Fractures that need immediate transport	Fractures that do not need immediate transport
Open fractures	Clavicle fractures
Angulated or displaced fractures	Suspected nondisplaced proximal humerus
Suspected femoral or tibial fractures	fractures
Suspected cervical spine fractures	Rib fractures
Fractures with neural or vascular compromise	Fractures of the hands and feet
Fractures associated with severe pain	Suspected avulsion fractures

Table 5
Ordinary materials that may be used for fracture splinting

Materials for padding	Rigid materials	Materials for securing
Towel	Cardboard	Athletic tape
T-shirt	Magazines	Nonadhesive wrap
Handkerchief	IV board	Masking tape
Napkin	Craft sticks	Duct tape
Roll gauze		Handkerchief
Diaper		
Pillow		

Dislocations

Dislocations commonly encountered in athletes include proximal interphalangeal joint dislocations, anterior glenohumeral dislocations, and posterior-medial elbow dislocations. Before and after any attempt at reduction, even an unsuccessful attempt, a thorough neural and vascular examination should be performed. Interphalangeal joint dislocations are most often dorsal in which the distal segment is displaced dorsal with respect to the proximal phalanx. These dislocations are best reduced by firmly grasping the distal segment, gently applying distal traction while increasing the dorsal angulation, and then using the thumb of the other hand to gently nudge the proximal end of the distal segment over the end of the proximal phalanx.

Debate on whether to reduce large joint dislocations, such as the shoulder and elbow, in the field centers on the risk of worsening or causing neurovascular compromise, and the consequences of delay. Reduction in the field may relieve neurovascular compromise, present a much easier reduction attempt before swelling and spasm set in, and obviate the need for sedation and anesthesia with their attendant risks. Factors influencing the decision to reduce shoulder and elbow dislocations are listed in Table 6. A variety of maneuvers may be used for reducing both shoulder and elbow dislocations. These maneuvers should be practiced regularly.

Table 6
Comparison of shoulder and elbow dislocations

Shoulder	Elbow
Low risk of associated fracture	Slightly higher risk of associated fracture
Low risk of neural or vascular compromise	Much higher risk of neural or vascular compromise
Amenable to multiple reduction attempts without further damage	Allow a single, gentle, but deliberate attempt at reduction

Anaphylaxis

Anaphylaxis in an athlete usually occurs when a previously sensitized athlete comes in contact with an allergen, most often an insect sting (hymenoptera). Less often, an athlete suffers exercise-induced anaphylaxis, which usually occurs in an individual with a history of atopy and in the setting of vigorous activity, often within 2 to 4 hours of ingesting an allergen, most commonly wheat.[7]

Administration of epinephrine 1:1000 is the mainstay of anaphylaxis treatment. The team physician may carry epinephrine in 1 of 3 forms: an autoinjector, a prefilled syringe, or a vial of epinephrine 1:1000 and injection supplies. Evidence favors the use of the autoinjector. Although it is more expensive, studies indicate that therapeutic levels are achieved more rapidly when epinephrine is administered by autoinjector than subcutaneously by syringe.[8] As soon as anaphylaxis is suspected, EMS should be activated. During the anaphylactic attack, the athlete's vital signs should be monitored continuously. If the patient is able to swallow and has an adequate airway, diphenhydramine (1-2 mg/kg, up to 50 mg) should be administered, if available, and albuterol given by inhaler and facemask. Emergency medical services should be summoned as soon as the epinephrine has been administered.

Breathing Problems

On the field, it may be difficult to determine whether dyspnea with exertion is being caused by asthma or some other problem. The most common cause of shortness of breath in an athlete is inadequate conditioning for the amount of exertion the athlete is being asked to perform. In most cases, the athlete with asthma and shortness of breath will have a history of asthma and associated chest discomfort. The differential diagnosis of dyspnea with exertion includes, but is not limited to, cardiac causes (angina, arrhythmia), another primary pulmonary cause (pneumonia), gastroesophageal reflux, anxiety (hyperventilation), paradoxical vocal cord dysfunction, and sickle cell crisis (which may occur even in individuals with sickle cell trait). The first goal is to make an assessment about the chest discomfort: does it seem anginal (crushing or pressure-like quality, high intensity, radiating into the neck or left arm, associated with nausea, presyncope)? Next, the chest should be auscultated. If clear breath sounds are heard and the patient is moving air well, the cause likely is not pulmonary. If wheezing is heard or if breath sounds are faint while the patient's respiratory effort is increased, a rescue dose of a short-acting bronchodilator should be administered immediately via spacer. If not available, the team physician should continuously monitor the athlete's respiratory status and activate EMS. If shortness of breath occurs suddenly and is accompanied by stridor instead of wheezing, the cause may be paradoxical vocal cord motion, also known as vocal cord dysfunction (VCD).[9] Individuals with VCD may have a history of treatment for suspected asthma, often with little success. The diagnosis of VCD often can be made by taking a careful history and later confirmed by office-based testing.

Heat Illness

The team physician should be alert for the possibility of 3 types of heat illness that require emergency treatment: heat stroke, sickle cell crisis, and hyponatremic dehydration.

The patient with heat stroke is no longer able to dissipate body heat through intrinsic mechanisms (sweating, vasodilation), resulting in an increased core temperature that initiates a cascade of pathophysiologic processes that ultimately may result in seizures, shock, cardiac arrest, and death. The patient with heat stroke will appear hot and lethargic with altered mental status. The only reliable method for assessing core temperature in an exercising athlete is by rectal thermometer.[10] Core temperature greater than 104°F (40°C) indicates that immediate whole-body cooling, most effectively accomplished by whole-body ice water immersion, is necessary. If a tub of sufficient size or a sufficient quantity of water an ice is not available, treatment should proceed as follows: remove as much clothing as possible, wet the entire skin, apply ice bags over areas where large blood vessels are close to the skin (neck, axillary, groin, popliteal fossa), elevate the legs, provide evaporative cooling with a fan or someone fanning the athlete with a towel, and activate EMS.

An athlete with sickle cell trait may develop sickling under conditions of heavy exertion in high-humidity conditions, resulting in acidosis, hypovolemia, and muscle hypoxia. The athlete in sickle cell crisis can be distinguished from the athlete with exercise-associated muscle cramps by the clinical findings listed in Table 7.[11] The athlete suspected of having a sickle cell crisis should be removed from further activity, cooled immediately, given oral hydration, and transported as quickly as possible to an emergency medical facility.

Hyponatremic dehydration usually occurs because of a combination of heavier than average sodium losses through sweat and overhydration with plain water or other dilute fluids.[12] Hyponatremia may present as heat exhaustion; the athlete has mild symptoms and has been hydrating. The team physician should have a

Table 7
Distinguishing characteristics of exercise-associated muscle cramps and sickle crisis

Exercise-associated muscle cramps	Sickle cell crisis
Increased muscle tone (tetany)	Muscle tone is normal or decreased
Onset after a prolonged period of exertion	Onset may occur early in the training session
Main complaint is pain	Athlete complains of pain and profound weakness
Significant dyspnea usually not present	Dyspnea and chest pain may be present

high index of suspicion in the athlete with signs and symptoms of heat exhaustion whose symptoms are not responding, or are worsening, despite oral rehydration.[13] The athlete who seems to be rehydrated (full stomach, producing urine) but is still having symptoms (headache, nausea, abdominal or muscle cramping) should have point-of-service testing of serum electrolytes (if available) or be transported to an emergency medical facility for assessment of electrolyte status.[14]

CONFIDENTIALITY AND RECORD-KEEPING

Confidentiality

The team physician should be thoroughly familiar with both federal and state legislation governing protection of confidential health information, including both the Health Insurance Portability and Accountability Act (HIPAA), which governs health information generated and stored by health care facilities and physicians, and the Federal Educational Rights and Privacy Act (FERPA), which governs the privacy of educational records, including medical information that is part of a student-athlete's school health record.[15]

HIPAA establishes a set of national standards and requirements that protect the privacy and security of individually identifiable health records. Initially applicable only to health information kept electronically, many entities and jurisdictions more broadly apply the HIPAA privacy standards to personally identifiable health information kept in any form. In brief, individually identifiable health information that is stored electronically or is used as part of an electronic transaction (eg, billing) is considered protected health information (PHI) under HIPAA.

If a team physician is employed by a school or college, the medical information generated in a physician-patient encounter is not considered PHI under HIPAA. However, the medical information is governed by FERPA if the school directly receives any federal funding. Schools that do not directly receive federal funding, such as many private schools, are not covered by FERPA. Usually, information in student medical records may be disclosed to other physicians without the explicit consent of the patient or parent if the information is being disclosed for treatment purposes only. If the team physician is employed by an entity distinct from the school or college and the physician transmits the student-athlete's medical information electronically, stores it electronically, or uses it as part of some transaction, the student-athlete's medical information is considered PHI under HIPAA.

Technically, student-athlete medical information that is not stored or transmitted electronically is not governed by HIPAA. Traditionally, this is the grounds by which team physicians are permitted to convey medical information to trainers and coaches on the sideline for treatment purposes (eg, providing an assessment of an athlete's condition for the purposes of immediate treatment or activity modification). However, many sports governing bodies, schools, colleges, and other entities require that communication of medical information, even under sideline conditions, be afforded the same measure of protection as PHI. They are now requiring student-athletes to sign a consent before sport participation that allows members of the health care team, including the team physician, athletic trainers, therapists, and coaches, to share information regarding the athletes.

Coaches are not licensed health care professionals. Although the team physician has traditionally considered coaches to be vital members of the athlete's health care team, the legal grounds for providing an athlete's health information to coaches is unclear. Many schools require parents to sign a consent allowing the coach to serve *in loco parentis* ("in place of the parent") in cases of emergency, thus allowing the coach access to the athlete's health information in urgent situations.

The most prudent course for the team physician is to be familiar with the school's or club's regulations regarding personal medical information because most schools have had their legal counsel address privacy issues since the HIPAA became law in 1996. If the club or school does not have unique privacy guidelines, the team physician should use judgment in disseminating an athlete's medical information and should work with the club or school to establish written privacy policies.

Maintaining Records on the Field

It is highly desirable for the team physician to maintain some type of treatment record on the field, not only for diagnosis and treatment that takes place after the contest but also for legal protection. Previously, some team physicians used a portable tape recorder. However, today's "smartphones" provide several functions that can be used for on-the-field record-keeping, such as typed notes and voice recording. Some electronic health records (EHRs) provide "apps" that allow record-keeping from a smartphone, although the limitation of these apps is that the physician must be able to create a patient health record instantly, which would require consent from the athlete or the athlete's guardian, or must have the athlete's health record already in place. Using a dedicated EHR for a specific team or event likely would be successful only if enrollment in the EHR was mandatory for all participants.[16]

Preparticipation Physical Evaluation

Issues related to the preparticipation physical evaluation (PPE) are important to the team physician. Conditions that may be prevented through proper preparticipation screening and education include ACL injuries, heat illness, and infectious diseases.

INJURY AND ILLNESS PREVENTION

Anterior Cruciate Ligament Injury

It is important that the team physician supervising or conducting the PPE be aware that obtaining an injury history and even performing a screening orthopedic examination have not been shown to be effective in preventing injuries.[17]

However, recent research has shown that certain movement patterns may place an athlete at risk for anterior cruciate ligament (ACL) injury, and these patterns may be identified through preseason screening.[18] Specifically, athletes who land from a jump with excessive knee valgus and limited hip and knee flexion are more likely to suffer ACL injuries. Preseason balance screening may also predict ankle injuries in high school athletes.[19] In the near future, functional screening could be increasingly incorporated into the PPE, although a recent hypothetical analysis using data from previous research suggests that applying ACL prevention training to unselected groups of athletes may be more cost-effective than screening for athletes with abnormal jump-landing patterns.[20]

The team physician should work with the team's athletic trainers and strength and conditioning specialists to incorporate an ACL prevention training program into the routine training regimen.

Heat Illness

The keys to preventing heat illness are education, awareness, and preparation. The team physician can play an important role in educating players, coaches, and parents on the signs and symptoms of heat illness. Communicating with athletic directors and event officials when heat conditions are hazardous can enable event staff to ensure that athletes remain well hydrated and that athletes with symptoms receive immediate care. Knowing the sickle cell trait status of athletes is helpful, as is knowing the health status of all athletes with a chronic disease (eg, diabetes, thyroid disease, epilepsy). This knowledge can help ensure that physicians are adequately prepared to care for these athletes. A useful practice for a team is pre- and post-practice weigh-ins, which enable athletes to accurately assess their level of dehydration.[21]

Infectious Diseases

It is important for teams to practice good hygiene with regard to water bottles. Not sharing water bottles or asking athletes not to put their mouths on the water bottles should be a standard policy. Razor blades and shavers should not be shared. Receptacles should be placed prominently wherever sharps are being used by medical staff. Weight training equipment and braces should be cleaned on a regular basis. Medical staff should follow Occupational Safety and Health Administration (OSHA) procedures whenever a sharps exposure has occurred with potential exposure of body fluids.

Yearly influenza immunization as a team may significantly reduce morbidity, including lost playing time, caused by influenza.

The team physician should raise awareness that athletes with impetiginous lesions may easily infect other teammates, possibly with methicillin-resistant *Staphylococcus aureus* (MRSA), and should encourage athletes to bring any such lesions to the attention of the team physician or the team athletic trainers.

DRUG TESTING

Some team physicians will be asked to assist with a drug testing program for athletes. Drug testing at the international and Olympic levels are primarily designed to identify use of performance-enhancing drugs. Drug testing at the professional and college levels may be designed to identify street drug use. Drug testing at the high school level is governed by each state and is variable. The governing bodies decide on the list of banned substances, and these lists can vary greatly. Some drug testing programs are administered to athletes on a random basis, whereas others are based on suspicion.[22] If testing is based on suspicion, it must be made clear to the athletes that the medical staff (including the team physician and the athletic training staff) is not involved in selecting athletes for testing based on suspicion. This will preserve the physician-patient or athletic trainer-athlete relationship so that an athlete who wants to confide in a health care professional will feel safe doing so.

Most drug testing programs use urine testing. At the international level there is a trend toward using blood tests as well. The specimen collection should be observed by a same-gender witness to prevent tampering with the sample. A urine specimen usually is divided into an "A" bottle and a "B" bottle for a retest in the event of an appeal of a positive test. Chain of custody procedures must be used during the entire process to ensure the specimens are secure until they reach the laboratory.

Most testing programs use inexpensive screening tests and then run a suspected positive test result through a more rigorous confirmatory test. It is helpful to talk to the toxicologist or laboratory director about the process. In most situations, a false-positive result is virtually impossible.

Procedures for handling a positive drug test vary with the organization. Penalties are determined by the governing body. There usually is an appeal process so that the athlete can request testing on the "B" specimen to determine whether the results are accurate.

Any school or team that has a drug testing program for street drugs should also have a student assistance program to help the athlete with a potential drug-dependence problem.[23] Access to an alcohol and other drug specialist is an imperative part of any drug testing program to assist with assessments and initiate treatment when necessary.

TRAVEL ISSUES

Sometimes the team physician will be asked to travel with the team. This may require a change in supplies for the medical bag and should be coordinated with the athletic trainers. It is most helpful to have a "little bit of everything."

There are 2 legal issues to consider when acting as a team physician in the United States. First, because medical licenses are issued by the state, a team physician who cares for a team outside of its home state but does not have a license in the other state is practicing medicine without a license and could face legal ramifications.[24] Some states have recently passed legislation to allow team physicians from other states to treat athletes while they are visiting out-of-state venues.[25] The exception is the US Olympic Training Center in Colorado Springs, Colorado, which enlists the help of volunteer physicians from around the country. The Olympic Training Center has an agreement with the Colorado Licensing Board to provide volunteer physicians with a temporary license to practice medicine in Colorado while they are volunteering for the US Olympic Committee.

The second issue is the prescribing of controlled drugs. In the past, physicians traveled with controlled drugs in the medical bag. Team physicians must be reminded that their Drug Enforcement Administration (DEA) permit is only good for a local hospital and clinic and is not valid when they are practicing outside that jurisdiction. When traveling, arrangements should be made with the host team physician to provide any prescription for a controlled medicine in the event an injury warrants it.

When traveling to another venue, it is always important for the team physician to discuss emergency planning with the host medical team. Where is the closest AED? Who will make the 911 call in the case of an emergency? Will the team physician receive a cell phone signal at the new venue? Where is the closest hospital?

When traveling out of state and overnight, it is important to know the location of the nearest pharmacy and the hours it is open. In some states, it will be necessary for a host physician to write the prescription. This arrangement should be discussed before the trip.

BUILDING A PRACTICE AS A TEAM PHYSICIAN

Serving as a team physician to a club team, high school, or college can be an effective and rewarding strategy for building a sports medicine practice. The team physician's primary responsibility in treating teams, specifically covering athletic events, is to provide conscientious assessment of sports injuries and to recommend prudent follow-up and treatment. The team physician should offer his services to further evaluate the athlete's injury but should make it clear that the choice of follow-up physician is entirely up to the athlete and the athlete's guardian. The federal laws collectively known as the "Stark Laws," which prohibit physicians from referring patients to ancillary care facilities (eg, imaging, physical therapy) in which referring physicians have a financial interest, do not expressly prohibit team physicians from referring injured team members exclusively to their practice. However, exclusive referral of all injured players on a team to the team physician's practice is considered unethical and will not be looked on favorably by athletes, guardians, and coaches. Above all, the team physician's main focus should be to attend to injury and illness on the team.

References

1. Boyd JL. Understanding the politics of being a team physician. *Clin Sports Med*. 2007;26:161-172
2. Kincaid JE. Coaches, a missing link in the health care system (letter). *Am J Dis Child*. 1992;146:1130
3. Herring SA, Kibler WB, Putukian M. Sideline preparedness for the team physician: a consensus statement—2012 update. *Med Sci Sport Exerc*. 2012;44:2442-2445
4. Buettner CM. The team physician's bag. *Clin Sports Med*. 1998;17:365-373
5. Everline C. Application of an online team physician survey to the consensus statement on sideline preparedness: the medical bag's highly desired items. *Br J Sports Med*. 2011;45:559-562
6. Waninger KE, Swartz EE. Cervical spine injury management in the helmeted athlete. *Curr Sports Med Rep*. 2011;10:45-49
7. Robson-Ansley P, Du Toit G. Pathophysiology, diagnosis and management of exercise-induced anaphylaxis. *Curr Opin Allergy Clin Immunol*. 2010;10:312-317
8. Simons FE, Roberts JR, Gu X, Simons KJ. Epinephrine absorption in children with a history of anaphylaxis. *J Allergy Clin Immunol*. 1998;101:33-37
9. Al-Alwan A, Kaminsky D. Vocal cord dysfunction in athletes: clinical presentation and review of the literature. *Phys Sports Med*. 2012;40:22-27
10. American College of Sports Medicine, Armstrong LE, Casa DJ, et al. Exertional heat illness during training and competition. *Med Sci Sports Exerc*. 2007;39:556-572
11. Eichner ER. Sickle cell trait in sports. *Curr Sports Med Rep*. 2010;9:347-351
12. Montain SJ, Sawka MN, Wenger CB. Hyponatremia associated with exercise: risk factors and pathogenesis. *Exerc Sports Sci Rev*. 2001;29:113-117

13. O'Brien KK, Montain SJ, Corr WP, et al. Hyponatremia associated with overhydration in U.S. Army trainees. *Milit Med.* 2001;166:405-410

14. Seigel AJ, d'Hemecourt P, Adner MM, et al. Exertional dysnatremia in collapsed marathon runners: a critical role for point-of-care testing to guide appropriate therapy. *Am J Clin Path.* 2009;132:336-340

15. Joint Guidance on the Application of the Family Educational Rights and Privacy Act (FERPA) and the Health Insurance Portability and Accountability Act of 1996 (HIPAA) to Student Health Records. Washington, DC: US Department of Health and Human Services and US Department of Education; 2008

16. Wells HJ, Higgins GL, Baumann MR. Implementing an electronic point-of-care medical record at an organized athletic event: challenges, pitfalls, and lessons learned. *Clin J Sports Med.* 2010;20:377-378

17. Garrick JG. Preparticipation orthopedic screening evaluation. *Clin J Sports Med.* 2004;14:123-126

18. Hewett TE, Myer GD, Ford KR, et al. Biomechanical measures of neuromuscular control and valgus loading of the knee predict anterior cruciate ligament injury risk in female athletes. *Am J Sports Med.* 2005;33:492-501

19. McGuine TA, Greene JJ, Best T, Leverson G. Balance as a predictor of ankle injuries in high school basketball players. *Clin J Sports Med.* 2000;10:239-244

20. Swart E, Redler L, Fabricant PD, et al. Prevention and screening programs for anterior cruciate ligament injuries in young athletes. A cost-effectiveness analysis. *J Bone Joint Surg Am.* 2014;96:705-711

21. Bergeron MF, McKeag DB, Casa DJ, et al. Youth football: heat stress and injury risk. *Med Sci Sports Exerc.* 2005;37:1421-1430

22. James-Burdumy S, Goesling B, Deke J, Einspruch E. The effectiveness of mandatory-random student drug testing: a cluster randomized trial. *J Adolesc Health.* 2012;50:172-178

23. Landry GL, Kokotailo PK. Drug screening in the athletic setting. *Curr Probl Pediatr.* 1994;24:344-359

24. Simon LM, Rubin AL. Traveling with the team. *Curr Sports Med Rep.* 2008;7:138-143

25. Viola T, Carlson C, Trojian TH, Anderson J. A survey of state medical licensing boards: can the traveling team physician practice in your state? *Br J Sports Med.* 2013;47:60-62

Adolesc Med 026 (2015) 18–38

Preparticipation Physical Evaluation

Michele LaBotz MD, FAAP[a]*;
David Bernhardt, MD, FAAP[b]

*InterMed Sports Medicine, South Portland, Maine; [b]University of Wisconsin
School of Medicine and Public Health, Madison, Wisconsin*

The preparticipation physical evaluation (PPE) has been part of the American youth sport experience for decades and has undergone significant evolution over time. However, concerns remain about the value and efficacy of this evaluation as a screening tool for young athletes. This article reviews the rationale, content, and logistics of these examinations. Topics of particular interest that are covered include the potential role of the electrocardiogram (ECG) and augmented cardiac screening in detecting conditions that may predispose to sudden death, as well as ongoing controversy regarding the role of sickle cell screening in the athletic population.

The primary objectives of the PPE are to screen for conditions that may be life-threatening or disabling, or may predispose to injury or illness.

Understanding that the PPE is often the athlete's only encounter with a physician, secondary objectives related to the promotion of general health and well-being include (1) determining the athlete's general health, (2) serving as the adolescent's entry point into the health care system, (3) providing anticipatory guidance, (4) updating immunizations, and (5) the final and least important objective from a medical viewpoint, fulfilling legal, insurance, and sport league requirements.

Although these evaluations are ubiquitous at all levels of athletic participation, there is a paucity of evidence on their true benefit and ability to achieve the objectives listed. The largest published review on the topic identified a limited number of pertinent original research articles, and these were all population-based clinical studies (type II evidence).[1] Those authors concluded that PPEs

---

*Corresponding author
E-mail address: mlabotz@gmail.com

were problematic in their implementation and uniformity, and they lacked the needed sensitivity and specificity to effectively detect many significant issues affecting young athletes. However, that study was published in 2004, and since then the PPE has changed significantly, with introduction of a new format and enhanced efforts at improving standardization of this examination.[2] At this time, there is no published research on the result of these changes on the effectiveness of the PPE.

The current recommended format for the PPE was developed by a consortium of medical societies (American Academy of Pediatrics [AAP], American Academy of Family Physicians, American College of Sports Medicine, American Medical Society for Sports Medicine, American Orthopedic Society for Sports Medicine, and American Osteopathic Academy of Sports Medicine) and was published in 2010 by the AAP in the 4th edition of *PPE Preparticipation Physical Evaluation*. This monograph reviews in detail how to obtain an appropriate history and examination and how to determine clearance for athletic participation. Sample forms for history, physical examination, special needs consideration, and clearance can be found at the end of this article, or downloaded from www.aap.org/en-us/professional-resources/practice-support/Documents/Preparticipation-Physical-Exam-Form.pdf. These forms essentially represent current best practice in performance of the PPE.

PREPARTICIPATION PHYSICAL EVALUATION SETTING

The recommended setting for the PPE is within the athlete's medical home.[2] The medical home provides full access to the athlete's past medical history, family history, and medical record, and provides the best opportunity for appropriate follow-up on any issues that are identified. In addition, the athlete's interaction with a known physician may provide an opportunity for greater disclosure than might otherwise occur if the examination were performed by a stranger.

However, in spite of this recommendation many PPEs occur in other locations, including urgent care clinics and pharmacies. Although these situations may be more convenient and less expensive and still offer a private examination, the providers typically do not have access to or knowledge of the athlete's medical record. In addition, the proficiency of the provider and the uncertainty of follow-up make this a less than ideal setting for the PPE.

Many schools provide "mass physicals." These are often facilitated by the school's licensed athletic trainer (or team physician) and may involve multiple practitioners with specific areas of interest or expertise. The athletes often progress through multiple stations, which assess different aspects of the evaluation. Advantages of these mass physicals include cost, convenience, and expertise of practitioners in performing appropriate assessments, as well as seamless integration with medical practitioners at the school. Shortcomings of this environment include incomplete knowledge of the medical history, lack of access to medical records, lack of privacy, and examination conditions that may be suboptimal (eg, noisy settings that may compromise auscultation). It is important that the final step of the mass physical process includes a thorough review of all history and examination findings by a qualified physician for clearance determination.

PREPARTICIPATION PHYSICAL EVALUATION PHYSICIANS

Preparticipation physical evaluations ideally should be performed by a physician or qualified practitioner who is familiar with all components of the evaluation, including the medical and athletic implications of findings on a multisystem physical examination.[2] Some states and organizations allow PPEs to be performed by nonphysician personnel, and although this may mitigate difficulties in areas with a shortage of physician providers, nonphysicians may lack the scope of training to address many of the medical issues faced by young athletes. In these cases, there should be a low threshold for consultation with a physician about any areas of uncertainty. Given the importance of the history in detecting issues on the PPE, it is particularly important that appropriate standardized history forms be used when nonphysician personnel are performing the evaluation.

PREPARTICIPATION PHYSICAL EVALUATION TIMING

The timing of the PPE must be close enough to the athletic season to reflect the athlete's current health status, yet far enough in advance to allow for additional assessment, consultation, or treatment of any issues that might be identified during the evaluation. Expert recommendation is for these assessments to be performed at least 4 to 6 weeks before the start of preseason practice.[2,3]

When considering frequency of the PPE, it is important to recognize that for many adolescents, this evaluation is their only nonacute contact with the health care system, and that for many families, this becomes their de facto preventive health care visit. One 2010 study looked at claims data over a 4-year interval for more than 40,000 continuously insured adolescents in Minnesota.[4] Among this population of adolescents aged 13 to 17 years, 30% had no preventive care visits, and about 40% had a single preventive care visit during this time period. This can be contrasted to the AAP recommendation for annual health maintenance visits throughout adolescence.

The frequency of required PPEs typically is determined by the state or sporting organization. These often are required on an annual basis, but some states and organizations mandate evaluations only every 2 to 3 years. Current expert recommendations are that an evaluation be performed every 2 years in preadolescent athletes and every 2 to 3 years in adolescents.[2] History updates and problem-focused evaluations should be performed annually in the interim.

The PPE has a lot of overlap with the content of child and adolescent annual health maintenance examinations. With the Affordable Care Act assuring coverage for annual preventive visits throughout childhood and adolescence, the benefits of incorporating the PPE into an annual health maintenance visit include possible improvements in (1) cost- and time-efficiency for families, patients, and practitioners; (2) streamlined school and activity-related paperwork for practitioners; (3) opportunities for counseling on physical activity and healthy lifestyle choices; and (4) adherence with recommendations for annual preventive care visits.

Some jurisdictions (including New Jersey and the District of Columbia) have "universal child health forms" that encompass all information pertinent to school and activity participation, including sports clearance, immunizations, special care plans, allergies, emergency plans, dietary restrictions, special equipment, behavioral issues, and medical conditions.

PREPARTICIPATION PHYSICAL EVALUATION HISTORY OVERVIEW

It is generally recognized that the history is often the most significant part of the whole examination. Therefore, accuracy in completion of the history form is key. A 1999 study compared PPE history forms completed by athletes with forms completed by parents.[5] The study found that only 20% of these forms were in complete agreement, and that differences in cardiovascular, neurologic, musculoskeletal, and weight-related histories accounted for almost 60% of all discrepancies. Although it is common for athletes to provide an incomplete history form or one that they completed without parental oversight, both athletes and parents need to be involved in completing the family and medical history. History forms require a parental signature for all athletes younger than 18 years, and physician review of the history, ideally with both athlete and parent, is important.

The current recommended history form is contained in *PPE: Preparticipation Evaluation*, 4th edition. Any variation on this format must include all components contained on that form.

SYSTEM-BASED HISTORY AND EXAMINATION REVIEW

General Health

The history includes queries on the overall health of the athlete. Previous hospitalizations, athletic restrictions, and the status of ongoing health issues need to be reviewed. Most stable, chronic medical conditions are compatible with athletic participation. Obesity is one of the most common conditions seen in the PPE. Arguably, the obese child or adolescent may gain particular benefit from sports participation. However, there is concern that these athletes may be at greater risk for a variety of issues, including heat-related illness[6] and lower extremity injury.[7] Insulin-dependent diabetics may need to adjust their diet, monitoring, and insulin dose to accommodate the demands of training and competition, and their athletic trainer or coach should be aware of their diagnosis. Examiners should consult the AAP statement on medical conditions and sports participation in the young athlete for further guidance.[8]

Cardiac

Although one of the primary objectives of the PPE is to prevent sudden cardiac death (SCD), there is no evidence that performing a standard history and physical examination actually reduces the risk of SCD. The sudden unexpected death of a healthy-appearing athlete causes significant hysteria among the general public and leads to the misperception that the screening examination will detect all conditions that could lead to SCD. However, knowing that the incidence of SCD is very low and that the leading causes of SCD often are silent, detection of these conditions is challenging.

The exact incidence of SCD in athletes in the United States is unknown. Over a 26-year period (1986-2011), 13 cases of sudden death were reported among high school student-athletes related to physical exertion, during competition or at practice.[9] Based on the size of the population studied, the calculated incidence among high school student-athletes is 0.7 per 100,000 person-years. In a study of collegiate athletes, over a 5-year period the incidence of sudden death was 2.3 per 100,000 person-years.[10] A more recent study of college student-athletes over a 10-year study period found 64 deaths likely were related to a cardiac condition, resulting in a rate of 1.2 per 100,000 person-years.[11] In both studies of collegiate populations, the risk of cardiovascular death was more common in black athletes than in white athletes.

The most common causes of SCD in the United States are hypertrophic cardiomyopathy, coronary artery anomalies, and aortic rupture associated with Marfan syndrome. Hypertrophic cardiomyopathy and aberrant coronary arteries often are silent conditions that are asymptomatic until SCD occurs. Other causes of SCD include myocarditis, arrhythmogenic right ventricular dysplasia, aortic stenosis, and ion channel disorders such as long QT syndrome, short QT syndrome, Brugada syndrome, and familial catecholaminergic polymorphic ventricular tachycardia.

The detailed cardiac history form published in the PPE monograph attempts to be more comprehensive than the previous history form.[12] A positive answer on the monograph screening questions should alert the provider to more thoroughly assess for a possible cardiac problem, including possible diagnostic testing or a referral to a pediatric cardiologist. Personal and family history is crucial in identifying a proportion of asymptomatic athletes at risk for SCD because the physical examination often is normal in most conditions that lead to SCD. An accurate history makes parent input vital in completing this portion of the form.

Use of a standardized history form allows for a collection of a detailed cardiac screening history in a timely manner. Symptoms associated with exercise, including chest pain, pressure, tightness, or discomfort, may indicate ischemia caused by a number of conditions. Exertional syncope at the finish line is fairly common and often benign; occurrence during exercise, however, may also indicate a cardiac condition and warrants further diagnostic testing. Most cases of syncope in athletes usually do not occur during exercise and usually are not associated with a cardiac etiology.[13]

A detailed family history may also identify the asymptomatic athlete with an unsuspected cardiac condition. The standardized form in the monograph questions the athlete and parents about a family history of sudden death before age 50, which indicates that, absent trauma, the death likely was cardiac related and may be familial. In addition, a family history of syncope, near-syncope, drowning, near-drowning, unexplained motor vehicle accidents, unexplained seizure activity, or sudden infant death syndrome may indicate an ion channel disorder.

The PPE should include blood pressure measurement, a detailed cardiac examination, including auscultation for heart murmurs in the supine and seated positions, palpation of the point of maximal impulse, and palpation of femoral pulses. In addition, the practitioner should look for physical examination findings consistent with Marfan syndrome.[14] Definitive diagnosis of Marfan syndrome relies on fulfillment of the Ghent criteria, which were updated in 2010.[14] Aortic root dilation and ectopia lentis (lens dislocation) are cardinal features of Marfan syndrome and, if present in combination, are sufficient for a definitive diagnosis. Otherwise, various combinations of family history, fibrillin-1 (FBN1) mutations, and history and physical examination findings can also be indicative of a Marfan diagnosis. Diagnostic tools and calculators have been published online by The Marfan Foundation (www.marfan.org/resources/professionals/marfandx). Suspicious findings should lead to a referral to a geneticist for confirmation and a cardiologist for evaluation of aortic root dilation.

Despite widespread acceptance by many different organizations, including the American Heart Association and the AAP, there is no evidence demonstrating the PPE is effective in meeting 1 of the primary objectives, namely, reducing the risk of sudden death in the athletic population. One also must keep in mind that other causes of death in the high school and collegiate athletic populations are more widespread. In a study of death in collegiate athletes by Maron et al,[11] the cause was not cardiac related in 65%. Other causes to consider include suicide, drugs, trauma, drowning, sickle cell trait (SCT), and heat stroke.

There continues to be a push for the widespread use of ECG in the screening for cardiac abnormalities associated with SCD. When making a decision regarding use of cardiac screening, one must consider the population to screen and the frequency of screening, the cost-effectiveness of this type of testing, the reliability of the actual test, along with the sensitivity, specificity, and predictive value of the test. If pediatricians and primary care physicians are recommending exercise for all patients, one must consider the possibility that ECG screening would be needed for *all* patients because everyone would be considered an athlete. At this time, there is a lack of infrastructure for screening everyone with ECG. There is no evidence suggesting that a one-time screening is adequate, and we do not have any scientific evidence suggesting that annual or biennial screening is adequate. Diagnostic accuracy of physician ECG interpretation is questionable, especially among primary care physicians and general cardiologists compared to physicians who are "experts" trained in ECG reading in terms of the causes of sudden death.[15] In addition, there is a lack of evidence-based ECG standards for young athletes. Based on the lack of trained ECG interpreters and the limited accuracy and interpretation of the studies, the false-positive rate would remain unacceptable, leading to an increasing number of tests and cost. At this time, until more evidence to the contrary becomes available, the assessment tool of choice continues to be a detailed history using a standardized form, physical examination, and use of other tests as medically indicated.

Musculoskeletal

Musculoskeletal injuries, particularly in the knee and ankle, are some of the most common issues in young athletes and are the most common reasons for restricting sports activity.[3] Although it can be difficult to sort out which of these injuries merit ongoing concern, it is important to consider that previous musculoskeletal injury is one of the best predictors of future musculoskeletal injury. The history should attempt to delineate injuries or conditions that cause current symptoms or that previously required the athlete to miss practice or competition; the athlete be sent for imaging, physical therapy, or surgery; or the athlete wear a cast, brace, or orthotic device. Particular attention should be paid to previous fractures or dislocations. Stress fractures may be a marker for an athlete with inadequate dietary intake and possible development of the female athlete triad (see *The Female Athlete Triad: Energy Deficiency, Physiologic Consequences and Treatment*, pp. 116-142).

If the musculoskeletal history is completely negative, then the general musculoskeletal screening examination (also known as the 2-minute screening examination) can be performed.[2] A more detailed, focused examination of an injured area should be performed for those regions with previous or ongoing issues. In addition, a number of authors have discussed the potential benefits of a more comprehensive musculoskeletal assessment to detect deficiencies that may hinder athletic performance or increase injury risk.[16-18] This may include general assessment of fundamental movement patterns or focused examinations of body areas under greater stress for each sport. For example, a swimmer or pitcher may warrant a more detailed shoulder and elbow evaluation, whereas a soccer or basketball player may require more attention to the knee and ankle.

Pulmonary

Asthma and exercise-induced bronchoconstriction (EIB) are often the primary considerations in young athletes with breathing complaints. However, a 2012 study of a sample of athletes referred to a tertiary care asthma center reported that 70% were subsequently diagnosed with vocal cord dysfunction (VCD), 52% were subsequently diagnosed with EIB, and 31% had both conditions coexisting.[19] Vocal cord dysfunction was more common in younger athletes and females. A history of poor response to typical asthma medications should lead to questions related to medication adherence and exploration of other possible causes of breathing complaints associated with exercise (VCD, cardiac causes, deconditioning, other pulmonary disease).

An appropriate pulmonary history includes questions about personal and family history of asthma and use of asthma medications, as well as presence of cough, wheeze, or other breathing issues, particularly during or after exercise. If asthma is identified, ready access at all times to rescue medications must be emphasized to the patient and family. This may require obtaining an additional inhaler for the athlete to keep in a sideline bag or with the licensed athletic trainer or coaching staff.

The pulmonary examination in athletes at rest typically is normal, even in athletes with known asthma and EIB. If wheezing or other findings are present at rest, the athlete requires further evaluation. If the history suggests obstructive airway disease, many physicians will often make a presumptive diagnosis of asthma or EIB if a therapeutic trial of beta-2 agonists provides symptomatic relief. Field challenge testing with portable spirometry or peak flows can be performed as well. If beta-2 agonists do not reverse symptoms or if hoarseness or stridor is present, then VCD must be considered. For athletes who are competing at the national level and are subject to US Anti-Doping Agency (USADA) oversight, use of beta-2 agonists is regulated.[20] Albuterol is currently allowed up to a maximum of 1600 mcg/day (14 puffs per day of a standard 108 mcg/puff inhaler). Athletes using dosages greater than this must complete a therapeutic use exemption form, which requires documented reductions in FEV_1 with spirometry testing. Information on the therapeutic use exemption process can be found at www.usada.org/substances/tue/policy.

Gastrointestinal and Genitourinary

Sport-specific gastrointestinal or genitourinary concerns include symptomatic hernias, organomegaly, and missing kidneys or testicles. History should inquire about groin or abdominal pain or bulges, as well as any known missing organs. Recent history of infectious mononucleosis should prompt careful assessment for hepatomegaly or splenomegaly. Studies looking at detection of splenomegaly on physical examination generally show much more specificity than sensitivity, and accuracy is improved in lean patients and in those who have not eaten for several hours before assessment.[21] The negative likelihood ratios for palpation (0.41) and percussion (0.48) in detecting splenomegaly suggest that normal physical examination findings are not good at ruling out an enlarged spleen.[21]

In the past, ultrasounds were commonly ordered for athletes with spleno-megaly resulting from infectious mononucleosis. However, because of the large variation in baseline spleen size, current recommendations are clinical follow-up of these patients rather than ultrasound assessment.[22] Several recent studies have investigated baseline spleen sizes in the athletic population, and if normative values are determined then the current recommendations may change.[23,24]

The genitourinary examination is not part of the PPE for females but is per-formed for males to assess for 2 normal, descended testicles without irregu-larity or masses. This examination requires a private setting, with an offer for a chaperone if the athlete prefers. Evaluation for inguinal hernias need be performed only if symptoms are reported.[2] Symptomatic hernias require additional evaluation, but athletic participation often can be continued as symptoms allow.

Dermatology

The history should inquire about current sores or skin-related issues, as well as a history of herpes or methicillin-resistant *Staphylococcus aureus* (MRSA) infec-tions. Most skin-related issues do not necessarily pose a danger to the athlete but are of greater concern because of potential spread to teammates or competitors. This is of greatest concern in wrestling and martial arts but also is of potential consequence in any contact sport or in team situations with shared training equipment or locker room facilities.

The physical examination needs to include a visual survey of the areas that are exposed or that might come into contact with other athletes during training or competition. Any open sores or lesions must be adequately covered by the uni-form or dressed in a fashion that cannot be dislodged during athletic participa-tion. The National Collegiate Athletic Association (NCAA) describes appropriate wound covering as gas-impermeable dressing, pre-wrap, and well-anchored stretch tape. If lesions cannot be adequately covered, then the athlete cannot be cleared to participate in contact sports. Certain skin infections require addi-tional consideration before clearance. Table 1 reviews current recommendations from the National Federation of State High School Associations.[25] Scholastic wrestlers with skin lesions often require written medical release to return to par-ticipation. A recommended form can be found at www.nfhs.org/media/869160/ wrestling_skin_lesion_form_2014-15.pdf.

Table 1
Summary of current National Federation of State High School Association (NFHS) recommendations for skin infection treatment and return to sport participation

Infection	Recommended treatment	Criteria for return to participation	Other
Herpes infections (*Herpes gladiatorum*)	Oral antivirals	Initial outbreak: no participation for minimum of 10 days after treatment initiated. If generalized symptoms (fever, lymphadenopathy) need treatment for 14 days. Recurrent infections: if antivirals used, must be on medication for 120 hours and lesions "noncontagious."	Location typically head/face/neck. Initial outbreaks may take up to 2 weeks to resolve. Recurrent outbreaks typically are shorter and less severe. Herpes lesions considered "noncontagious": all lesions dry and with well-adherent scabs, no new lesions preceding 48 hours, no local lymphadenopathy. Consider prophylactic oral antivirals for athletic season.
Other herpes infections (cold sores, zoster infections)	Oral antivirals	All lesions noncontagious Primary outbreaks: 10-14 days on antivirals Recurrent outbreaks: at least 5 days of antiviral treatment	
Molluscum contagiosum	Curettage and hyfrecation	Cover with bio-occlusive dressing	May wrestle immediately after treatment
Verruca vulgaris	No treatment required by NFHS	Should be covered if prone to bleeding or abrasion	Considered not highly contagious
Tinea infections *Tinea corporis* (ringworm)	Oral or topical antifungals	72 hours on antifungal	May return when no longer contagious and lesions covered with bio-occlusive dressing
Tinea capitus	Oral antifungals	2 weeks on antifungal	
Scabies, head lice	Topical	24 hours after starting treatment	
Bacterial infections (eg, impetigo, folliculitis, carbuncles)	Oral antibiotics	72 hours on antibiotic with clinical improvement All lesions scabbed over, no discharge, no lesions past 48 hours	If new lesions develop or drain after 72 hours, methicillin-resistant *Staphylococcus aureus* should be considered

Derived from McCorkle R, Thomas B, Suffaletto H, Jehle D. Normative spleen size in tall healthy athletes: implications for safe return to contact sports after infectious mononucleosis. *Clin J Sport Med.* 2010;20(6):413-415.

Neurologic

The neurologic history covers a spectrum of potential intracranial as well as cervical issues in the athlete. Injuries that produce sensory or motor symptoms in any of the extremities suggest possible cervical spine pathology. Transient unilateral upper extremity symptoms suggest a possible "burner" or "stinger," which is a relatively common traction or compression injury to the upper nerve roots. A recent survey study of football players at the high school, collegiate, and professional levels revealed that more than 50% of these players reported sustaining a stinger during their athletic careers.[26] Isolated stingers that resolve fairly quickly do not warrant restriction as long as the cervical and neurologic examinations are normal. Athletes who report recurrent stingers, especially multiple stingers within a single season, or those with persistent symptoms should be considered for additional evaluation and imaging to assess for possible cervical nerve root compromise that may predispose the athlete to repeat injury.[27]

An athlete who presents with a history of posttraumatic symptoms in bilateral upper extremities or with any lower extremity involvement suggests probable cervical spinal cord neuropraxia, also known as transient quadriparesis. These injuries are much less common than stingers affecting about 0.17 in 100,000 football players at the high school level.[28] Any athlete with this history warrants imaging for evaluation of cervical spinal stenosis, including cervical spine radiographs with flexion and extension, as well as magnetic resonance imaging to assess for "functional reserve" (ie, cerebrospinal fluid surrounding the cord).[28] Given the rarity of these injuries there are few data supporting return to play decision-making. Expert opinion currently supports return to play for athletes with normal imaging studies and full return of neurologic function after a single episode of transient quadriparesis. There is some debate about the role of any identified cervical stenosis on spinal injury, but current evidence seems to indicate that stenosis does not predispose to injury per se but may portend a poorer prognosis once an injury has occurred.[28] In spite of this information, given the gravity of cervical spine injuries, physicians and parents often will choose a conservative course for the young athlete and refrain from return to collision sports after an episode of transient quadriparesis.

The *PPE: Preparticipation Physical Evaluation*, 4th edition, history form asks about previous concussions, but it also asks about specific symptoms after head injury in an attempt to increase the sensitivity for detecting concussive events that may have been unrecognized. Concussions, or mild traumatic brain injuries, are the most common intracranial injury in young athletes, representing almost 9% of all sports injuries in high school athletes.[29] Athletes with a concussion history should be asked specifically about the mechanism of injury as well as the type and duration of postconcussive symptoms.[30] A history of significant symptoms following relatively trivial mechanisms of injury may signify a pattern of vulnerability to injury that may warrant additional caution.

In some schools, baseline computerized neuropsychologic testing is obtained during the PPE, particularly for athletes participating in contact/collision sports. Although this testing is not considered an essential part of concussion management,[30] having baseline information can be helpful when interpreting postinjury test results, particularly in athletes with attention-deficit/hyperactivity disorder or a learning disability whose test results may not follow population norms.

Clearance for return to sport for any athlete reporting a concussion history requires full resolution of symptoms and return to prior levels of cognitive function. The physical examination in athletes reporting a history of concussion should be normal, including a nonfocal neurologic examination. A common concern that arises during the PPE is counseling and clearing athletes with a previous history of multiple concussions or prolonged postconcussion recovery. These decisions are highly individualized, and there is no absolute threshold. Disqualification should be considered for any athlete with a history of prolonged postconcussive symptoms (ie, >3 months) or with 3 or more concussions within a single season.[29]

Vision

Any history of significant eye injury or other issue that may affect visual acuity needs further review. The physical evaluation includes assessment of acuity, as well as pupil reactivity and extraocular muscle function. For athletes with corrective lenses, acuity should be checked with and without correction. For children older than 6 years, "best acuity" (ie, with corrective lenses if needed) worse than 20/30 should be evaluated further.[31] Athletes with best corrected vision of 20/40 or worse in either eye are considered functionally "one-eyed," and current recommendations are mandatory eye protection regardless of selected sport. Both the AAP and the American Academy of Ophthalmology are united in recommending against participation by athletes with this condition in boxing and full contact martial arts, and in exercising great caution when clearing these athletes for wrestling. About 20% of the population has anisocoria at baseline, and this condition should be documented to prevent future concern if a head injury evaluation is warranted.

Nutrition and Weight

Athletes should be questioned about any weight-related or dietary concerns. These are common issues, and athletes can be susceptible to these influences for the sake of their sport. The history should specifically ask about any ongoing dietary restrictions or efforts to gain or lose weight. This is of particular interest in athletes participating in wrestling and other weight-classified sports. Most wrestlers undergo a process of weight certification at least 6 weeks before the start of their season. This involves an assessment of body composition and calculations to determine the minimum weight class in which each wrestler may participate for the season. These calculations typically are based on a body fat percentage of 7% for boys and 12% for girls and an allowable weight loss of 1.5% body weight per week until that minimum is obtained. For athletes whose "natural" body weight falls below these allowed percentiles, a physician may write a letter of clearance stating that the athlete may participate safely at his lower natural weight.

Female Athletes

The recommended history form contains several questions regarding age of menarche and menstrual frequency. Oligomenorrhea or delayed menarche is a potential marker for female athletes with inadequate caloric intake. The relationship between caloric intake, menstrual function, and bone health is known as the female athlete triad. Athletes who have positive responses to PPE history questions should be screened further.

Hematologic

There has been recent controversy over the potential benefit of screening young athletes for SCT. Children and adolescents who are homozygous for sickle cell hemoglobin often become too symptomatic and too anemic to continue sports participation into high school, but SCT is seen in up to 4% of Division I college football players.[32] Military studies have demonstrated a 30-fold increased risk for sudden death in recruits with SCT, and a recent review of 10 years of mortality data in NCAA Division I college football players showed that 10 of 16 deaths during conditioning were attributable to SCT.[32] Current theories attribute these deaths to hypoxemia, lactic acidosis, hyperosmolarity, and red cell dehydration during high levels of exertion, which can lead to sickling within the microcirculation. Although all 50 states currently screen newborns for sickle hemoglobin, several lawsuits against the NCAA have prompted the association to require all athletes to undergo screening unless they provide proof of prior sickle cell screening or sign a waiver. This is an area of ongoing debate. Ideally pediatricians should be aware of the sickle cell status of young athletes undergoing PPE, but at present there are no universal recommendations for screening at the precollegiate level, and the American Society of Hematology currently does not support sickle cell testing as a prerequisite for athletic participation.[33]

Special Needs Athletes

No single form can encompass all the issues that need consideration in athletes with cognitive or physical impairments. The examiner needs to have a good understanding of the athlete's baseline medical status and any potential associated issues that may affect sports participation. Special needs athletes and their parent or guardian should complete the standard PPE history form as well as the supplemental history form contained in the 4th ed PPE monograph.[2] The physical should include all components of the standard PPE, with additional attention paid to any system that may be directly or indirectly affected by the disability. Table 2 outlines several common issues that arise during the PPE in special needs athletes.[34]

Table 2
Summary of common issues in special needs athletes

Spinal cord injury/ wheelchair athletes	• Overuse syndromes of upper extremities common: carpal tunnel syndrome (50%-75%), ulnar nerve entrapment at wrist (Guyon tunnel), rotator cuff impingement and tendinitis, biceps tendinitis.
	• Pressure sores: many sports wheelchairs elevate knees relative to buttocks, increasing risk of skin breakdown over sacrum and ischial tuberosities. These issues may be asymptomatic if sensory loss is present.
	• Athletes with lesions above T6 should be asked about history of autonomic dysreflexia. This phenomenon is caused by loss of inhibition of the sympathetic nervous system, which leads to acute and potentially life-threatening sympathetic response. Triggers are stimuli from below level of lesion, such as urinary tract or other infection, bowel or bladder distention, tight garments, and variety of other noxious stimuli. Some athletes self-induce autonomic dysreflexia in order to enhance performance.
	• Athletes with lesions above T8 are at particular risk for both heat and cold injury as a result of impairment of sudomotor and vasomotor activity below the lesion.
Amputee athletes	• Prosthetics and orthotics checked for fit and wear.
	• Friction and pressure lead to skin breakdown and irritation, and adventitial bursae formation. Sensory loss is common and may be asymptomatic.
Hydrocephalus and shunt	• Most common sport-related issues are broken shunt catheters and shunt dysfunction.
	• 90% of pediatric neurosurgeons allow unrestricted noncontact sport participation. Head gear or helmets are recommended for contact sports participation.
Down syndrome	• 15% have atlantoaxial instability (AAI). Most are asymptomatic, and there is controversy over the significance of asymptomatic AAI as a risk factor for future AAI symptoms.
	• Currently, the Special Olympics requires athletes with Down syndrome to undergo physical and radiographic evaluation for AAI (flexion and extension cervical spine images). Some experts recommend rescreening every 3-5 years.
	• Athletes with radiographic AAI (cervical hyperextension, "radical flexion," direct pressure over cervical spine) are prohibited from participating in sports. However, athletes with radiographic AAI who are asymptomatic and want to participate in "at-risk" sports may do so after completion of a waiver. This includes signatures of the athlete, parent/guardian, and 2 licensed medical professionals.
	• Variety of other associated conditions with Down syndrome (eg, about 50% have received surgical treatment for congenital heart disease).

Derived from Patel D, Greydanus DE. Sport participation by physically and cognitively challenged young athletes. *Pediatr Clin N Am.* 2010;57:795-817.

Clearance

The primary objective of the PPE is to determine clearance status for sport participation. This should be determined by a qualified provider who has reviewed findings from the entire history and physical examination. The emphasis during the PPE is often on detecting conditions that might limit or disqualify an athlete from sport participation. However, given the myriad benefits of sports activity for children and adolescents, it is just as important that examiners not disqualify an athlete unless there is a compelling medical reason.[35] When considering clearance status, the guidelines in Table 3 should help guide decision-making.

Clearance status can and should change at any point if problematic historical information is subsequently revealed or upon development of new injuries or medical conditions.

Information regarding clearance status can be released to the school without further authorization and need only state that clearance has been rescinded, unless the patient and family have given permission to release more details related to the specific reason or change. Further information can only be released in accordance with HIPAA regulations and requires appropriately signed releases. This will depend on the state and the PPE setting.

It is critical that team personnel (athletic trainer or team physician) be aware of an athlete's allergies, tetanus status, and certain medical conditions (eg, diabetes, asthma).When this information is not available, a member of the coaching staff

Table 3
Guidelines for determining clearance for sports participation

---

- Will the issue of concern place the athlete or other participants at risk for injury or illness?
- Does the condition allow for safe participation in some sports, even though other sports might pose significant risk?
- Will the athlete be able to participate to some degree in conditioning or practice situations while undergoing treatment?

Clearance for sport participation is not an "all or nothing" proposition, and it is important to recognize that sport participation is not without some risk. The multiple benefits of sport participation must be weighed against the risk for any given athlete, and it is important to recognize that some degree of risk will always be present. Most young athletes will be cleared for full participation without restriction, but the following categories allow for individualization of clearance recommendations:

- Cleared for all sports without restriction
- Cleared for all sports without restriction with recommendations for further evaluation or treatment for issues identified during the preparticipation physical evaluation
- Not cleared pending further evaluation
- Not cleared for certain sports
- Not cleared for any sports

From Bernhardt DT, Roberts WO, eds. *PPE: Preparticipation Physical Evaluation.* 4th ed. Elk Grove Village, IL: American Academy of Pediatrics; 2010, with permission.

may need to serve as a medical contact. The PPE clearance form example provided at the end of this article includes line items for this information, but a separate release form will often be required.

SUMMARY

Preparticipation physical evaluations are often a challenge for physicians. A recent study examined the PPE in clinical practice among pediatricians and family physicians in the state of Washington.[36] Unfortunately, many physicians in this study perceived significant barriers to effective performance of the PPE. These barriers included uncertainty about how to perform the PPE, the relative importance of each PPE component, and the lack of a standardized approach and time for appropriate performance of the PPE. Although these concerns are shared by physicians beyond the borders of Washington, those who are aware of the information contained in the PPE monograph are able to use current best practices to enhance the effectiveness and efficiency of this examination and report greater comfort and satisfaction with these evaluations.[36]

References

1. Wingfield K, Matheson GO, Meeuwisse WH. Preparticipation evaluation: an evidence-based review. *Clin J Sport Med*. 2004;14(3):109-122
2. Bernhardt DT, Roberts WO, eds. *PPE: Preparticipation Physical Evaluation*. 4th ed. Elk Grove Village, IL: American Academy of Pediatrics; 2010
3. Conley KM, Bolin DJ, Carek PJ, et al. National Athletic Trainers' position statement: preparticipation physical examinations and disqualifying conditions. *J Athl Train*. 2014;49(1):102-120
4. Nordin JD, Solberg LI, Parker ED. Adolescent primary care visit patterns. *Ann Fam Med*. 2010;8(6):511-516
5. Carek PJ, Futrell M, Hueston WJ. The preparticipation physical examination history: who has the correct answers? *Clin J Sports Med*. 1999;9(3):124-128
6. Kerr ZY, Casa DJ, Marshall SW, Comstock RD. Epidemiology of exertional heat illness among U.S. high school athletes. *Am J Prev Med*. 2013;44(1):8-14
7. McHugh MP. Oversized young athletes: a weighty concern. *Br J Sports Med*. 2010:44:45-49
8. Rice SG; American Academy of Pediatrics Council on Sports Medicine and Fitness. Medical conditions affecting sports participation. *Pediatrics*. 2008;121(4):841-848
9. Maron BJ, Haas TS, Ahluwalia A, Rutten-Ramos SC. Incidence of cardiovascular sudden deaths in Minnesota high school athletes. *Heart Rhythm*. 2013;10(3):374-377
10. Harmon KG, Asif IM, Klossner D, Drezner JA. Incidence of sudden cardiac death in National Collegiate Athletic Association athletes. *Circulation*. 2011;123(15):1594-1600
11. Maron BJ, Haas TS, Murphy CJ, Ahluwalia A, Rutten-Ramos S. Incidence and causes of sudden death in U.S. college athletes. *J Am Coll Cardiol*. 2014;63(16):1636-1643
12. Maron BJ, Thompson PD, Ackerman MJ, et al. Recommendations and considerations related to preparticipation screening for cardiovascular abnormalities in competitive athletes: 2007 update: a scientific statement from the American Heart Association Council on Nutrition, Physical Activity, and Metabolism: endorsed by the American College of Cardiology Foundation. *Circulation*. 2007;115(12):1643-1645
13. Colivicchi F, Ammirati F, Santini M. Epidemiology and prognostic implications of syncope in young competing athletes. *Eur Heart J*. 2004;25(19):1749-1753
14. Loeys BL, Dietz HC, Braverman AC, et al. The revised Ghent nosology for the Marfan syndrome. *J Med Genet*. 2010;47:476-485

15. Magee C , Kazman J, Haigney M, et al. Reliability and validity of physician ECG interpretation for athletes. *Ann Noninvasive Electrocardiol.* 2014;19(4):319-329
16. Cook G, Burton L, Hoogenboom B. Pre-participation screening: the use of fundamental movements as an assessment of function—part 1. *N Am J Sports Phys Ther.* 2006;1(2):62-72
17. Sanders B, Blackburn TA, Boucher B. Preparticipation screening: the sports physical therapy perspective. *Int J Sports Phys Ther.* 2013;8(2):180-193
18. Wilkerson GB, Giles JL, Seibel DK. Prediction of core and lower extremity strains and sprains in collegiate football players: a preliminary study. *J Athl Train.* 2012;47(3):264-272
19. Hanks CD, Parsons J, Benninger C, et al. Etiology of dyspnea in elite and recreational athletes. *Phys Sportsmed.* 2012;40(2):28-33
20. World AntiDoping Agency 2014 Prohibited List. Published November 2013. Available at: www.wada-ama.org/en/resources/science-medicine/prohibited-list#.U_0TSRZ1IXq. Accessed August 26, 2014
21. Grover SA, Barkun AN, Sackett DL. Does this patient have splenomegaly? In: Simel DL, Rennie D, eds. *The Rational Clinical Examination: Evidence-Based Clinical Diagnosis.* New York: McGraw-Hill Medical; 2009:605-614
22. American Medical Society for Sports Medicine. Five things physicians and patients should question. Choosing Wisely campaign. Available at: www.amssm.org/Content/pdf%20files/Choosing_Wisely.pdf. Accessed August 26, 2014
23. Hosey RG, Mattacola CG, Kriss V, et al. Ultrasound assessment of spleen size in collegiate athletes. *Br J Sports Med.* 2006;40(3):251-254
24. McCorkle R, Thomas B, Suffaletto H, Jehle D. Normative spleen size in tall healthy athletes: implications for safe return to contact sports after infectious mononucleosis. *Clin J Sport Med.* 2010;20(6):413-415
25. National Federation of State High School State Associations. NFHS medical release form for wrestler to participate with skin lesions 2014-15. Available at: www.nfhs.org/media/882323/wr_skin_lesion_form-clean.pdf. Accessed August 27, 2014
26. Starr HM Jr, Anderson B, Courson R, Seiler JG. Brachial plexus injury: a descriptive study of American football. *J Surg Orthop Adv.* 2014;23(2):90-97
27. Standaert CJ, Herring SA. Expert opinion and controversies in musculoskeletal and sports medicine: stingers. *Arch Phys Med Rehab.* 2009;90(3):402-406
28. Concannon LG, Harrast MA, Herring SA. Radiating upper limb pain in the contact sport athlete: an update on transient quadriparesis and stingers. *Curr Sports Med Reports.* 2012;11(1):28-34
29. Halstead ME, Walter KD; American Academy of Pediatrics Council on Sports Medicine and Fitness. Clinical report: sport-related concussion in children and adolescents. *Pediatrics.* 2010;126(3):597-615
30. McCrory P, Meeuwisse WH, Aubry M, et al. Consensus statement on concussion in sport: the 4th International Conference on Concussion in Sport held in Zurich, November 2012. *Br J Sports Med.* 2013;47:250-258
31. American Academy of Pediatrics, American Association of Certified Orthoptists, American Association for Pediatric Ophthalmology and Strabismus, American Academy of Ophthalmology. Policy statement: eye examination in infants, children and young adults by pediatricians. *Pediatrics.* 2003;111:902-907. Reaffirmed May 2007
32. Eichner ER. Sickle cell trait in sports. *Curr Sports Med Rep.* 2010;9(6):347-351
33. Thompson AA. Sickle cell trait testing and athletic participation: a solution in search of a problem? *Hematology Am Soc Hematol Educ Program.* 2013;2013(1):632-637
34. Patel D, Greydanus DE. Sport participation by physically and cognitively challenged young athletes. *Pediatr Clin N Am.* 2010;57:795-817
35. Athletic preparticipation examinations for adolescents. Report of the Board of Trustees. Group on Science and Technology, American Medical Association. *Arch Pediatr Adolesc Med.* 1994:148(1):93-98
36. Madsen NL, Drezner JA, Salerno JC. The preparticipation physical evaluation: an analysis of clinical practice. *Clin J Sport Med.* 2014;24(2):142-149

■ PREPARTICIPATION PHYSICAL EVALUATION
HISTORY FORM

(Note: This form is to be filled out by the patient and parent prior to seeing the physician. The physician should keep this form in the chart.)

Date of Exam _____

Name _____ Date of birth _____

Sex _____ Age _____ Grade _____ School _____ Sport(s) _____

Medicines and Allergies: Please list all of the prescription and over-the-counter medicines and supplements (herbal and nutritional) that you are currently taking

_____

_____

_____

Do you have any allergies?   ☐ Yes ☐ No   If yes, please identify specific allergy below.
☐ Medicines   ☐ Pollens   ☐ Food   ☐ Stinging Insects

Explain "Yes" answers below. Circle questions you don't know the answers to.

GENERAL QUESTIONS	Yes	No	MEDICAL QUESTIONS	Yes	No
1. Has a doctor ever denied or restricted your participation in sports for any reason?			26. Do you cough, wheeze, or have difficulty breathing during or after exercise?		
2. Do you have any ongoing medical conditions? If so, please identify below: ☐ Asthma ☐ Anemia ☐ Diabetes ☐ Infections Other: _____			27. Have you ever used an inhaler or taken asthma medicine?		
			28. Is there anyone in your family who has asthma?		
3. Have you ever spent the night in the hospital?			29. Were you born without or are you missing a kidney, an eye, a testicle (males), your spleen, or any other organ?		
4. Have you ever had surgery?			30. Do you have groin pain or a painful bulge or hernia in the groin area?		
HEART HEALTH QUESTIONS ABOUT YOU — Yes — No			31. Have you had infectious mononucleosis (mono) within the last month?		
5. Have you ever passed out or nearly passed out DURING or AFTER exercise?			32. Do you have any rashes, pressure sores, or other skin problems?		
6. Have you ever had discomfort, pain, tightness, or pressure in your chest during exercise?			33. Have you had a herpes or MRSA skin infection?		
7. Does your heart ever race or skip beats (irregular beats) during exercise?			34. Have you ever had a head injury or concussion?		
8. Has a doctor ever told you that you have any heart problems? If so, check all that apply: ☐ High blood pressure ☐ A heart murmur ☐ High cholesterol ☐ A heart infection ☐ Kawasaki disease Other: _____			35. Have you ever had a hit or blow to the head that caused confusion, prolonged headache, or memory problems?		
			36. Do you have a history of seizure disorder?		
9. Has a doctor ever ordered a test for your heart? (For example, ECG/EKG, echocardiogram)			37. Do you have headaches with exercise?		
			38. Have you ever had numbness, tingling, or weakness in your arms or legs after being hit or falling?		
10. Do you get lightheaded or feel more short of breath than expected during exercise?			39. Have you ever been unable to move your arms or legs after being hit or falling?		
11. Have you ever had an unexplained seizure?			40. Have you ever become ill while exercising in the heat?		
12. Do you get more tired or short of breath more quickly than your friends during exercise?			41. Do you get frequent muscle cramps when exercising?		
HEART HEALTH QUESTIONS ABOUT YOUR FAMILY — Yes — No			42. Do you or someone in your family have sickle cell trait or disease?		
13. Has any family member or relative died of heart problems or had an unexpected or unexplained sudden death before age 50 (including drowning, unexplained car accident, or sudden infant death syndrome)?			43. Have you had any problems with your eyes or vision?		
			44. Have you had any eye injuries?		
14. Does anyone in your family have hypertrophic cardiomyopathy, Marfan syndrome, arrhythmogenic right ventricular cardiomyopathy, long QT syndrome, short QT syndrome, Brugada syndrome, or catecholaminergic polymorphic ventricular tachycardia?			45. Do you wear glasses or contact lenses?		
			46. Do you wear protective eyewear, such as goggles or a face shield?		
			47. Do you worry about your weight?		
15. Does anyone in your family have a heart problem, pacemaker, or implanted defibrillator?			48. Are you trying to or has anyone recommended that you gain or lose weight?		
			49. Are you on a special diet or do you avoid certain types of foods?		
16. Has anyone in your family had unexplained fainting, unexplained seizures, or near drowning?			50. Have you ever had an eating disorder?		
BONE AND JOINT QUESTIONS — Yes — No			51. Do you have any concerns that you would like to discuss with a doctor?		
17. Have you ever had an injury to a bone, muscle, ligament, or tendon that caused you to miss a practice or a game?			**FEMALES ONLY**		
			52. Have you ever had a menstrual period?		
18. Have you ever had any broken or fractured bones or dislocated joints?			53. How old were you when you had your first menstrual period?		
19. Have you ever had an injury that required x-rays, MRI, CT scan, injections, therapy, a brace, a cast, or crutches?			54. How many periods have you had in the last 12 months?		
20. Have you ever had a stress fracture?			**Explain "yes" answers here**		
21. Have you ever been told that you have or have you had an x-ray for neck instability or atlantoaxial instability? (Down syndrome or dwarfism)			_____		
22. Do you regularly use a brace, orthotics, or other assistive device?			_____		
23. Do you have a bone, muscle, or joint injury that bothers you?			_____		
24. Do any of your joints become painful, swollen, feel warm, or look red?			_____		
25. Do you have any history of juvenile arthritis or connective tissue disease?			_____		

I hereby state that, to the best of my knowledge, my answers to the above questions are complete and correct.

Signature of athlete _____ Signature of parent/guardian _____ Date _____

■ PREPARTICIPATION PHYSICAL EVALUATION
THE ATHLETE WITH SPECIAL NEEDS: SUPPLEMENTAL HISTORY FORM

Date of Exam _____

Name _____ Date of birth _____

Sex _____ Age _____ Grade _____ School _____ Sport(s) _____

1. Type of disability		
2. Date of disability		
3. Classification (if available)		
4. Cause of disability (birth, disease, accident/trauma, other)		
5. List the sports you are interested in playing		

	Yes	No
6. Do you regularly use a brace, assistive device, or prosthetic?		
7. Do you use any special brace or assistive device for sports?		
8. Do you have any rashes, pressure sores, or any other skin problems?		
9. Do you have a hearing loss? Do you use a hearing aid?		
10. Do you have a visual impairment?		
11. Do you use any special devices for bowel or bladder function?		
12. Do you have burning or discomfort when urinating?		
13. Have you had autonomic dysreflexia?		
14. Have you ever been diagnosed with a heat-related (hyperthermia) or cold-related (hypothermia) illness?		
15. Do you have muscle spasticity?		
16. Do you have frequent seizures that cannot be controlled by medication?		

Explain "yes" answers here

_____

_____

_____

_____

_____

Please indicate if you have ever had any of the following.

	Yes	No
Atlantoaxial instability		
X-ray evaluation for atlantoaxial instability		
Dislocated joints (more than one)		
Easy bleeding		
Enlarged spleen		
Hepatitis		
Osteopenia or osteoporosis		
Difficulty controlling bowel		
Difficulty controlling bladder		
Numbness or tingling in arms or hands		
Numbness or tingling in legs or feet		
Weakness in arms or hands		
Weakness in legs or feet		
Recent change in coordination		
Recent change in ability to walk		
Spina bifida		
Latex allergy		

Explain "yes" answers here

_____

_____

_____

_____

_____

I hereby state that, to the best of my knowledge, my answers to the above questions are complete and correct.

Signature of athlete _____ Signature of parent/guardian _____ Date _____

■ PREPARTICIPATION PHYSICAL EVALUATION
PHYSICAL EXAMINATION FORM

Name _____ Date of birth _____

PHYSICIAN REMINDERS
1. Consider additional questions on more sensitive issues
   - Do you feel stressed out or under a lot of pressure?
   - Do you ever feel sad, hopeless, depressed, or anxious?
   - Do you feel safe at your home or residence?
   - Have you ever tried cigarettes, chewing tobacco, snuff, or dip?
   - During the past 30 days, did you use chewing tobacco, snuff, or dip?
   - Do you drink alcohol or use any other drugs?
   - Have you ever taken anabolic steroids or used any other performance supplement?
   - Have you ever taken any supplements to help you gain or lose weight or improve your performance?
   - Do you wear a seat belt, use a helmet, and use condoms?
2. Consider reviewing questions on cardiovascular symptoms (questions 5–14).

EXAMINATION

Height		Weight		☐ Male ☐ Female			
BP	/	(/)	Pulse	Vision R 20/	L 20/	Corrected ☐ Y ☐ N	

MEDICAL	NORMAL	ABNORMAL FINDINGS
Appearance • Marfan stigmata (kyphoscoliosis, high-arched palate, pectus excavatum, arachnodactyly, arm span > height, hyperlaxity, myopia, MVP, aortic insufficiency)		
Eyes/ears/nose/throat • Pupils equal • Hearing		
Lymph nodes		
Heart [a] • Murmurs (auscultation standing, supine, +/- Valsalva) • Location of point of maximal impulse (PMI)		
Pulses • Simultaneous femoral and radial pulses		
Lungs		
Abdomen		
Genitourinary (males only) [b]		
Skin • HSV, lesions suggestive of MRSA, tinea corporis		
Neurologic [c]		
MUSCULOSKELETAL		
Neck		
Back		
Shoulder/arm		
Elbow/forearm		
Wrist/hand/fingers		
Hip/thigh		
Knee		
Leg/ankle		
Foot/toes		
Functional • Duck-walk, single leg hop		

[a] Consider ECG, echocardiogram, and referral to cardiology for abnormal cardiac history or exam.
[b] Consider GU exam if in private setting. Having third party present is recommended.
[c] Consider cognitive evaluation or baseline neuropsychiatric testing if a history of significant concussion.

☐ Cleared for all sports without restriction

☐ Cleared for all sports without restriction with recommendations for further evaluation or treatment for _____
_____

☐ Not cleared

      ☐ Pending further evaluation

      ☐ For any sports

      ☐ For certain sports _____

         Reason _____

Recommendations _____

I have examined the above-named student and completed the preparticipation physical evaluation. The athlete does not present apparent clinical contraindications to practice and participate in the sport(s) as outlined above. A copy of the physical exam is on record in my office and can be made available to the school at the request of the parents. If conditions arise after the athlete has been cleared for participation, the physician may rescind the clearance until the problem is resolved and the potential consequences are completely explained to the athlete (and parents/guardians).

Name of physician (print/type) _____ Date _____

Address _____ Phone _____

Signature of physician _____ , MD or DO

■ PREPARTICIPATION PHYSICAL EVALUATION
CLEARANCE FORM

Name _____ Sex ☐ M ☐ F   Age _____   Date of birth _____

☐ Cleared for all sports without restriction

☐ Cleared for all sports without restriction with recommendations for further evaluation or treatment for _____

_____

☐ Not cleared

      ☐ Pending further evaluation

      ☐ For any sports

      ☐ For certain sports _____

      Reason _____

Recommendations _____

_____

_____

_____

_____

_____

_____

I have examined the above-named student and completed the preparticipation physical evaluation. The athlete does not present apparent clinical contraindications to practice and participate in the sport(s) as outlined above. A copy of the physical exam is on record in my office and can be made available to the school at the request of the parents. If conditions arise after the athlete has been cleared for participation, the physician may rescind the clearance until the problem is resolved and the potential consequences are completely explained to the athlete (and parents/guardians).

Name of physician (print/type) _____ Date _____

Address _____ Phone _____

Signature of physician _____ , MD or DO

EMERGENCY INFORMATION

Allergies _____

_____

_____

_____

_____

_____

Other information _____

_____

_____

_____

_____

_____

_____

_____

_____

_____

Adolesc Med 026 (2015) 39–52

Concussion in Teenage Athletes

Kevin D. Walter, MD, FAAP[a]*;
Mark E. Halstead, MD, FAAP[b]

[a]Medical College of Wisconsin, Children's Hospital of Wisconsin, Milwaukee, Wisconsin;
[b]Washington University School of Medicine, St. Louis Children's Hospital, St. Louis, Missouri

Over the last decade, concussions occurring during sports have been an area of intense interest among medical professionals and the media. A media-proclaimed "concussion crisis" now exists, spawning significant increases in published research on the topic, a proliferation of devices and gear in an attempt to reduce the risk of sustaining a concussion and improving the likelihood of detecting a concussion, and increased anxiety among parents about letting their children participate in contact sports or return to contact sports after a concussion.

Since 2010, several leading organizations (American Academy of Pediatrics, American Academy of Neurology, American Medical Society for Sports Medicine, Concussion in Sport Group) have published clinical reports or position statements on sport-related concussion.[1-4] Despite these numerous guidelines, a study by Carl and Kinsella[5] found that pediatricians in Illinois were knowledgeable about concussions but demonstrated poor knowledge of recently passed legislation and the consensus guidelines for sport-related concussion.

Despite reporting knowledge of concussive injuries, pediatricians believe that there are barriers to providing adequate care to patients with concussions.[6] Barriers include inadequate training and time to educate patients about their injuries. Further educational efforts of pediatricians and the development of resources to support their daily practice may help physicians with their comfort and ability in managing concussions appropriately.

*Corresponding author
E-mail address: KWalter@chw.org

DEFINITION

Concussions are often defined by the development of a constellation of symptoms and signs that are present after a traumatic blow to the head. The Concussion in Sport Group defines a concussion, based on expert opinion, as a "complex pathophysiological process affecting the brain, induced by biomechanical forces."[4] This group also includes 5 features of concussions that involve a direct blow, rapid onset of symptoms, functional rather than structural disturbances to the brain, graded set of clinical symptoms, and grossly normal neuroimaging studies.[4]

Although no universally accepted definition exists, a consensus group developed evidence-based indicators of concussion from a systematic review of the literature. These indicators of concussion include observed and documented confusion immediately after the event; impaired balance within 1 day after injury; slower reaction time within 2 days after injury; and impaired verbal learning and memory within 2 days after injury.[7]

BIOMECHANICS AND PATHOPHYSIOLOGY

Existing studies of head injury biomechanics are inadequate in identifying thresholds for injury in youth.[8] Biomechanical sensors placed in helmets and on the skin currently are being used to conduct further research in order to define direction and age-related injury thresholds. At this time, biomechanical information obtained from sensors has no validated clinical value.

Cerebral physiology may be adversely affected for weeks by the neurometabolic cascade occurring after a concussion.[9] In 2001, Giza and Hovda[9] coauthored a definitive article on the neurometabolic cascade that occurs after a concussion. The primary components of this cascade include abrupt neuronal depolarization, ionic shifts, increased glucose metabolism coupled with decreased cerebral blood flow, and release of excitatory neurotransmitters that lead to impaired axonal function.

EPIDEMIOLOGY

The Centers for Disease Control and Prevention (CDC) estimates that 1.6 to 3.8 million concussions occur in sports and recreational activities each year.[10] Because in most cases athletes who sustain concussions must report their symptoms and injury, it is believed that most epidemiologic figures underestimate the total burden of concussion.[11,12] McCrea et al[12] noted that athletes did not report their injury because of fear of removal from participation and because they were unsure if they had a concussion. The Institute of Medicine (IOM) proposed that variable research definitions of concussion and less than ideal youth injury surveillance systems also hamper the accuracy of epidemiologic studies.[8]

Many recent studies have shown that the rate of reported concussion is increasing over time. Data from the National Collegiate Athletic Association (NCAA) Injury Surveillance System showed that overall reported concussion rates doubled from the school years 1988 to 1989 to 2003 to 2004.[13] A study of public high schools showed a 4-fold increase in reported concussions from the school years 1997 to 1998 to 2007 to 2008.[14] Studies have also shown increased visits to emergency departments (EDs) for concussion in children and adolescents aged 19 years and younger.[15,16]

Research has shown that collegiate athletes had higher overall rates of concussion than high school athletes in the same sport.[17] However, the IOM report found a lack of data to determine the variations of concussion rates across the pediatric age range.[8] It has been speculated that the immaturity of the developing central nervous system, a larger head-to-body ratio, less neck and shoulder strength, a larger subarachnoid space in which the brain can move, and differences in cerebral blood volume are potential reasons for increased susceptibility to concussions for youth compared to adult athletes.[8] Also relative to adults, children demonstrate more widespread and prolonged metabolic sensitivities after head injury, which may result in more severe and persistent symptoms.[8] Concussion rates are higher during competition than practice, with the exception of cheerleading, which carries an elevated risk during practice.[13,17,18]

Females frequently are reported to have a higher rate of concussion than males when they participate in the same sport (eg, soccer) and in sports such as lacrosse and ice hockey, which are non-contact for females.[8] Contact and collision sports carry the highest incidence of concussion.[8] Common high school and private club contact sports include football, ice hockey, soccer, lacrosse, wrestling, and basketball. In addition, athletes with a history of previous concussions are 2 to 5.8 times more likely to sustain a subsequent concussion, although the reasons why they are more susceptible are unclear.[1,3,8]

SIDELINE ASSESSMENT

For many young athletes, medical practitioners are not available on the sideline to perform injury assessments during practice or competition. Therefore, educational efforts aimed at athletes, parents, and coaches are critical to help improve awareness and recognition of concussion. A further difficulty is that symptoms may not become apparent for a few hours after the injury, which may delay identification of the injury.[4] Signs are problems that can be observed in an injured athlete, whereas symptoms are what the athlete reports about how he feels (Table 1).

Some schools and private club teams have athletic trainers to provide care on the sidelines and help with concussion management. In some states, athletic trainers care for concussed athletes independently, but many recommend that injured athletes seek out a physician for further care. A good relationship and open com-

Table 1

Signs and Symptoms of Concussion Relevant to Sideline Assessment

---

Signs observed
    Appears dazed or stunned (glassy eyed)
    Is confused about position or assignment on the field
    Forgets play or instruction
    Is unsure of score or opponent
    Moves clumsily or has poor balance
    Answers questions slowly
    Loses consciousness (even briefly)
    Shows mood, behavior, or personality changes
    Cannot recall events before hit or fall
    Cannot recall events after hit or fall
Symptoms reported by athlete
    Headache or "pressure" in head
    Nausea or vomiting
    Balance problems or dizziness
    Double or blurry vision
    Sensitivity to light or noise
    Feels sluggish, hazy, foggy, or groggy
    Concentration or memory problems
    Confusion
    Feels more emotional, nervous, or anxious
    Does not "feel right" or is "feeling down"

From Institute of Medicine and National Research Council. *Sports Related Concussions in Youth: Improving the Science, Changing the Culture.* Washington, DC: The National Academies Press; 2013:99.

munication with community athletic trainers is important because the athletic trainer may have information that the athlete is withholding in an attempt to appear recovered. Also, the athletic trainer may be able to provide oversight to improve the athlete's transition back to school and sport.

Any athlete who has sustained a blow to the head or a jolt should be watched closely and questioned about concussion. If there are any signs or symptoms, the athlete should be immediately removed from play for a thorough evaluation for concussion by a medical practitioner. The mantra for someone with a suspected concussion is "when in doubt, sit them out."[8]

In order to help with the evaluation of a suspected concussion, most practitioners use the Sport Concussion Assessment Tool, 3rd edition (SCAT3), on the sideline.[4] This is a free, standardized tool for concussion evaluation of injured athletes 13 years and older (available at bjsm.bmj.com/content/47/5/259.full.pdf+html). The SCAT3 includes instructions for use, and advice and education for the athlete. It allows the practitioner to record a brief medical history and includes a checklist for signs and symptoms. There are sections to provide the Glasgow Coma score (GCS); the Maddocks score, which tests an athlete's orientation to place and time; and a cognitive assessment. There are also prompts to record physical examination findings for neck evaluation, balance assessment, and coordination assessment. Because athletes may not be honest about their injury and symptoms, the SCAT3 can provide valuable objective information about the injury. It also can be used in clinic to ensure a thorough evaluation is completed.

Athletes with a suspected concussion should be evaluated for a cervical spine injury. If the athlete displayed loss of consciousness, cervical spine precautions and immobilization are paramount. Any athlete with deterioration or concern for cervical spine injury should be transported to an ED.

Athletes with suspected or known concussions should continue to be monitored for several hours after the injury to assess for possible deterioration. Any deterioration may herald the need for referral to the ED. Referral to the ED is warranted if an athlete experiences repeated vomiting, severe or progressively worsening headache, seizure activity, unsteady gait or slurred speech, weakness or numbness in the extremities, unusual behavior, signs of a basilar skull fracture, or altered mental status resulting in a GCS less than 15.[1]

CLINICAL EVALUATION

The diagnosis of concussion is primarily made based on the history of trauma and the presence of a constellation of symptoms (Table 2). Physical examination should include a thorough neurologic evaluation, balance and coordination testing, and cognitive testing. These evaluations are present on the SCAT3.[4] Using all of these evaluation tools can increase the sensitivity and specificity of concussion diagnosis.[2,3]

A variety of symptom checklists can be used to track symptoms over time. The Post-Concussion Symptom Scale is a validated, 22-item, Likert scale tool that is commonly used.[19] The Balance Error Scoring System (BESS) is a good method to assess postural stability but often requires a preinjury assessment to identify changes.[4,8]

Quantitative electroencephalography and event-related potential procedures can detect differences between concussed and non-concussed individuals, but further research is needed to define the role of those tests in clinical care.[8] There is no evidence that serum biomarkers are valuable for identification of concussion in pediatric and adolescent patients.[8]

Computerized neurocognitive tests have become very popular. Research has shown variable results on their effectiveness in diagnosing concussion.[8] All commercial test platforms have studies indicating acceptable reliability, but there are studies that have demonstrated less than adequate reliability.[8] Many sports med-

Table 2
Concussion symptoms

Somatic
Headache
Blurry vision
Dizziness
Fatigue
Drowsiness
Sensitivity to light
Sensitivity to noise
Balance problems
Nausea or vomiting shortly after the injury
Cognitive
Difficulty thinking clearly
Feeling slowed down
Difficulty concentrating
Difficulty remembering new information
Emotional
Irritability
Sadness
Feeling more emotional
Nervousness or anxiety
Sleep
Sleeping more than usual
Sleeping less than usual
Trouble falling asleep

From CDC. Injury prevention and control: traumatic brain injury. Available at: www.cdc.gov/concussion/signs_symptoms.html. Accessed October 11, 2014.

icine specialists advocate baseline testing, although not all agree that it is indicated. Baseline or preinjury computerized testing, if performed, should be obtained in the preseason. This allows the practitioner to compare postinjury test results to assess for changes in cognitive function. Practitioners require training and experience to proctor and interpret. Tests may be best interpreted by a neuropsychologist. Use of neurocognitive testing is further discussed in the acute management section.

Neuroimaging

Conventional neuroimaging, such as computed tomography (CT) and magnetic resonance imaging (MRI), can be obtained to assess for structural damage in the brain, such as skull fracture or intracranial hemorrhage. These imaging modalities often are normal in concussion and do not contribute to the diagnostic or prognostic value.[20] Routine use of CT in concussion places patients at risk for unnecessary radiation exposure. If neuroimaging is needed, most experts recommend CT scan within the first 48 hours after injury and MRI after 2 days.

Magnetic resonance imaging enables the detection of lesions such as cerebral contusion, petechial hemorrhage, white matter injury, and Chiari malformations that may be missed on CT scan.[20]

Kupperman et al[21] enrolled 42,412 children in a study through the Pediatric Emergency Care Applied Research Network (PECARN) to establish predictive rules for CT scan use in patients younger than 18 years presenting with a GCS of 14 or 15 and within 24 hours after head trauma. The rules were based on the risk of clinically important traumatic brain injury (ciTBI), which was defined as hospital admission for longer than 2 nights, neurosurgery intervention, intubation for more than 24 hours, or death from brain injury. Computed tomographic scan was recommended for adolescent patients presenting with a GCS of 14 or other signs of altered mental status (agitation, somnolence, repetitive questioning, or slow response to verbal communication), or signs of basilar skull fracture, because this group had a 4.3% risk of ciTBI. Patients with a GCS of 15 and a history of loss of consciousness, vomiting, severe headache, or severe mechanism of injury carried a 0.9% risk of ciTBI. Observation in the ED versus CT scan was recommended for this intermediate-risk group. The remainder of the patients without the risk factors discussed carried a less than 0.05% risk of ciTBI, and observation was recommended.

Studies of other advanced imaging modalities, such as diffusion tensor imaging, functional MRI, positron emission tomography, and magnetic resonance spectroscopy, have shown differences between concussed and nonconcussed individuals.[20] However, these imaging modalities have no clinical indications at this time, and further research is needed, especially in the pediatric and adolescent populations.

ACUTE MANAGEMENT

In high school athletes, approximately 70% will be symptom-free by 1 week after the injury, and 90% will be symptom-free by 3 weeks.[22] With this rapid resolution, concussion is an ideal injury that can be managed by a patient's primary physician. Proper knowledge of early treatment recommendations and knowing when referral to a specialist is needed will help the adolescent physician manage most concussive injuries.

After an acute concussion, the mainstay of recommended treatment has been rest, both physical and cognitive. It would be impossible to practice complete cognitive rest, as often described, without the person being in a comatose state. Recommendations range from so-called "cocoon therapy," in which an athlete is removed from all stimulus and kept in a darkened environment for several days, to an approach of little to no rest from physical and cognitive activity. Unfortunately, expert opinion has prevailed, with little research supporting one approach over another.

Over the past year, some research has suggested that extremes of rest are not as beneficial as a more moderate approach.[23] A prospective cohort study demonstrated the longest recovery in patients who did not reduce their cognitive activity level at all. Those with mild to severe reductions in cognitive load recovered much faster after their concussion.[24] This suggests that failing to reduce cognitive activity at all is detrimental to recovery.

In a retrospective study of collegiate athletes, those who engaged in school and some level of physical activity performed the best on neurocognitive testing up to 1 month after injury.[25] Those who did not participate in school or physical activity and those with full school and full activity performed the worst on neurocognitive testing. This finding again suggests that extremes may be detrimental to neurocognitive performance.

From a practical standpoint, it seems reasonable that some level of activity would be beneficial to the athlete. Because these athletes usually are removed from sport after diagnosis, their typical social networks are disrupted. Often the athlete is advised not to text or use computers, and perhaps to remain home from school, which isolates the athlete from normal social situations. It would not be unusual for an athlete to quickly become depressed, further complicating the recovery and making it more difficult for the physician to determine whether the prolonged symptoms are the result of the depression or the concussion.

Ideally, early after the concussion, physical rest is necessary because the athlete does not feel well and physical activity often worsens symptoms. As symptoms begin to decrease, it would be reasonable to start short durations of 20 minutes or less of light cardiovascular activity, provided the symptoms do not worsen during this phase. Once symptoms have returned to the athlete's baseline level for 24 hours, progression on a return to play protocol (see Return to Play Program section) could be initiated.

Cognitive adjustments may be necessary for the athlete in the early phases while recovering from a concussion. These adjustments should be symptom-based and may vary on a day-to-day basis. Adjustments may include a reduced workload, additional time to complete tests or assignments, audio books for those with reading difficulties, and allowing breaks in the day if symptoms worsen. Further detailed information on the concept of returning to learning may be found in the American Academy of Pediatrics clinical report published in 2013 (see Table 3).[26]

Athletes with prolonged (>3-4 weeks) symptoms, severe symptoms, or a history of multiple concussions should be considered for a referral to a specialist. Several factors have been proposed as modifiers for recovery from a concussion, including previous history of concussion, severity and number of reported symptoms, and preexisting mood, psychological, or migraine disorders.[3] Athletes with a history of these modifiers may also be considered for referral to a specialist.

Table 3
Resources for Returning to Learning

American Academy of Pediatrics Returning to Learning Following a Concussion Clinical Report: pediatrics.aappublications.org/content/132/5/948.full
Centers for Disease Control and Prevention Heads Up Program: www.cdc.gov/concussion/ HeadsUp
National Federation of State High School Associations: www.nfhs.org
SCAT3, British Journal of Sports Medicine: bjsm.bmj.com/content/47/5/259.full.pdf+html
Virginia Tech Football Helmet Ratings: www.sbes.vt.edu/helmet.php

---

MEDICATION USE

Limited data are available on the utility of medication use after a concussion. Regular use of over-the-counter analgesics may contribute to chronic medication overuse headaches, which would cloud the assessment of recovery after a concussion.[27] Amantadine may be helpful in reducing cognitive deficits and symptom reporting.[28] Further research is needed on the utility of various medications and supplements in the management of concussion.

NEUROCOGNITIVE TESTING

Neurocognitive testing may be an adjunct to concussion assessment. Consensus statements have stressed that most concussions can be managed without neurocognitive testing and that neurocognitive testing is only 1 tool in concussion management and return to play decision-making.[1,3,4]

Typical testing is performed through 1 of several computerized assessments. Traditional pencil-and-paper testing for an acute concussion is not as practical given the longer time to complete testing batteries and the limited availability of neuropsychologists. Formal neuropsychologic testing may be warranted for the athlete with prolonged symptoms.

Several factors can have an effect on the test, independent of a concussion. These include sleep, group versus individual testing, overall effort, and prior computer use.[29-32] Knowledge of and accounting for these variables when conducting baseline and postinjury assessments is important.

RETURN TO PLAY PROGRAM

In order to begin a return to play protocol (Table 4), an athlete must be back at the baseline level of symptoms for at least a full day. In addition, the athlete should be off all medications used to treat symptoms and should be fully functional in school. If the athlete remains symptom-free while working through the entire return to play protocol, he or she can be considered ready to return to play

Table 4
Concussion rehabilitation/stepwise return to play

Rehabilitation stage	Functional exercise
1. No activity	Complete physical and cognitive rest
2. Light aerobic activity	Walking, swimming, stationary cycling at 70% maximum heart rate; no resistance exercises
3. Sport-specific exercise	Specific sport-related drills but no head involvement
4. Noncontact training drills	More complex drills; may start light resistance training
5. Full-contact practice	After medical clearance, participate in normal training
6. Return to play	Normal game play

Each stage in concussion rehabilitation should last no less than 24 hours with a minimum of 5 days required to consider a full return to competition. If symptoms recur during the rehabilitation program, the athlete should stop immediately. Once the athlete has been asymptomatic for at least another 24 hours, he should return to the previous asymptomatic level and try to progress again. The athlete should contact his physician if symptoms recur. Any athlete with multiple concussions or prolonged symptoms may require a prolonged concussion rehabilitation program, which ideally is created by a physician experienced in concussion management.

From Halstead ME, Walter KW; American Academy of Pediatrics Council on Sports Medicine and Fitness. Clinical report: sport-related concussion in children and adolescents. *Pediatrics.* 2010;126:597-615.

in full competition. If symptoms increase during the protocol, the athlete should stop physical exertion and not progress without medical clearance. In these instances, care should be taken to ensure that the concussion has truly resolved before allowing the athlete to resume the protocol. Adjustments to the protocols may be considered in the athlete with recurrent concussions or prolonged symptoms after a concussion.

PREVENTION

It is unlikely that concussions can be completely prevented in sports. Over the last few years, increased efforts have been made to modify protective gear, particularly with regard to helmet design. Rule changes in sport seem to occur on an annual basis in an attempt to reduce the risk of concussion. Educational efforts continue in an attempt to bring more awareness and recognition of this injury.

The influence of helmet design on concussion risk is controversial. A recent retrospective study comparing 2 Riddel football helmets demonstrated a significant risk reduction of concussive injuries in athletes who wore the newer Revolution helmet compared to the older VSR4 helmet.[33] On the other hand, a prospective study showed that the risk of sustaining a concussion and the severity of a concussion were not associated with a specific football helmet brand.[34] A systematic review found an overall reduction on head injuries, but not necessarily concussion risk, with helmet use during skiing, snowboarding, and bicycling.[35]

Mouth guard use in sports is known to produce a significant reduction in orofacial injuries but has not consistently demonstrated a consistent reduction in concussion risk.[36] However, a small study of high school football players found the athletes had a reduction in concussion incidence with the use of a custom mandibular orthotic.[37] Yet another study found a higher incidence of concussion in athletes who wore custom mouth guards compared to stock mouth guards.[34] Further research is needed to evaluate the protective equipment and concussion risk.

In a study of high school athletes, those with more neck strength were found to have a lower risk of concussion, suggesting a possible area for concussion reduction efforts.[38]

Education should continue to be a part of all prevention measures. Multiple studies continue to demonstrate deficiencies in knowledge and attitudes toward concussions by parents, athletes, and coaches despite increased media attention and educational efforts.[39-41] Athletes may not follow recommendations or may avoid disclosing their symptoms after a concussion in order to continue sport participation.[42,43] Further efforts should be made toward determining the optimal educational formats and materials for concussion education.

Many of the governing bodies for each individual sport have created concussion educational programs and policies for their members. Resources for families and adolescents include the National Federation of State High School Associations (see Table 3) and each state's interscholastic athletic association that governs high school athletics.

LEGISLATION

As of February 2014, all 50 states had passed some form of legislation relating to sport concussions. Most of the laws include 3 components modeled after the Zackery Lystedt law, which was passed in the state of Washington in 2009. These components are education, often for parents and athletes but may include coaches and other individuals; removal from play after a suspected concussion; and written clearance from a qualified health care professional, the type of which varies by state, before the athlete can return to play.

After implementation of the law in the state of Washington, concussion knowledge of coaches was found to be good, but athlete and parent knowledge was poor.[44] Symptom reporting after a suspected concussion was also found to be poor among athletes after implementation of the law.[45] Further education efforts for athletes likely are necessary as part of this legislation to help improve the knowledge base as well as to emphasize the importance of symptom reporting.

CONCLUSION

Sport-related concussion is a common injury among adolescent athletes. Despite increasing concussion awareness, underreporting of injury still is likely because athletes may not disclose their symptoms in an attempt to continue playing. In addition, many concussion signs and symptoms can overlap with other medical and mental health conditions, which can complicate diagnosis and management. Neuroimaging studies are generally normal in concussion but may be needed to assess for more significant intracranial injury. Athletes with concussion need cognitive and physical rest to recover. No athlete should return to play while still symptomatic, nor should any athlete return to play on the same day. Computerized concussion testing has become more prevalent but remains only 1 tool that may be helpful with concussion management. Athletes with multiple concussions, prolonged recovery, or complicating medical conditions should be referred to a specialist for further management. Education and increasing awareness are the cornerstones of reducing risk because protective equipment does not appear to modify concussion risk at this time. Physicians should understand the concussion law for their state. It is imperative that further research be done to improve and refine diagnostic and management strategies.

References

1. Halstead ME, Walter KW; American Academy of Pediatrics Council on Sports Medicine and Fitness. Clinical report: sport-related concussion in children and adolescents. *Pediatrics.* 2010;126: 597-615
2. Giza CC, Kutcher JS, Ashwal S, et al. Summary of evidence-based guideline update: evaluation and management of concussion in sports: report of the Guideline Development Subcommittee of the American Academy of Neurology. *Neurology.* 2013;80:2250-2257
3. Harmon KG, Drezner J, Gammons M, et al. American Medical Society for Sports Medicine position statement: concussion in sport. *Clin J Sport Med.* 2013;23:1-18
4. McCrory P, Meeuwisse W, Aubry M, et al. Consensus statement on concussion in sport—the 4th International Conference on Concussion in Sport held in Zurich, November 2012. *Clin J Sport Med.* 2013;23:89-117
5. Carl RL, Kinsella SB. Pediatricians' knowledge of current sports concussion legislation and guidelines and comfort with sports concussion management: a cross-sectional study. *Clin Pediatr (Phila).* 2014;53:689-697
6. Zonfrillo MR, Master CL, Grady MF, et al. Pediatric providers' self-reported knowledge, practices, and attitudes about concussion. *Pediatrics.* 2012;130:1120-1125
7. Carney N, Ghajar J, Jagoda A, et al. Concussion guidelines step 1: systematic review of prevalent indicators. *Neurosurgery.* 2014;75(Suppl 1):S3-S15
8. Institute of Medicine and National Research Council. *Sports Related Concussions in Youth: Improving the Science, Changing the Culture.* Washington, DC: The National Academies Press; 2013
9. Giza CC, Hovda DA. The neurometabolic cascade of concussion. *J Athl Train.* 2001;36:228-235
10. Langlois JA, Rutland-Brown W, Wald MM. The epidemiology and impact of traumatic brain injury: a brief overview. *J Head Trauma Rehabil.* 2006;21(5):375-378
11. Daneshvar DH, Nowinski CJ, McKee A, Cantu RC. The epidemiology of sport-related concussion. *Clin Sports Med.* 2011;30:1-17
12. McCrea M, Hammeke T, Olsen G, Leo P, Guskiewicz K. Unreported concussion in high school football players: implications for prevention. *Clin J Sport Med.* 2004;14:13-17

13. Hootman J, Dick R, Agel J. Epidemiology of collegiate injuries for 15 sports: summary and recommendations for injury prevention initiatives. *J Athl Train*. 2007;42:311-319

14. Lincoln A, Caswell S, Almquist J, et al. Trends in concussion incidence in high school sports: a prospective 11-year study. *Am J Sports Med*. 2011;39:958-963

15. Bakhos LL, Lockhart GR, Myers R, Linakis JG. Emergency department visits for concussion in young child athletes. *Pediatrics*. 2010;126:e550-e556

16. Gilchrist J, Thomas KE, Xu L, McGuire LC, Coronado V. Nonfatal traumatic brain injuries related to sports and recreation activities among persons ≤19 years—United States, 2001-2009. *MMWR*. 2011;60:1337-1342

17. Gessel LM, Fields SK, Collins CL, Dick RW, Comstock RD. Concussions among United States high school and collegiate athletes. *J Athl Train*. 2007;42:495-503

18. Marar M, McIlcain N, Fields S, Comstock R. Epidemiology of concussions among United States high school athletes in 20 sports. *Am J Sports Med*. 2012;40:747-755

19. Lovell MR, Collins MW. Neuropsychological assessment of the college football player. *J Head Trauma Rehabil*. 1998;13:9-26

20. Apps JN, Walter KD, eds. *Pediatric and Adolescent Concussion: Diagnosis, Management, and Outcomes*. New York: Springer; 2012:81-91

21. Kupperman N, Holmes JF, Dayan PS, et al. Identification of children at very low risk of clinically-important brain injuries after head trauma: a prospective cohort study. *Lancet*. 2009;374:1160-1170

22. McKeon JM, Livingston SC, Reed A, et al. Trends in concussion return-to-play timelines among high school athletes from 2007 to 2009. *J Athl Train*. 2013;48:836-843

23. Thomas DG, Apps JN, Hoffman RG, McCrea M, Hammeke T. Benefits of strict rest after acute concussion: a randomized controlled trial. *Pediatrics*. 2015;135(2):213-223

24. Brown NJ, Mannix RC, O'Brien MH, et al. Effect of cognitive activity level on duration of post-concussion symptoms. *Pediatrics*. 2014;133:e299-e304

25. Majerske CW, Mihalik JP, Ren D, et al. Concussion in sports: postconcussive activity levels, symptoms, and neurocognitive performance. *J Athl Train*. 2008;43:265-274

26. Halstead ME, McAvoy K, Devore CD, et al. Returning to learning following a concussion. *Pediatrics*. 2013;132:948-957

27. Heyer GL, Idris SA. Does analgesic overuse contribute to chronic post-traumatic headaches in adolescent patients? *Pediatr Neurol*. 2014;50:464-468

28. Reddy CC, Collins M, Lovell M, Kontos AP. Efficacy of amantadine treatment on symptoms and neurocognitive performance among adolescents following sport-related concussion. *J Head Trauma Rehabil*. 2013;28:260-265

29. McClure DJ, Zuckerman SL, Kutscher SJ, Gregory AJ, Solomon GS. Baseline neurocognitive testing in sports-related concussion: the importance of a prior night's sleep. *Am J Sports Med*. 2014;42:472-478

30. Moser RS, Schatz P, Neidzwski K, Ott SD. Group versus individual administration affects baseline neurocognitive testing. *Am J Sports Med*. 2011;39:2325-2330

31. Hunt TN, Ferrara MS, Miller LS, Macciocchi S. The effect of effort on baseline neuropsychological test scores in high school athletes. *Arch Clin Neuropsychol*. 2007;22:615-621

32. Iverson GL, Brooks BL, Ashton VL, Johnson LG, Gualtieri CT. Does familiarity with computers affect computerized neuropsychological testing performance? *J Clin Exp Neuropsychol*. 2009;31:594-604

33. Rowson S, Duma SM, Greenwald RM, et al. Can helmet design reduce the risk of concussion in football? *J Neurosurg*. 2014;120:919-922

34. McGuine T, Brooks A, Hetzel S, Rasmussen J, McCrea M. The association of the type of football helmet and mouth guard with the incidence of sport related concussion in high school football players. *Ortho J Sport Med*. 2013;1(4 Suppl 1). Published September 20, 2013. doi:10.1177/2325967113S00027

35. Benson BW, Hamilton GM, Meeuwisse WH, McCrory P, Dvorak J. Is protective equipment useful in preventing concussion? A systematic review of the literature. *Br J Sports Med*. 2009;43(Suppl 1):i56-i67

36. Knapik JJ, Marshall SW, Lee RB, et al. Mouthguards in sport activities: history, physical properties and injury prevention effectiveness. *Sports Med.* 2007;37:117-144

37. Singh GD, Maher GJ, Padilla RR. Customized mandibular orthotics in the prevention of concussion/ mild traumatic brain injury in football players: a preliminary study. *Dent Traumatol.* 2009;25:515-521

38. Collins CL, Fletcher EN, Fields SK, et al. Neck strength: a protective factor reducing risk for concussion in high school sports. *J Prim Prev.* 2014;35:309-319

39. Mannings C, Kalynych C, Joseph MM, Smotherman C, Kraemer DF. Knowledge assessment of sports-related concussion among parents of children aged 5 to 15 years enrolled in recreational tackle football. *J Trauma Acute Care Surg.* 2014;77(3 Suppl 1):S18-S22

40. Cournoyer J, Tripp BL. Concussion knowledge in high school football players. *J Athl Train.* 2014;49:654-658

41. White PE, Newton JD, Makdissi M, et al. Knowledge about sports-related concussion: is the message getting through to coaches and trainers. *Br J Sports Med.* 2014;48:119-124

42. Mrazik M, Perra A, Brooks BL, Naidu D. Exploring minor hockey players' knowledge and attitudes towards concussion: implications for prevention. *J Head Trauma Rehabil.* February 28, 2014 [Epub ahead of print]

43. Register-Mihalik JK, Guskiewicz KM, McLeod TC, et al. Knowledge, attitude and concussion-reporting behaviors among high school athletes: a preliminary study. *J Athl Train.* 2013;48:645-653

44. Chrisman SP, Schiff MA, Chung SK, Herring SA, Rivara FP. Implementation of concussion legislation and extent of concussion education for athletes, parents, and coaches in Washington State. *Am J Sports Med.* 2014;42:1190-1196

45. Rivara FP, Schiff MA, Chrisman SP, et al. The effect of coach education on reporting of concussions among high school athletes after passage of a concussion law. *Am J Sports Med.* 2014;42:1197-1203

Adolesc Med 026 (2015) 53–78

Musculoskeletal Injuries
Not to Miss in Teens

Leda A. Ghannad, MD[a]; Andrew M. Watson, MD, MS[b];
Alison Brooks, MD, MPH[c]; Cynthia R. LaBella, MD[d]*

[a]Pediatric Sports Medicine Fellow, Division of Orthopaedic Surgery and Sports Medicine,
Ann & Robert H. Lurie Children's Hospital of Chicago, Chicago, Illinois; [b]Clinical Instructor,
Departments of Orthopedics and Pediatrics, Division of Sports Medicine, University of Wisconsin–
Madison, Madison, Wisconsin; [c]Assistant Professor, Departments of Orthopedics and Pediatrics,
Division of Sports Medicine, University of Wisconsin–Madison, Madison, Wisconsin;
[d]Associate Professor of Pediatrics, Division of Orthopaedic Surgery and Sports Medicine,
Ann & Robert H. Lurie Children's Hospital of Chicago, Chicago, Illinois

Adolescence is a period of rapid musculoskeletal growth and with this growth comes an increased susceptibility to injuries unique to this age group. The purpose of this article is not to provide a comprehensive review of all musculoskeletal injuries that can be sustained during adolescence but rather to focus on those conditions that necessitate early diagnosis and management to improve outcomes and decrease morbidity. Topics discussed include the diagnosis and management of upper and lower extremity ligamentous injuries, neurovascular injuries, traumatic fractures, stress fractures, and other high-risk bone lesions.

HAND INJURIES

Hand injuries are common in the pediatric population and have a substantial effect on sports participation and activities of daily living. Fractures constitute a large portion of pediatric hand injuries, with mechanism and location varying based on patient age.[1] Young children are more susceptible to crush injuries involving the distal phalanx, with soft tissue involvement. In contrast, adolescents are more likely to sustain proximal phalanx and metacarpal fractures during sports activities.[2] Teenagers between 13 and 15 years of age are at highest risk, and males are more likely than females to sustain a sports-related frac-

---

*Corresponding author
E-mail address: CLabella@luriechildrens.org

ture.[1-3] History often reveals a low-energy injury to the hand, and physical examination shows swelling and tenderness at the digit.[3] Diagnosis of phalangeal fractures requires dedicated posteroanterior and lateral radiographs of the digit in question.[2] Hand views may provide inadequate visualization of the phalanx, leading to underdiagnosis, whereas misdiagnosis results primarily from misinterpretation of the normal epiphyses as a fracture.[2] Management of finger fractures in children and adolescents often is nonsurgical and involves splinting and immobilizing the digit.[1] However, in cases of intra-articular fractures, displaced phalangeal neck fractures, and malrotated fractures, orthopedic referral and surgical management with internal fixation often are necessary.[1]

Seymour Fracture

Crush injuries to the distal phalanx, commonly caused by jamming a finger in a door, demand special attention because of increased morbidity from frequent soft tissue and nail bed involvement.[4] In addition to radiographs of the digit to evaluate for fracture, careful examination under magnification or local anesthesia by a specialist, such as an orthopedic or plastic surgeon, may be necessary to determine the extent of soft tissue and nail bed involvement.[5] A Seymour fracture includes juxtaepiphyseal fracture of the terminal phalanx, laceration of the nail bed, and flexion deformity of the digit (Figure 1).[6] These injuries have a high risk for complications, including growth disturbance of the distal phalanx, limited distal interphalangeal (DIP) joint range of motion, abnormal or absent nail growth, infection, and amputation.[4,6] Uncomplicated closed fractures can be managed with irrigation, closed reduction, and splinting in extension for 2 to 4 weeks.[4,6] A short course of oral antibiotics should be considered in cases of severe soft tissue damage or a delay in treatment of more than 6 hours.[6] Open fractures require surgical management with presurgical intravenous antibiotics, debridement, open reduction, nail bed repair, and nail plate fixation, followed by a short course of oral antibiotics.[6] Given the complexity of nail bed injuries,

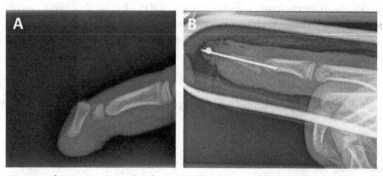

Fig 1. Seymour fracture. **A:** Lateral radiograph of digit demonstrating a fracture-dislocation of the distal phalanx involving the physis and a flexion deformity. **B:** Postoperative lateral radiograph of the digit in the same patient after pinning and nail bed repair. (Images courtesy of Ann & Robert H. Lurie Children's Hospital of Chicago Department of Radiology.)

practitioners unfamiliar with these cases should consider immediate referral to the emergency room for evaluation by a specialist.

Scaphoid Fracture

As in adults, the scaphoid is the most commonly injured carpal bone in children.[7] Most fractures result from a fall onto an outstretched hand on a firm surface, often during sports such as skateboarding, bicycling, or basketball. In younger children this force more commonly results in injury to the distal forearm, but as physes close and the carpal bones ossify, scaphoid fractures increase in frequency. As a result, a scaphoid fracture is rare in children younger than 8 years, and peak incidence in children occurs around 15 years of age.[8] Because the blood supply to the scaphoid arises distally, the middle and proximal poles are entirely dependent on retrograde blood flow for perfusion and are susceptible to non-union or avascular necrosis after injury. Therefore, early identification of scaphoid fractures is important to reduce the risk of complications.[7,9]

Patients will present with radial wrist pain and reduced range of motion after a fall onto an outstretched hand. Examination reveals tenderness at the anatomic snuffbox with or without overlying swelling, and pain with scaphoid compression (axial loading of the first metacarpal with the wrist in radial deviation). Pain will also typically be elicited by full wrist flexion, extension, and radial deviation. Care should be taken to examine the forearm, hand, and elbow because these structures may be injured concomitantly.[9]

The initial imaging modality of choice is plain radiographs, including anteroposterior (AP), lateral, oblique, and scaphoid (AP in pronation and ulnar deviation) views (Figure 2). Individuals with negative initial radiographs but high

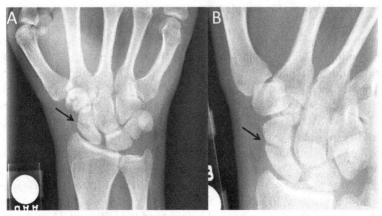

Fig 2. Scaphoid fracture. **A:** Posteroanterior radiograph of the wrist. *Arrow* points to a midpole scaphoid fracture. **B:** Scaphoid view radiograph of the same wrist. Note ulnar deviation of metacarpals in this view. (Image courtesy of Northwestern Memorial Hospital Department of Radiology.)

clinical suspicion should be placed in a short arm thumb spica cast or splint and re-evaluated with repeat radiographs in 2 weeks.[7] If radiographs remain negative and symptoms have resolved, immobilization can be discontinued and an alternate diagnosis should be considered. If symptoms persist but radiographs are negative, magnetic resonance imaging (MRI) can provide a definitive diagnosis.[9] Alternatively, adolescent athletes with more urgent need for definitive diagnosis may undergo MRI at the initial evaluation if radiographs are negative. Management of patients with a confirmed, non-displaced scaphoid fracture depends on the location. Injuries to the distal third can be managed with a short arm thumb spica cast for 4 to 6 weeks, whereas injuries to the middle and proximal third typically require a long arm thumb spica cast for 6 to 8 weeks. Scaphoid fractures with displacement, non-union, or other associated carpal injuries should be referred to an orthopedic surgeon.[7]

Mallet Finger

Mallet finger is caused by disruption of the extensor tendon at the DIP joint during forced flexion of an extended finger, which often occurs during athletic participation as a result of contact with another player, a ball, or the ground.[10,11] Physical examination reveals DIP flexion deformity with loss of active DIP extension. Bruising or swelling may be present, and tenderness at the dorsal DIP joint suggests a phalangeal fracture.[12] Radiographs of the digit are needed to rule out associated avulsion fracture at the base of the distal phalanx where the extensor tendon inserts.[11] Management of closed injuries is conservative and involves continuous splinting of the DIP joint in extension for 4 to 8 weeks, followed by an additional 4 to 6 weeks of nighttime splinting. Open injuries and those associated with a large distal phalanx fracture with physeal or articular involvement require surgical referral for irrigation, debridement, or pinning of the fracture fragment.[10]

Central Slip Rupture (Boutonniere Deformity)

The central slip is formed by the distal portion of the extensor digitorum communis tendon as it inserts onto the base of the middle phalanx.[10] Injury to the central tendon, also known as a boutonniere injury, can occur because of hyperextension of the proximal interphalangeal (PIP) joint, laceration, crush injury, or fracture-dislocation of the PIP joint.[10,12] Examination reveals swelling with tenderness at the base of the middle phalanx.[10] Radiographs of the digit are needed to evaluate for associated fracture at the base of the middle phalanx.[10] If radiographs are unremarkable, the Elson test can be performed to determine whether the central slip is intact by placing the PIP joint in 90 degrees of flexion and observing active motion of the PIP and DIP joints when resistance is applied to the middle phalanx (Figure 3).[12] With an intact central slip, the patient should be able to extend the PIP but be unable to extend the DIP joint. However, if the central slip is ruptured, the patient will be unable to extend the PIP but extension or hyperextension of the DIP will occur.[12] Closed central slip injuries can be

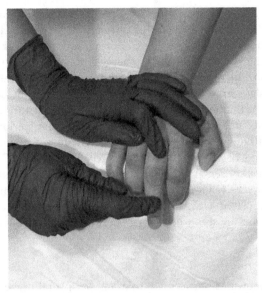

Fig 3. Normal Elson test. The proximal interphalangeal joint is placed in 90 degrees of flexion while resistance is applied to the middle phalanx to evaluate for central slip rupture.

managed conservatively by splinting the PIP joint in extension for 4 to 6 weeks, followed by 4 to 6 weeks of nighttime splinting.[10,12] The patient can be instructed to perform active DIP flexion exercises to promote proper positioning of the lateral bands, which extend from the distal extensor digitorum communis tendon.[12] Surgical referral is needed for open injuries, fracture-dislocations, lacerations of the central slip, and large displaced avulsion fractures.[10]

Jersey Finger

Jersey finger is caused by avulsion of the flexor digitorum profundus at the distal phalanx.[11] A common mechanism of this injury is catching the finger in an opponent's jersey, causing hyperextension of the DIP joint while in active flexion.[13] Examination reveals swelling and tenderness at the DIP with inability to flex the DIP joint. Radiographs of the digit are needed to evaluate for bony avulsion.[13] Suspected cases of jersey finger require immediate referral for surgical evaluation because early repair leads to improved outcomes.[11,13]

Ulnar Collateral Ligament injury (Skier's Thumb)

The ulnar collateral ligament (UCL) of the thumb crosses the metacarpophalangeal (MCP) joint and functions to support the MCP joint against valgus and volar stress.[14,15] Injury to the UCL occurs because of valgus stress on an abducted thumb. The injury can be acute, known as skier's thumb, or chronic, known as gamekeeper's thumb.[14] Injuries can involve a sprain, partial, or complete UCL rupture (Figure

4). With complete UCL rupture the distal portion of the torn UCL can become trapped under the adductor aponeurosis, causing a Stener lesion (Figure 4).[15] Physical examination is notable for swelling, bruising, and tenderness along the MCP joint of the thumb. A palpable mass is sometimes present at the MCP joint in cases of a Stener lesion.[15] Increased laxity and absence of a firm end point can be appreciated through valgus stress testing of the thumb (Figure 5).[14,15] Before stress testing, radiographs of the thumb are recommended to assess for fracture at the base of the proximal phalanx and for volar subluxation.[15] If clinical suspicion for fracture is high and initial radiographs are negative, radiographs with valgus stress on the thumb, ultrasound, or MRI should be considered.[14] Treatment of UCL sprains and partial ruptures is conservative, with immobilization using a thumb spica cast or splint for 2 to 8 weeks, followed by range of motion and strengthening exercises.[14,15] Complete or displaced UCL tears require prompt surgical evaluation because improved outcomes are seen when surgery occurs within 3 to 4 weeks of injury.[14,15]

STINGERS

Stingers, also known as burners, are transient peripheral nerve injuries caused by traction or direct trauma to the brachial plexus or cervical nerve roots.[16] Injury most commonly occurs during contact sports and can be the result of compression from direct pressure on Erb's point located just superior to the clavicle and posterior to the sternocleidomastoid muscle, compression from forceful neck extension and lateral flexion toward the affected arm, or a stretch injury resulting from forceful shoulder depression and neck lateral flexion toward the

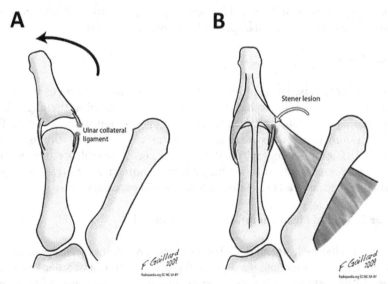

Fig 4. **A:** Ulnar collateral ligament (UCL) rupture. *Arrow* indicates direction of valgus force during UCL stress testing. **B:** Stener lesion. (Reproduced with permission. Images by Dr Frank Gaillard, Radiopaedia.org.)

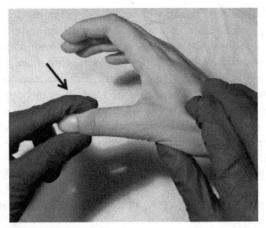

Fig 5. Valgus stress test of thumb to evaluate for ulnar collateral ligament injury. *Arrow* indicates direction of force.

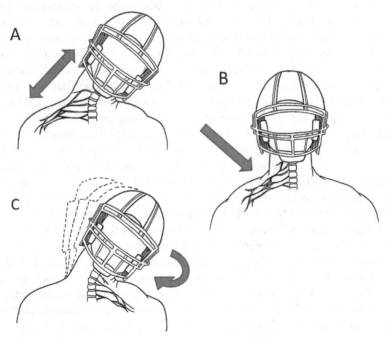

Fig 6. Stingers mechanism of injury. **A:** Stretch injury. **B:** Direct pressure to Erb's point. **C:** Forceful neck extension and lateral flexion. (Images by Tina Chan.)

contralateral arm (Figure 6).[16] Patients present with transient unilateral upper extremity pain and paresthesias, with or without muscle weakness, most often in the C5-C6 distribution, which lasts for seconds to minutes.[16,17] Bilateral symptoms, even if transient, may indicate cervical spinal cord injury and warrant immediate spine stabilization and transfer to the emergency department (ED) for further evaluation.[16,17] Patients with unilateral symptoms can be evaluated on the field with physical examination of the cervical spine for tenderness and range of motion, followed by a complete neurologic examination.[16] If physical examination is unremarkable and the patient's symptoms have resolved, then no further evaluation is necessary, and the patient may return to play the same day.[16] If examination reveals cervical spine tenderness or neurologic changes, then the patient should be referred to the ED for cervical spine imaging.[16] Additionally, patients with prolonged symptoms lasting more than a few minutes or a history of 2 or more stingers should be evaluated further, before returning to play, with cervical spine radiographs or MRI to identify foraminal or spinal stenosis that may predispose athletes to nerve root or spinal cord injury.[16,17]

VASCULAR OR NERVE INJURY AFTER SHOULDER DISLOCATION

Adolescent and young adult males involved in contact sports are the highest-risk population for shoulder dislocations.[18] The most common mechanism of injury involves forceful external rotation and abduction of the arm causing anterior glenohumeral joint dislocation. The patient presents with shoulder pain and the arm held in external rotation and abduction. An uncommon but serious complication of anterior shoulder dislocation is a vascular injury, so a careful neurovascular examination should be performed both before and after reduction. The axillary artery is most at risk for injury. Decreased distal pulses and axillary hematoma are signs of potential vascular injury and warrant angiography and surgical consultation.[18] The presence of a vascular injury should raise suspicion for concomitant brachial plexus or peripheral nerve injury.[18] Brachial plexus injury produces deficits in more than 1 peripheral nerve distribution. Focal peripheral nerve injury most often involves the axillary nerve, which is injured in up to 10% of cases of anterior shoulder dislocations, and produces focal deltoid and teres minor weakness with proximal lateral arm numbness. On physical examination the strength of the deltoid muscle is tested with resisted shoulder abduction, and the teres minor is tested with resisted external rotation while the arm is adducted and the elbow is flexed to 90 degrees. Nerve injury often is incomplete, and prognosis for recovery is good.[18] After physical examination, radiographs of the shoulder, including anteroposterior and axillary views, should be considered, if available, to confirm the diagnosis and rule out humeral fracture.[18] If fracture and vascular injury are ruled out, then reduction may be attempted. Postreduction immobilization in a sling may be considered for comfort, followed by physical therapy to restore range of motion and strength. Patients younger than 20 years are at high risk for recurrent dislocation and may benefit from consultation with an orthopedic surgeon regarding long-term prognosis and management.[18]

SPONDYLOLYSIS

Spondylolysis refers to a defect in the pars interarticularis, the portion of the vertebral lamina between the inferior and superior articular facets (Figure 7).

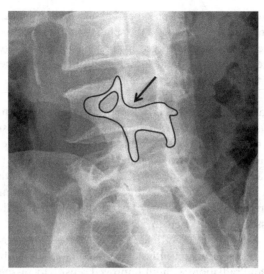

Fig 7. Oblique radiograph of the lumbar spine outlining normal "Scottie dog" appearance. *Arrow* indicates location of pars interarticularis where spondylolysis lesions can be appreciated. (Reproduced with permission. Image by Drs Frank Gaillard and Ayush Goel, et al, Radiopaedia.org.)

Although the defect may be congenital or result from degeneration, dysplasia, or trauma, stress fracture of the pars interarticularis is a common cause of lower back pain (LBP) in adolescent athletes. While spondylolysis has been found in 6% to 8% of the general population with LBP,[19] the prevalence in adolescents participating in certain sports may be as high as 47% to 63%.[19-21]

Spondylolysis occurs most commonly in the lumbar spine. The injury results from activities that incorporate a significant amount of repetitive lumbar extension and rotation, such as gymnastics, diving, football, and volleyball.[22] During extension, the pars interarticularis undergoes a shear stress as a result of the downward force of the proximal vertebra on the superior articulating facet and the upward force of the distal spinal segment on the inferior articular facet. Over time, repetitive stress can result in a stress reaction and ultimately fracture.[23] Although most lesions are unilateral, bilateral lesions can develop and lead to spondylolisthesis, in which the vertebral body translates anteriorly with respect to the adjacent distal vertebral body, potentially resulting in pain and neurologic symptoms. Identification of spondylolysis is important because early, active lesions may be amenable to healing, whereas older lesions are more likely to lead to chronic non-union and increased risk of spondylolisthesis.[23,24]

Adolescents with spondylolysis typically present with several weeks of LBP without radiating symptoms or neurologic deficits. Although typically not preceded by a specific incident or trauma, the pain develops insidiously after a period of increased activity and is exacerbated by extension and rotation. Physical examination reveals tenderness to palpation on and alongside the spinous process of the affected vertebra. Range of motion of the spine typically is normal, but extension is painful.[24] The "stork," or one-legged hyperextension, test (Figure 8) may also elicit pain, although sensitivity and specificity of the test have been found to be only 50% to 55% and 45% to 65%, respectively.[25]

Radiographs have been the initial imaging modality of choice, and identification of spondylolysis on radiographs is definitive. However, the sensitivity of radiographs is poor, and which views to include are currently a source of controversy. Anteroposterior films may demonstrate indirect evidence of spondylolysis, including lateral deviation of the spinous process away from the affected side because of lengthening of the affected pars from recurrent injury and healing. Lateral films are necessary to evaluate for spondylolisthesis. Although oblique films have classically been used to identify a pars fracture, represented by a lucency at the neck of the "Scottie dog" (Figure 7), false-negative results are common, and it has been recently suggested that their addition results in increased cost and radiation, without improved sensitivity or specificity.[26-28]

Similarly, opinions vary regarding the best imaging modality for suspected spondylolysis with negative radiographs. Computed tomography (CT) provides the best anatomic detail of a fracture (Figure 9) but may fail to identify a stress reac-

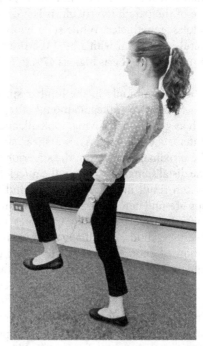

Fig 8. Stork test. Patient is asked to stand on 1 leg and hyperextend her lower back. Examiner should stand behind patient to offer support. A positive test elicits low back pain.

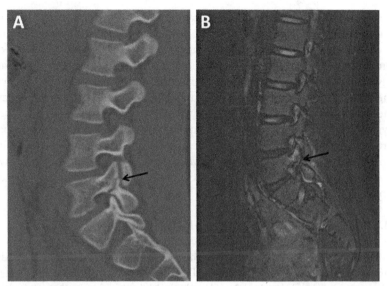

Fig 9. Spondylolysis. **A:** Computed tomography of the lumbar spine (sagittal bone window). *Arrow* points to L5 pars lytic defect. **B:** Magnetic resonance imaging of the lumbar spine (sagittal STIR) in the same patient. *Arrow* points to edema in the L5 par interarticularis. (Images courtesy of Ann & Robert H. Lurie Children's Hospital of Chicago Department of Radiology.)

tion. Single photon emission computed tomography (SPECT) scans have been shown to be sensitive for the detection of early lesions, and some authors suggest the use of initial SPECT scan, followed by CT, if positive.[23,29] Others argue for the use of thin-slice MRI (Figure 9) as the preferred imaging modality for suspected spondylolysis with negative radiographs because of the lack of radiation and the ability to identify other potential soft tissue sources of pain.[24,30] Finally, some authors suggest that routine follow-up CT imaging be performed at 4 months to document healing,[31] whereas others recommend that repeat imaging be limited to those who do not improve with initial conservative measures.[26]

Initial management of spondylolysis is conservative and includes limiting activities to a pain-free level and guided physical therapy to improve core strength and hamstring flexibility. For patients with lesions that appear chronic and thus unlikely to heal with a bony union, activity restriction is simply continued until resolution of pain. Patients with evidence of early, active lesions are restricted from activity for at least 3 months and then gradually returned to activity once pain-free thereafter. Ideal timing of physical therapy in either case is unclear, with some suggesting immediate initiation,[31] initiation at 6 to 8 weeks for stress reactions,[24] or deferral until full clinical resolution of symptoms.[24,26,31]

The use of antilordotic bracing also is controversial. Although initial longitudinal studies demonstrated good outcomes with the use of braces in adults[32] and children,[33] these studies did not include control groups for comparison.[32,33]

Other research found similar bony healing among patients treated with and without braces.[34,35] Currently there is no consensus regarding the use of antilor-dotic bracing. Some authors suggest that braces should be used routinely for 6 months after diagnosis,[31] whereas others suggest that they be reserved for those individuals who do not respond to initial management.[26,31] Finally, electrical bone stimulation has been suggested as an adjunct to therapy in refractory cases, although evidence is limited to only a few case reports.[36] Although rarely neces-sary, surgical intervention may be required for those with increasing pain, increasing neurologic symptoms, progressive listhesis, or persistent pain or limi-tation after 6 to 9 months of conservative management. Surgical outcomes typi-cally are good, with most patients able to return to sport in an average of 7 months.[37]

PELVIC APOPHYSEAL AVULSION FRACTURES

Avulsion fractures of the pelvis are common injuries that occur at secondary ossification sites in adolescent athletes. Typical locations include the iliac crest at the insertion of the abdominal muscles, the ischial tuberosity at the origin of the hamstring, the anterior superior iliac spine (ASIS) at the origin of the sartorius and tensor fascia lata, the anterior inferior iliac spine (AIIS) at the origin of the rectus femoris muscle, the lesser trochanter at the insertion of the iliopsoas, and the greater trochanter at the insertion of the gluteal muscles and lateral rotators of the hip. Fusion of these apophyses occurs in the late teens to mid-20s. Before this period the tensile strength of the physis is less than that of the attached muscle and tendon, making it susceptible to injury during explosive move-ments.[38] Location of avulsion fractures is based on the mechanism of injury. Forceful hip extension during a sprint can cause an avulsion fracture of the ischial tuberosity at the origin of the hamstring, a kick with hip extension to sud-den flexion can avulse the ASIS at the origin of the sartorius, and a kick with hip hyperextension and knee flexion can cause avulsion of the AIIS at the origin of the rectus femoris. Failure to identify and properly manage pelvic avulsion frac-tures can result in persistent pain and non-union.[39]

Patients often describe a pop and sudden onset of pain during a maximal effort such as sprinting or kicking. Physical examination reveals a focal area of bony tenderness and sometimes overlying swelling. Passive stretch or contraction of the attached muscle will elicit pain and reveal weakness.[38,39] An AP radiograph of the pelvis is sufficient to identify most avulsion fractures (Figure 10). If radio-graphs are negative but significant clinical suspicion persists, patients can be treated conservatively, or a CT or MRI can be ordered for definitive diagnosis.[38]

Most pelvic avulsion fractures respond well to conservative management, with resolution and return to activity within 8 to 10 weeks. Initial management involves complete rest, ice, analgesia, and crutches for those with pain with ambulation. Physical therapy can be initiated once pain subsides for restoration

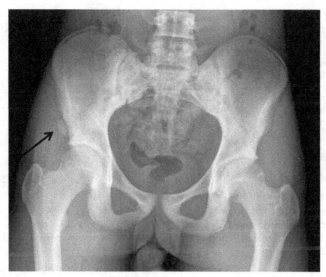

Fig 10. Anterior superior iliac spine (ASIS) avulsion fracture. Anteroposterior radiograph of the pelvis. *Arrow* points to a subacute right ASIS avulsion fracture. (Image courtesy of Ann & Robert H. Lurie Children's Hospital of Chicago Department of Radiology.)

of active range of motion, muscle strengthening, and supervised gradual return to play once range of motion, flexibility, and strength are normal and pain-free. Repeat radiographs typically are not needed for patients with good clinical recovery. Surgical referral can be considered for those with significant displacement of the apophyseal fragment (typically >2 cm) or failure to improve with conservative treatment.[8]

SLIPPED CAPITAL FEMORAL EPIPHYSIS

Slipped capital femoral epiphysis (SCFE) is a hip disorder seen in adolescents defined by the disruption of the proximal femoral epiphyseal plate with displacement of the femoral head relative to the femoral neck and shaft. The incidence is 10 per 100,000 adolescents in the United States, with 60% of cases affecting males.[40] The etiology is unknown but is thought to be caused by either an abnormally high load across a normal physis, as seen in obese adolescents, or a normal load across an abnormally weak physis in children with a metabolic disorder or chronic illness.[41] Patients present with poorly localized pain in the hip, groin, thigh, or knee, and they may present with a limp. Physical examination reveals restricted hip internal range of motion. Diagnosis is confirmed by radiographs of the pelvis, including AP and lateral frog-leg views (Figure 11).[40] Early surgical management is recommended to prevent the progression of the slip and to decrease long-term complications such as osteoarthritis.[40] Choice of procedure depends on the severity of the slip. It may involve bilateral fixation

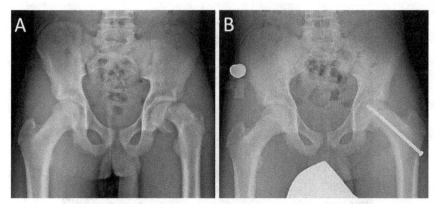

Fig 11. Slipped capital femoral epiphysis (SCFE). **A:** Anteroposterior (AP) radiograph of the pelvis depicting an unstable left SCFE. **B:** Postoperative AP radiograph of the pelvis in the same patient after pinning. (Images courtesy of Ann & Robert H. Lurie Children's Hospital of Chicago Department of Radiology.)

because 20% to 50% of patients with unilateral SCFE develop bilateral symptoms over time.[40] There is an association between SCFE and various endocrinopathies, most commonly hypothyroidism and growth hormone deficiency. In a 2013 systematic review, Witbreuk et al[41] concluded that universal testing for endocrinopathies is not indicated in all children with SCFE but should be considered in younger patients (girls <10 years and boys <12 years) and in children below the 10th percentile for height.

ANTERIOR CRUCIATE LIGAMENT TEAR

The anterior cruciate ligament (ACL) plays an important role in the stability of the knee by primarily preventing anterior translation of the tibia relative to the femur. Anterior cruciate ligament injuries have become increasingly common in the pediatric population, with adolescent females representing the population at highest risk.[42] ACL injuries usually occur during sports, and 70% to 80% occur without contact with another player, such as landing from a jump, rapid deceleration, or change of direction.[42] The acute mechanism of injury, report of hearing a "tear" or a "pop," and the presence of a large effusion and initial inability to bear weight are highly suggestive of an ACL tear. Patellar dislocations and intra-articular fractures also can cause large effusions and should be considered part of the differential diagnosis. Physical examination of acute ACL tears reveals a large hemarthrosis, decreased knee range of motion, and a positive Lachman test. The Lachman test evaluates the integrity of the ACL. It is performed by flexing the injured knee to 30 degrees, stabilizing the lower thigh in place with 1 hand, and pulling the proximal tibia anteriorly with the other hand to assess for excess anterior translation and lack of a firm endpoint (Figure 12). The Lachman test has been shown to have better specificity and sensitivity compared to the anterior drawer test, which involves flexing the injured knee to 90 degrees and pulling the tibia anteriorly with 2 hands

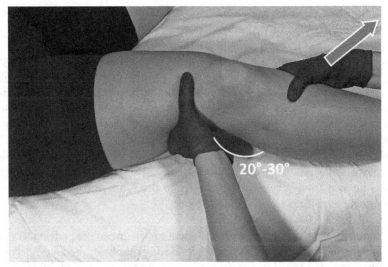

Fig 12. Lachman test to evaluate integrity of the anterior cruciate ligament. Knee is flexed 20 to 30 degrees. *Arrow* indicates direction of force pulling proximal tibia anteriorly.

to assess for laxity while stabilizing the patient's foot with the examiner's body.[43] Anteroposterior and lateral radiographs of the knee should be performed to rule out fracture and are often followed by an MRI of the knee to evaluate for concurrent injuries to the meniscus and other ligaments.[42] Most pediatric patients undergo early surgical ACL reconstruction because of knee instability, inability to participate in desired sports, and increased risk of additional intra-articular injuries and early-onset arthritis with a torn ACL.[42] Surgical approach depends on skeletal maturity and is followed by a minimum of 6 months of intensive rehabilitation.[42] Children who have sustained an ACL tear are at increased risk for developing osteoarthritis by the time they reach young adulthood, regardless of whether the ACL is surgically repaired. Given the morbidity of this condition, recent focus has been on prevention strategies, including implementation of neuromuscular training programs that have been shown to significantly decrease the risk of ACL injury, especially among female adolescent athletes.[42]

ANKLE SYNDESMOTIC INJURIES

Ankle sprains are the most common sports-related injuries in adolescents.[44,45] Syndesmosis injury (or high ankle sprain), which may be present in 10% to 20% of cases, can lead to ankle instability and increased risk of recurrent injury. The distal tibiofibular syndesmosis is made up of the anterior and posterior inferior tibiofibular ligaments, the inferior transverse ligament, and the interosseous membrane. Syndesmotic injury is particularly common during activities that involve rigid immobilization of the ankle, such as skiing and hockey, and typically occurs during an internal rotation of the leg and body on a planted, dorsiflexed foot.[44-47] Less commonly, the syndesmosis may be injured from a plantarflexion-inversion mechanism.[48,49]

Pain is often present over the anterior or posteromedial ankle and is increased with weight bearing. The syndesmosis can be palpated at the anterior ankle between the tibia and fibula, noting how far tenderness extends proximally from the ankle joint.[44] Patients often will have a positive squeeze test (pain with lateral and medial pressure in the middle lower leg to compress the tibia and fibula). Pain with passive dorsiflexion and external rotation also is suggestive of syndesmotic injury, as is pain or increased laxity with anterior-posterior translation of the distal fibula relative to the contralateral side.[44] The proximal fibula also should be evaluated because severe injury to the syndesmosis may result in a Maisonneuve fracture of the proximal fibula.[8]

Although clinical findings often are sufficient for diagnosis of syndesmotic injuries, weight-bearing AP, mortise, and lateral radiographs of the ankle may help identify associated injuries, as associated avulsion fractures of the tibia may be identified in up to 50% of cases.[50] Increased space between the distal tibia and fibula of more than 6 mm on AP films is suggestive of severe syndesmotic injury

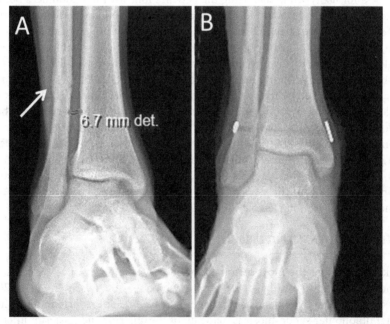

Fig 13. Ankle syndesmotic injury. **A:** Anteroposterior (AP) radiograph of the ankle showing more than 6-mm diastasis between the distal tibia and fibula. *Arrow* points to associated subacute fibular fracture. **B:** Postoperative AP radiograph of the ankle after fixation of the tibiofibular syndesmosis. (Images courtesy of Ann & Robert H. Lurie Children's Hospital of Chicago Department of Radiology.)

(Figure 13) and typically requires surgical management. Magnetic resonance imaging can be used to better define syndesmotic injury, although typically it is not necessary and the ability of MRI findings to predict clinical outcomes or meaningfully affect management decisions is unclear.[44]

Most syndesmotic injuries can be successfully managed with rest, anti-inflammatory measures, and elevation.[44] Immobilization in a walking boot or cast should be used by individuals with significant pain and difficulty ambulating. Patients unable to ambulate comfortably even in a cast or boot may require brief non–weight bearing and then partial weight bearing with crutches until ambulation is safe and comfortable. For individuals with less pain, an ankle brace may provide sufficient protection while allowing muscle activation to promote early rehabilitation.[44] Range of motion exercises should begin as early as possible but may be deferred for 1 to 2 weeks in those with severe injuries. Subsequent strength and sport-specific neuromuscular rehabilitation are important to restore balance and function, allow return to sport, and minimize the risk of reinjury.[44,51] Patients often have expectations of recovery based on prior experience with ankle injuries, but full recovery from high ankle sprains typically takes up to several weeks longer than lateral ankle sprains. Finally, surgical referral is indicated for individuals who demonstrate frank diastasis of more than 6 mm on radiographs because this likely represents a complete tear of the syndesmosis, which typically requires operative fixation for proper healing.[44]

OSTEOCHONDRITIS DISSECANS

Osteochondritis dissecans (OCD) is a focal idiopathic subchondral bone lesion thought to be caused by repetitive microtrauma that can be a cause of joint pain in adolescents.[52,53] It most commonly occurs in the elbow, knee, and ankle joints.[52,54] Lesions begin as focal softening of subchondral bone and can progress to fragmentation and formation of loose bodies.[53] Early diagnosis is essential to decrease morbidity and requires a high index of suspicion because presenting symptoms often are nonspecific.

The most common location for OCD is in the knee at the lateral border of the medial femoral condyle.[52,53] OCD of the knee can present with pain, swelling, and mechanical symptoms such as catching and locking.[52] Physical examination may reveal joint-line tenderness or effusion. Imaging is required for definitive diagnosis.[52] Radiographs of the knee should include AP, lateral, tunnel, and Merchant or sunrise views to allow for adequate visualization of the lateral aspect of the medial femoral condyle.[52,55,56] The tunnel (also known as notch) view is performed with the radiograph beam aimed posterior to anterior and the knee flexed at 30 to 40 degrees to accentuate the posterior femoral condyles where OCD is often found and is otherwise difficult to visualize on standard AP views of the knee. On radiographs, OCD appears as a lucent area in the subchondral bone with a well-demarcated sclerotic border (Figure 14). Magnetic resonance

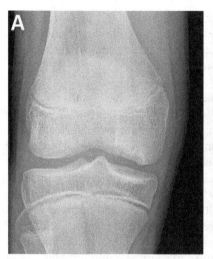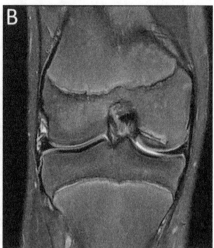

Fig 14. Osteochondritis dissecans (OCD). **A:** Anteroposterior (AP) radiograph of knee depicting an irregular lucent defect in the medial femoral condyle. **B:** Coronal T2 fat-saturated magnetic resonance imaging of the same knee showing unstable OCD with surrounding bone marrow edema and a linear fluid cleft deep to the lesion. (Images courtesy of Dr Jonathan Samet, Ann & Robert H. Lurie Children's Hospital of Chicago Department of Radiology.)

imaging can further characterize the lesion as stable or unstable (Figure 14). Management depends on skeletal maturity and the stability of the lesion.[52] Most skeletally immature patients with stable OCD lesions can be treated nonoperatively. Debate exists on the best protocol for conservative treatment and whether a period of non–weight bearing with or without immobilization with a cast or brace is necessary.[55,57] Most agree that strict avoidance of running, jumping, and impact activities for an average of 3 to 6 months is necessary to allow adequate healing.[55,57] Skeletally mature patients, those nearing skeletal maturity, and those with unstable lesions or loose bodies have little capacity to heal without surgical intervention.[52] Several surgical techniques exist and may include fixation or autologous chondrocyte implantation with bone grafting.[52]

The second most common location for OCD is the elbow at the capitellum. This lesion is most commonly seen in overhead athletes and those who bear weight through the arms, such as baseball players and gymnasts, respectively.[53] Patients present with complaints of diffuse elbow pain, swelling, and mechanical symptoms. Physical examination can reveal decreased elbow range of motion, tenderness to palpation of the posterolateral elbow, and effusion. Imaging is needed to differentiate OCD from other causes of elbow pain, such as Panner disease (osteochondrosis of the capitellum) and Little League elbow (medial epicondyle apophysitis).[53] Radiographs should include AP, lateral, oblique, or axial views.[53] Positive radiographs are followed by MRI to further characterize the lesion. Similar to OCD in the knee, stable lesions in skeletally immature athletes initially can be treated with rest from painful activities with or without bracing. In contrast to OCD at the knee, the capitellum has a tenuous blood supply that makes natural healing of an OCD lesion in the elbow more difficult.[53] Duration of rest is variable and can range from 6 weeks to 6 months. Repeat imaging often is not helpful in guiding return to sport because radiographic findings often lag behind resolution of symptoms.[53] Surgical treatment with fixation or reconstruction is recommended for those who do not respond to conservative treatment or those with unstable lesions or loose bodies.[53]

The third most common location for OCD is the medial talus in the ankle.[54,56] In contrast to knee and elbow lesions, 70% of OCD lesions in the talus are associated with a history of acute trauma such as an ankle sprain.[54] Patients present with complaints of pain, swelling, limited range of motion, or mechanical symptoms. Imaging begins with radiographs of the ankle, followed by MRI. Conservative treatment of stable lesions involves immobilization and non–weight bearing for 6 weeks.[58] Similar to knee and elbow OCD, surgical treatment with repair or reconstruction is considered for patients in whom conservative treatment is unsuccessful and for unstable lesions.[58]

HIGH-RISK STRESS FRACTURES

Stress fractures refer to injuries to bone that occur as a result of repetitive exposure to tensile or compressive forces with insufficient opportunity for recovery. These can result from an inability of normal bone to tolerate excessive stress or from normal stress placed on abnormally weakened bone (eg, secondary to infection, tumor, osteoporosis, or prolonged corticosteroid use).[59] During periods of rapid growth, long bones grow faster than the attached muscle-tendon units, placing an additional stress on the bone, which can predispose it to stress injury.[8] Sudden changes in the volume of stress experienced by the bone, such as during the onset of sport seasons, initially result in increased bone remodeling, making it temporarily more susceptible to injury. Continued repetitive stress on the vulnerable bone results in microtrauma, bone marrow edema, periosteal bone formation, and ultimately cortical fracture if the stress persists.[60] Multiple intrinsic and extrinsic risk factors for stress fractures have been identified, including decreased bone mass, lower body fat percentage and lean mass, anatomic factors (femoral anteversion, genu varum or valgum, tibial external rotation), poor nutrition, low fitness level, prior stress fracture, smoking, menstrual irregularity, and female gender.[59,61,62] Young female runners seem to be at greatest risk, likely because of overall energy imbalance leading to hormonal dysregulation and decreased bone density in the face of high training volume. Several of these factors are modifiable and represent important areas of both primary and secondary intervention to reduce the risk of stress fractures.

Stress fractures are generally classified as low risk or high risk based on the fracture site and the likelihood for non-union or fracture propagation. Examples of

high-risk stress fractures that may be missed in adolescents include the navicular, the base of the 5th metatarsal, and the superior cortex of the femoral neck.
Patients typically report insidious onset of pain in the affected area during periods of increased activity. Pain initially presents only during periods of prolonged
activity but gradually worsens until it is present even at rest.[61] Patients with fractures at the base of the 5th metatarsal typically have well-localized pain and focal
tenderness at the location of injury (Figure 15). Navicular stress fractures often
present with tenderness over the navicular bone, but symptoms may be vague,
with pain over the dorsomedial midfoot.[63] The femoral neck is more difficult to
evaluate because it may present with poorly localized pain in the hip, thigh, or

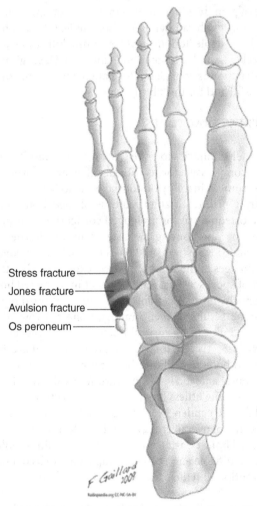

Fig 15. Fifth metatarsal fracture types by typical location. (Reproduced with permission. Image
by Dr Frank Gaillard, Radiopaedia.org.)

inguinal area and is difficult to directly palpate. Hip range of motion may induce pain but physical examination findings often are nonspecific, making a high degree of clinical suspicion important for any athlete presenting with insidious onset of activity-related groin or thigh pain.[61]

Plain radiographs are the initial imaging modality when stress fractures are suspected, and the views used depend on the specific location being evaluated. Although findings of periosteal reaction, cortical thickening, callous formation, or fracture line are diagnostic, radiographs may appear normal and can be insensitive for weeks to months after symptoms develop.[59] Although bone scans have been used as a sensitive secondary imaging modality for the detection of stress fractures, they are nonspecific and often fail to differentiate between stress fractures and other causes of increased bone turnover. As a result, MRI has become the standard for evaluating a suspected stress fracture. Magnetic resonance imaging findings can be graded based on the presence of periosteal edema, marrow edema, or a cortical fracture line, with higher grade injuries (those with severe edema or a fracture line) typically requiring a longer recovery period.[64]

Whereas most low-risk stress fractures will heal well with rest, physical therapy, and gradual, symptom-driven return to play, high-risk fractures initially should be managed with non–weight bearing and referral to an orthopedic or sports medicine specialist. Unlike the other metatarsal bones, stress fractures of the 5th metatarsal often result in nonunion and recurrence. Consequently, these fractures often are managed with screw fixation, especially in competitive athletes when a shorter recovery period is required.[62,63] Navicular fractures have a tendency for non-union and recurrence as well, although conservative measures with non–weight bearing and repeat radiographs may be undertaken initially. Screw fixation is indicated for failure of conservative measures, displaced fractures, or a need for a more immediate return to activity.[63] Given their propensity for propagation and displacement, fractures of the superior cortex, or tension side of the femoral neck, should be referred to an orthopedic surgeon for consideration of operative fixation.[60]

SALTER-HARRIS TYPE I PHYSEAL FRACTURES

In the immature skeleton, the epiphyseal plate, or physis, represents an area of relative weakness and frequent injury, and it accounts for 15% to 20% of all pediatric fractures.[8] Common sites of injury include the distal radius, femur, fibula, tibia, and lateral condyle of the elbow. Physeal injuries are commonly classified according to their radiographic appearance as initially described by Salter and Harris (Figure 16).[65] The physis represents an area of long bone growth in adolescents, and the risk of growth disruption increases from type 1 to type 5 fractures. Injuries to the growth plate should be readily identified and managed to reduce the risk of growth disruption and the development of angular deformity.[66,67]

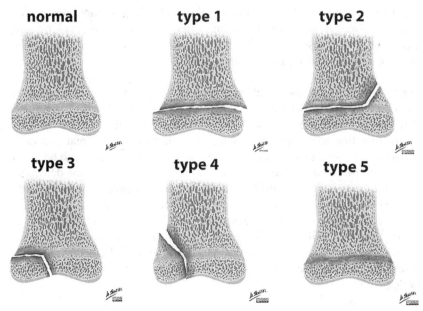

Fig 16. Salter-Harris classification. Shown from **left** to **right** are **top row:** normal physis; type 1—fracture through physis; type 2—fracture through physis and metaphysis; **bottom row:** type 3—fracture through physis and epiphysis; type 4—fracture through physis, metaphysis, and epiphysis; type 5—compression fracture of physis. (Reproduced with permission. Images by Dr Matt Skalski, Radiopaedia.org.)

Patients with physeal injuries present acutely after trauma with subsequent pain and swelling localized to the injured area. Range of motion often is limited because of swelling and pain. Localization of tenderness to palpation at the physis is paramount for proper diagnosis.[65] Examination should include a careful evaluation of the remainder of the extremity because injury to multiple areas from the same mechanism is not uncommon (eg, fractures to distal radius and supracondylar humerus after a fall onto an outstretched hand). Although radiographs are the imaging modality of choice, Salter-Harris type I fractures are a common diagnostic pitfall because they involve only the physis itself, without accompanying injury to the adjacent epiphysis or metaphysis, and thus radiographic findings may be subtle or absent.[68]

Non-displaced type 1 fractures may demonstrate only mild physeal widening and comparison to the contralateral side may be useful, but in some cases initial radiographs appear normal.[69] In these instances, tenderness over the physis on examination is sufficient for diagnosis. Follow-up radiographs 2 to 3 weeks after the initial injury typically demonstrate bony healing, thereby providing definitive diagnosis. Normal follow-up radiographs rule out physeal injury.[8]

Although the specific management will vary according to the site of injury, acute management of non-displaced type 1 fractures involves analgesia and immobilization in a splint or bivalve cast to accommodate swelling.[68] Definitive care involves immobilization and re-examination every 1 to 2 weeks until range of motion of the adjacent joint is painless and the affected area is no longer tender to palpation. Immobilization is discontinued at this time, but further protection during return to contact activities typically is continued for an additional 4 to 6 weeks. Children tolerate immobilization better than adults, and range of motion usually is quickly restored without the need for formal physical therapy. Repeat radiographs should be obtained at 6 months and 1 year to ensure normal bone growth.[8]

CONCLUSION

Adolescence is a period of increased susceptibility to musculoskeletal injuries because of the unique demands of the immature and growing musculoskeletal system. This article provided a brief description of the musculoskeletal injuries that require prompt diagnosis and treatment for adequate healing and the prevention of long-term complications. Given the complexity of these injuries, practitioners should not hesitate to collaborate with their orthopedic or sports medicine colleagues for assistance with diagnosis and management.

References

1. Liu EH, Alqahtani S, Alsaaran RN, et al. A prospective study of pediatric hand fractures and review of the literature. *Pediatr Emerg Care.* 2014;30(5):299-304
2. Chew EM, Chong AK. Hand fractures in children: epidemiology and misdiagnosis in a tertiary referral hospital. *J Hand Surg Am.* 2012;37(8):1684-1688
3. Wood AM, Robertson GA, Rennie L, Caesar BC, Court-Brown CM. The epidemiology of sports-related fractures in adolescents. *Injury.* 2010;41(8):834-838
4. Fairbairn N. No such thing as "just" a nail bed injury. *Pediatr Emerg Care.* 2012;28(4):363-365
5. Gellman H. Fingertip-nail bed injuries in children: current concepts and controversies of treatment. *J Craniofac Surg.* 2009;20(4):1033-1035
6. Krusche-Mandl I, Kottstorfer J, Thalhammer G, et al. Seymour fractures: retrospective analysis and therapeutic considerations. *J Hand Surg Am.* 2013;38(2):258-264
7. Anz AW, Bushnell BD, Bynum DK, Chloros GD, Wiesler ER. Pediatric scaphoid fractures. *J Am Acad Orthop Surg.* 2009;17(2):77-87
8. Harris SS, Anderson SJ; American Academy of Pediatrics, American Academy of Orthopaedic Surgeons. *Care of the Young Athlete.* 2nd ed. Elk Grove Village, IL: American Academy of Pediatrics; 2010
9. Elhassan BT, Shin AY. Scaphoid fracture in children. *Hand Clin.* 2006;22(1):31-41
10. Chauhan A, Jacobs B, Andoga A, Baratz ME. Extensor tendon injuries in athletes. *Sports Med Arthrosc.* 2014;22(1):45-55
11. Cheung K, Hatchell A, Thoma A. Approach to traumatic hand injuries for primary care physicians. *Can Fam Physician.* 2013;59(6):614-618
12. Lin JD, Strauch RJ. Closed soft tissue extensor mechanism injuries (mallet, boutonniere, and sagittal band). *J Hand Surg Am.* 2014;39(5):1005-1011
13. Goodson A, Morgan M, Rajeswaran G, Lee J, Katsarma E. Current management of Jersey finger in rugby players: case series and literature review. *Hand Surg.* 2010;15(2):103-107

14. Rhee PC, Jones DB, Kakar S. Management of thumb metacarpophalangeal ulnar collateral ligament injuries. *J Bone Joint Surg Am.* 2012;94(21):2005-2012
15. Ritting AW, Baldwin PC, Rodner CM. Ulnar collateral ligament injury of the thumb metacarpophalangeal joint. *Clin J Sport Med.* 2010;20(2):106-112
16. Concannon LG, Harrast MA, Herring SA. Radiating upper limb pain in the contact sport athlete: an update on transient quadriparesis and stingers. *Curr Sports Med Rep.* 2012;11(1):28-34
17. Dimberg EL, Burns TM. Management of common neurologic conditions in sports. *Clin Sports Med.* 2005;24(3):637-662, ix
18. Cutts S, Prempeh M, Drew S. Anterior shoulder dislocation. *Ann R Coll Surg Engl.* 2009;91(1):2-7
19. Micheli LJ, Wood R. Back pain in young athletes. Significant differences from adults in causes and patterns. *Arch Pediatr Adolesc Med.* 1995;149(1):15-18
20. Rossi F. Spondylolysis, spondylolisthesis and sports. *J Sports Med Phys Fitness.* 1978;18(4):317-340
21. Brooks BK, Southam SL, Mlady GW, Logan J, Rosett M. Lumbar spine spondylolysis in the adult population: using computed tomography to evaluate the possibility of adult onset lumbar spondylosis as a cause of back pain. *Skeletal Radiol.* 2010;39(7):669-673
22. Baker RJ, Patel D. Lower back pain in the athlete: common conditions and treatment. *Prim Care.* 2005;32(1):201-229
23. Leone A, Cianfoni A, Cerase A, Magarelli N, Bonomo L. Lumbar spondylolysis: a review. *Skeletal Radiol.* 2011;40(6):683-700
24. Kim HJ, Green DW. Spondylolysis in the adolescent athlete. *Curr Opin Pediatr.* 2011;23(1):68-72
25. Masci L, Pike J, Malara F, et al. Use of the one-legged hyperextension test and magnetic resonance imaging in the diagnosis of active spondylolysis. *Br J Sports Med.* 2006;40(11):940-946; discussion 946
26. Standaert CJ, Herring SA. Expert opinion and controversies in sports and musculoskeletal medicine: the diagnosis and treatment of spondylolysis in adolescent athletes. *Arch Phys Med Rehabil.* 2007;88(4):537-540
27. Beck NA, Miller R, Baldwin K, et al. Do oblique views add value in the diagnosis of spondylolysis in adolescents? *J Bone Joint Surg Am.* 2013;95(10):e65
28. Amato M, Totty WG, Gilula LA. Spondylolysis of the lumbar spine: demonstration of defects and laminal fragmentation. *Radiology.* 1984;153(3):627-629
29. Standaert CJ, Herring SA. Expert opinion and controversies in musculoskeletal and sports medicine: core stabilization as a treatment for low back pain. *Arch Phys Med Rehabil.* 2007;88(12):1734-1736
30. Campbell RS, Grainger AJ, Hide IG, Papastefanou S, Greenough CG. Juvenile spondylolysis: a comparative analysis of CT, SPECT and MRI. *Skeletal Radiol.* 2005;34(2):63-73
31. Micheli LJ, Curtis C. Stress fractures in the spine and sacrum. *Clin Sports Med.* 2006;25(1):75-88, ix
32. Steiner ME, Micheli LJ. Treatment of symptomatic spondylolysis and spondylolisthesis with the modified Boston brace. *Spine (Phila Pa 1976).* 1985;10(10):937-943
33. d'Hemecourt PA, Zurakowski D, Kriemler S, Micheli LJ. Spondylolysis: returning the athlete to sports participation with brace treatment. *Orthopedics.* 2002;25(6):653-657
34. Blanda J, Bethem D, Moats W, Lew M. Defects of pars interarticularis in athletes: a protocol for nonoperative treatment. *J Spinal Disord.* 1993;6(5):406-411
35. Jackson DW, Wiltse LL, Dingeman RD, Hayes M. Stress reactions involving the pars interarticularis in young athletes. *Am J Sports Med.* 1981;9(5):304-312
36. Stasinopoulos D. Treatment of spondylolysis with external electrical stimulation in young athletes: a critical literature review. *Br J Sports Med.* 2004;38(3):352-354
37. Debnath UK, Freeman BJ, Gregory P, et al. Clinical outcome and return to sport after the surgical treatment of spondylolysis in young athletes. *J Bone Joint Surg Br.* 2003;85(2):244-249
38. Gill KG. Pediatric hip: pearls and pitfalls. *Semin Musculoskelet Radiol.* 2013;17(3):328-338
39. Moeller JL. Pelvic and hip apophyseal avulsion injuries in young athletes. *Curr Sports Med Rep.* 2003;2(2):110-115

40. Aronsson DD, Loder RT, Breur GJ, Weinstein SL. Slipped capital femoral epiphysis: current concepts. *J Am Acad Orthop Surg.* 2006;14(12):666-679

41. Witbreuk M, van Kemenade FJ, van der Sluijs JA, et al. Slipped capital femoral epiphysis and its association with endocrine, metabolic and chronic diseases: a systematic review of the literature. *J Child Orthop.* 2013;7(3):213-223

42. LaBella CR, Hennrikus W, Hewett TE. Anterior cruciate ligament injuries: diagnosis, treatment, and prevention. *Pediatrics.* 2014;133(5):e1437-e1450

43. Ostrowski JA. Accuracy of 3 diagnostic tests for anterior cruciate ligament tears. *J Athlet Train.* 2006;41(1):120-121

44. Williams GN, Jones MH, Amendola A. Syndesmotic ankle sprains in athletes. *Am J Sports Med.* 2007;35(7):1197-1207

45. Gerber JP, Williams GN, Scoville CR, Arciero RA, Taylor DC. Persistent disability associated with ankle sprains: a prospective examination of an athletic population. *Foot Ankle Int.* 1998;19(10):653-660

46. Fritschy D. An unusual ankle injury in top skiers. *Am J Sports Med.* 1989;17(2):282-285; discussion 285-286

47. Wright RW, Barile RJ, Surprenant DA, Matava MJ. Ankle syndesmosis sprains in national hockey league players. *Am J Sports Med.* 2004;32(8):1941-1945

48. Hopkinson WJ, St Pierre P, Ryan JB, Wheeler JH. Syndesmosis sprains of the ankle. *Foot Ankle.* 1990;10(6):325-330

49. Milz P, Milz S, Steinborn M, et al. Lateral ankle ligaments and tibiofibular syndesmosis. 13-MHz high-frequency sonography and MRI compared in 20 patients. *Acta Orthop Scand.* 1998;69(1):51-55

50. Harper MC, Keller TS. A radiographic evaluation of the tibiofibular syndesmosis. *Foot Ankle.* 1989;10(3):156-160

51. Nussbaum ED, Hosea TM, Sieler SD, Incremona BR, Kessler DE. Prospective evaluation of syndesmotic ankle sprains without diastasis. *Am J Sports Med.* 2001;29(1):31-35

52. Carey JL, Grimm NL. Treatment algorithm for osteochondritis dissecans of the knee. *Clin Sports Med.* 2014;33(2):375-382

53. Nissen CW. Osteochondritis dissecans of the elbow. *Clin Sports Med.* 2014;33(2):251-265

54. Kessler JI, Weiss JM, Nikizad H, et al. Osteochondritis dissecans of the ankle in children and adolescents: demographics and epidemiology. *Am J Sports Med.* 2014;42(9):2165-2171

55. Pascual-Garrido C, Moran CJ, Green DW, Cole BJ. Osteochondritis dissecans of the knee in children and adolescents. *Curr Opin Pediatr.* 2013;25(1):46-51

56. Zbojniewicz AM, Laor T. Imaging of osteochondritis dissecans. *Clin Sports Med.* 2014;33(2):221-250

57. Polousky JD. Juvenile osteochondritis dissecans. *Sports Med Arthrosc.* 2011;19(1):56-63

58. Badekas T, Takvorian M, Souras N. Treatment principles for osteochondral lesions in foot and ankle. *Int Orthop.* 2013;37(9):1697-1706

59. Patel DS, Roth M, Kapil N. Stress fractures: diagnosis, treatment, and prevention. *Am Fam Physician.* 2011;83(1):39-46

60. Behrens SB, Deren ME, Matson A, Fadale PD, Monchik KO. Stress fractures of the pelvis and legs in athletes: a review. *Sports Health.* 2013;5(2):165-174

61. Heyworth BE, Green DW. Lower extremity stress fractures in pediatric and adolescent athletes. *Curr Opin Pediatr.* 2008;20(1):58-61

62. Pegrum J, Crisp T, Padhiar N. Diagnosis and management of bone stress injuries of the lower limb in athletes. *BMJ.* 2012;344:e2511

63. Gehrmann RM, Renard RL. Current concepts review: stress fractures of the foot. *Foot Ankle Int.* 2006;27(9):750-757

64. Nattiv A, Kennedy G, Barrack MT, et al. Correlation of MRI grading of bone stress injuries with clinical risk factors and return to play: a 5-year prospective study in collegiate track and field athletes. *Am J Sports Med.* 2013;41(8):1930-1941

65. Brown JH, DeLuca SA. Growth plate injuries: Salter-Harris classification. *Am Fam Physician.* 1992;46(4):1180-1184
66. Maffulli N, Longo UG, Spiezia F, Denaro V. Aetiology and prevention of injuries in elite young athletes. *Med Sport Sci.* 2011;56:187-200
67. Chambers HG. Ankle and foot disorders in skeletally immature athletes. *Orthop Clin North Am.* 2003;34(3):445-459
68. Perron AD, Miller MD, Brady WJ. Orthopedic pitfalls in the ED: pediatric growth plate injuries. *Am J Emerg Med.* 2002;20(1):50-54
69. Rogers LF, Poznanski AK. Imaging of epiphyseal injuries. *Radiology.* 1994;191(2):297-308

Adolesc Med 026 (2015) 79–99

Overuse and Overtraining Injuries in Teenage Athletes

Joel S. Brenner, MD, MPH, FAAP[a]*;
Amanda Weiss Kelly, MD, FAAP[b]

[a]*Medical Director, Children's Hospital of The King's Daughters' Sports Medicine Program, Director, Division of Sports Medicine and Adolescent Medicine, Associate Professor of Pediatrics, Eastern Virginia Medical School, Children's Specialty Group, PLLC, Norfolk, Virginia;* [b]*Division Chief, Pediatric Sports Medicine, UH Case Medical Center and Rainbow Babies and Children's Hospital, Program Director, Pediatric Sports Medicine, UH Case Medical Center, Associate Professor, Pediatrics, CWRU School of Medicine, Cleveland, Ohio*

Youth sports provide many benefits, including learning lifelong physical activity skills, peer socialization, teamwork, leadership, improving self-esteem, and allowing young athletes to have fun. Unfortunately, sports for teenagers have changed from adolescent-driven games and activities to adult-driven activities. Now a group of teenagers is less likely to congregate after school or on a weekend to play in a "pick-up" game, as was common practice in the 1970s and 1980s. Along with the paradigm shift of adults becoming the driving force came increased pressure to participate at a high level, specialize in a single sport early, and play year-round, sometimes on multiple teams. This has led to an increase in overuse injuries and overtraining. This article reviews the scope of the problem of overuse and overtraining injuries, discusses common overuse injuries using a case-based format, presents a few overtraining issues, and offers general prevention recommendations.

SCOPE OF THE PROBLEM

According to the 2008 National Council of Youth Sports' (NCYS) report on trends and participation in organized youth sports, 60 million youth aged 6 to 18 years participated in organized sports, with 66% being male and 34% female.[1] Of the 60 million reported, 44 million were unique youth participants (some youth

*Corresponding author
E-mail address: Joel.brenner@chkd.org

participated in more than 1 sport).[1] This is an increase from 45 million youth participants (32 million unique youth) in 1997, with the gender ratio remaining constant.[1] Figure 1 shows the increase in participation in organized youth sports from 1987 through 2008. According to the 2013 to 2014 high school athletics participation survey from the National Federation of High School Sports (NFHS), there were 7.8 million high school participants.[2] These statistics underestimate actual participation rates because they only capture those athletes who participate in organized sports surveyed or high schools that belong to the NFHS. Currently there are no data on how many young athletes play year-round or on multiple teams at the same time.

The actual incidence of overuse and overtraining injuries is difficult to assess because of the lack of uniformity and agreement throughout the literature in

Youth Participation

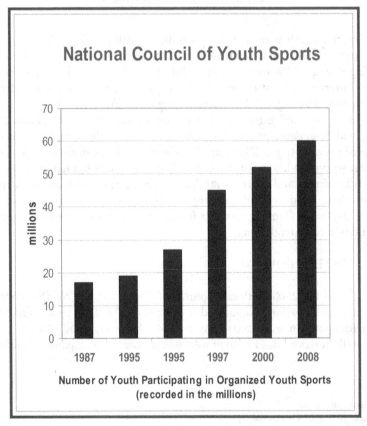

Fig 1. Increase in participation in organized youth sports from 1987 through 2008. (From National Council of Youth Sports. *Report on Trends and Participation in Organized Youth Sports.* Stuart, FL: National Council of Youth Sports; 2008.)

definitions used. According to some reports overuse injuries account for 46% to 50% of all athletic injuries.[3,4] Actual injury rates vary by age, gender, and sport.

Common Chronic Conditions in Adolescent Athletes

The following case-based descriptions of chronic injuries in adolescent athletes highlight the role of overuse in the injury of young athletes.

Case 1: Elbow Pain in a Pitcher

A 14-year-old right-handed pitcher presents with insidious onset of medial elbow pain over 6 weeks. He has noticed intermittent swelling and is concerned about the decreased velocity of his fastball. He currently is playing with 2 teams and pitches 2 to 4 games each week. Both teams keep strict pitch counts of fewer than 75 pitches per game. When he is not pitching, he plays catcher or third base.

On physical examination, he has mild soft tissue swelling of the medial epicondyle, pain with resisted wrist flexion, pronation of the forearm and grip strength testing, and pain at the medial epicondyle with valgus stress testing. He also has decreased strength with testing of the rotator cuff and core muscles. Radiographic examination demonstrates minimal widening of the medial epicondyle on the right compared to the left (Figure 2).

He was diagnosed with medial epicondyle apophysitis, also known as Little League elbow, a common condition among young throwers and other overhead athletes.

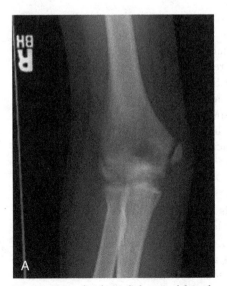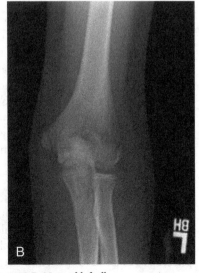

Fig 2. **A:** Injured right medial epicondyle with separation. **B:** Normal left elbow comparison.

Twenty-five percent of both pitchers and tennis players frequently complain of elbow pain.[5] Athletes with medial epicondyle apophysitis typically present with pain and, sometimes, mild swelling at the medial elbow and complaints of loss of power with throwing or overhead activities. Those with acute avulsions of the medial epicondyle apophysis report an event that caused a sudden increase in pain and significant swelling of the medial elbow.

Physical examination usually reveals tenderness to palpation of the medial epicondyle. There may be some loss of extension compared to the unaffected side. The ulnar nerve may be tender to palpation, and the Tinel test (the examiner taps the patient's ulnar nerve at the cubital tunnel posterior to the medial epicondyle, reproducing the symptoms) may be positive. Valgus stress of the elbow often elicits pain at the medial epicondyle.

Radiographic examination may reveal hypertrophy and separation or fragmentation of the medial epicondyle.[6] Comparison views of the unaffected side are useful in making the diagnosis.

Little League elbow is caused by repetitive valgus stress during the cocking and acceleration phases of throwing, which lead to physeal microtrauma.[7,8] Over time, fragmentation, hypertrophy, and separation of the apophysis can occur. Avulsion of the apophysis can occur acutely. Various studies have found that risk for elbow injury increases with total number of pitches per season, pitching with arm fatigue, pitching more than 8 months of the year, and playing outside of the league (eg, pitching in "showcases").[5,9] The risk of throwing breaking balls at an early age has not been clearly defined, with some investigators finding increased risk but others failing to do so.[5,9,10]

Relative rest and rehabilitation are the mainstays of treatment. Rest from all painful activities for 4 to 8 weeks usually allows for resolution of symptoms. During this period, rehabilitation to restore normal range of motion of the shoulder and elbow should take place. Strengthening and endurance exercises should focus on core, scapular, shoulder, and lower extremity musculature.[7] Also, improving the flexibility of the shoulders and hamstrings may allow for improved throwing mechanics.[11] Once the athlete is pain-free, an interval return to throwing program that gradually increases throwing distance, volume, and speed should be used to prevent reinjury upon return to pitching.

Case 2: Shoulder Pain in a Pitcher
A 13-year-old pitcher/catcher presents with several weeks of right shoulder pain. The onset of pain was insidious. He reports that his pain is over the anterior and lateral portions of his shoulder. His pain is associated with any type of throwing. He has been playing catcher and pitcher, but he has had to give up pitching because of his pain and decreased performance.

Physical examination reveals pain with palpation of the proximal humeral physis, increased passive external rotation on the right, and decreased internal rotation on the right compared to the left scapular winging with active range of motion. He has 4/5 strength with testing of the supraspinatus, infraspinatus, teres minor, and subscapularis on the right and 5/5 strength on the left. He has pain with all strength testing on the right.

Plain radiographs demonstrate widening of the proximal humeral physis on the right compared to the left (Figure 3), consistent with a Salter-Harris I injury of the proximal humeral physis, also known as Little League shoulder.

Little League shoulder is defined as a proximal humeral epiphysiolysis or stress fracture/Salter-Harris I fracture of the proximal humeral physis. It is caused by chronic repetitive microtrauma from rotational torques, which can be generated by the pitching motion but has also been identified in other overhead athletes who perform repetitive motion at the shoulder, including swimmers and volleyball players.[12,13] It is most common in overhead athletes aged 11 to 16 years.[13]

Physical examination typically reveals tenderness to palpation of the proximal humerus. Deficits in glenohumeral internal rotation may be present. Other less common findings include swelling of the proximal humerus and weakness of the rotator cuff, deltoid, or scapular stabilizers.[13] Radiographs show widening of the proximal humeral physis compared to the unaffected extremity.

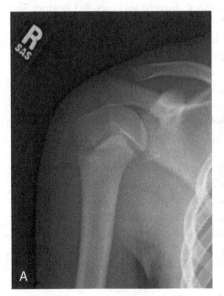
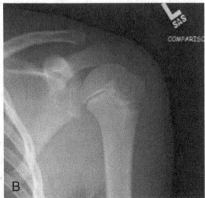

Fig 3. **A:** Salter-Harris I right proximal humeral physis, with widening of the physis. **B:** Normal left shoulder comparison.

Relative rest and rehabilitation are the mainstays of treatment. Rest from painful activities for 4 to 12 weeks usually allows for resolution of symptoms. During this period, rehabilitation to restore normal range of motion of the shoulder and elbow, and strengthening and increasing the endurance of supporting muscles should take place. Strengthening exercises should focus on core, scapular, shoulder, and lower extremity musculature.[7] Improving the flexibility of the shoulders and hamstrings may allow for improved throwing mechanics.[11] Once the athlete is pain-free, an interval return to throwing program should be used to prevent reinjury upon return to pitching.

Risk factors for shoulder pain in pitchers include number of pitches per game and season, pitching more than 8 months of the year, and pitching with arm fatigue.[5,9,14-16]

Case 3: Shoulder Pain in a Swimmer
A 16-year-old, year-round swimmer presents with several months of bilateral shoulder pain that has worsened over the last 3 to 4 weeks. She typically swims 1.5 hours per day with her summer team, but she has been increasing her time in the pool and yardage since returning to her school team in the fall. Butterfly stroke is the most painful, followed by freestyle. Most pain occurs during the pull-through phase of her stroke. Breaststroke and backstroke are pain-free.

On examination, she has poor posture, with her shoulders slumped forward. She has full range of motion of her shoulder, with mild pain during 90 to 120 degrees of abduction and scapular dyskinesis during abduction and forward flexion. She has decreased strength with testing of all of the rotator cuff muscles and pain with supraspinatus testing. On palpation, she has tenderness of the biceps tendon. She has pain with impingement testing. Stability testing reveals hyperlaxity with a positive sulcus sign and increased anterior and posterior glide of the humerus during load and shift testing. Radiographs of the shoulders are normal.

She was diagnosed with "swimmer's shoulder" with impingement. Physical therapy to improve rotator cuff muscle strength and endurance, posture, pectoralis tightness, scapular control, and core strength was prescribed. Her volume of swimming was reduced by 50%, and she rested from the butterfly stroke completely. She worked with her coaches to improve technique. She had significant improvement in her symptoms after 6 weeks and was able to gradually increase her volume of swimming over the next 6 weeks. She remained pain-free through the state meet. However, she stopped doing her home exercise program because she was pain-free. Her symptoms returned 4 months later, and she required another treatment course similar to the first, thus emphasizing the need to maintain a home exercise program.

Shoulder pain is the most common complaint in swimmers, with 40% to 90% experiencing shoulder pain.[17-20] The cause of shoulder pain in swimmers has been debated. Proposed causes include subacromial bursa impingement, supraspinatus tendinopathy, and biceps tendonitis.[17,20,21] Magnetic resonance imaging (MRI) has demonstrated that more than 1 of these diagnoses can be present concurrently in a given swimmer.[20]

Physical examination in swimmers with shoulder pain frequently reveals scapular dyskinesis and weakness of the rotator cuff muscles and core muscles. Pain with impingement testing also is common. Many swimmers have shoulder joint hyperlaxity. Whether the increased laxity is advantageous to swimmers by allowing them to be more successful and remain in the sport longer or the increased laxity is caused by the swimming itself is not clear.[20] However, increased laxity does seem to be correlated with impingement type pain.[20,21]

Treatment typically requires a reduction in training, although complete rest is rarely required. Physical therapy to improve rotator cuff strength, scapular control, posture, and core strength should be prescribed. The athlete should work with coaches to ensure good technique, concentrating on body roll and scapular retraction.[21] Once the athlete is pain-free, a gradual increase in training volume is permitted.

Risk factors for shoulder pain in swimmers include increased number of yards or hours swum per week, sudden increases in swimming volume or intensity, use of hand paddles, and poor posture, core strength, and scapular control.[20,21]

Case 4: Wrist Pain in a Gymnast

A 13-year-old level 7 (intermediate level) gymnast has complaints of 1 year of bilateral wrist pain. Initially, her pain was intermittent but has become more consistent and painful over the last month. Now she has pain with all upper extremity weight bearing at gymnastics, but the pain is worst with floor exercise and vault. She indicates that the dorsal aspect of the wrist is most painful.

On physical examination, the wrists have a normal appearance. She has mild limitations in extension of the left wrist compared to the right, and pain with active and passive extension of the wrists bilaterally. She has tenderness to palpation of the dorsal, distal radius and ulna, and diffuse tenderness of the dorsal wrist joint. She has pain in the dorsal wrist bilaterally with pushing her body off the table using her hands. Radiographs of the bilateral wrists demonstrate widening of the distal radial physes, and cystic and sclerotic changes of the physes of the bilateral distal radius and ulna (Figure 4).

She was diagnosed with a stress injury of the distal radial and ulnar physes, epiphysiolysis, or stress fracture/Salter-Harris I fracture of the distal radius and ulna, sometimes called "gymnast wrist." With 8 weeks of active rest, during which only upper extremity weight bearing was limited, she was pain-free. Physical therapy to improve core and upper body strength and proprioception was

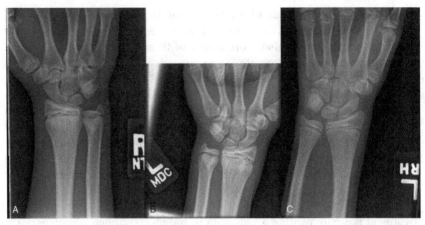

Fig 4. **A, B:** Bilateral widening of the distal radial and ulnar physes with cystic and sclerotic changes. **C:** Normal wrist.

also prescribed. A gradual return to upper extremity weight bearing over an 8-week period (bars followed by beam and finally floor and vault), using padded wrist supports (tiger paws), was permitted, and she was able to return without recurrence of pain. Coaches paid close attention to her mechanics with each activity, correcting any form errors that might have contributed to her injury (eg, elbow hyperextension). Repeat radiographs 7 months later were normal, with both the radial and ulnar physes still open.

A feature unique to gymnastics is use of the upper extremities for weight bearing, which predisposes the gymnast to wrist injuries uncommon in other sports. Wrist pain in skeletally immature gymnasts is common, with 50% of young, beginning, and midlevel gymnasts reporting wrist pain that can lead to significant time lost from training.[22,23] Possible causes include distal radial physeal injury, as described in this case, which typically presents with insidious onset of achy, dorsal wrist pain with weight bearing. Radiographs may demonstrate significant physeal changes, as in this case, or they may be normal. In cases with normal radiographs, MRI may be helpful in making the diagnosis. Most athletes respond to a period of rest, which can be several weeks to several months depending on the severity of injury and length of time symptoms have been present. Another relatively common cause of wrist pain in the young gymnast is dorsal impingement syndrome, a capsulitis caused by repetitive impingement of the wrist capsule during weight bearing (axial loading) with the wrist in extension. It should be considered a diagnosis of exclusion, after ruling out distal radial physeal injury.[22] It presents with symptoms similar to distal radial physeal injury. Pain usually resolves with rest and, depending on the severity of symptoms, a period of bracing.

Case 5: Knee Pain in a Basketball Player

A 14-year-old complains of the gradual onset of bilateral anterior knee pain for 4 to 5 months. His pain is increased with running and jumping, kneeling, and going up and down steps. He reports intermittent swelling below the patella.

On physical examination, he has tenderness to palpation of the tibial tubercle bilaterally, poor quadriceps and hamstring flexibility, and pain with full passive flexion of the knees and with resisted extension of the knees. Radiographs were normal with mild fragmentation of the tibial tubercle apophysis (Figure 5).

He was diagnosed with Osgood-Schlatter syndrome (OSS), and treatment recommendations included icing, analgesics, and exercises to improve flexibility,

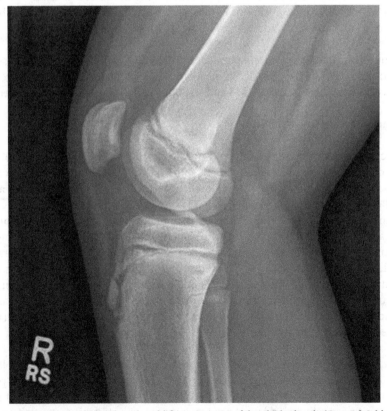

Fig 5. Normal knee radiograph with mild fragmentation of the tibial tubercle (Osgood-Schlatter syndrome).

balance, and strength. He was permitted to continue to participate in basketball as long as he was not having significant discomfort.

Osgood-Schlatter syndrome is a traction apophysitis resulting from repetitive microtrauma from the patellar tendon.[24] It is a common diagnosis in young athletes. Kujala et al[25] found that 21% of adolescents actively involved in sports had OSS compared to 4.5% of sedentary controls. It usually occurs in boys between the ages of 12 and 15 and in girls between the ages of 8 and 12 years. It is characterized by insidious onset of pain and swelling at the tibial tubercle that usually is worse with physical activity. Physical examination findings are similar to the case described, with mild soft tissue swelling, tenderness with palpation of the tibial tubercle, pain with resisted extension of the knee, and poor flexibility of the lower extremities. It is a self-limiting condition that typically improves with activity modifications, ice, analgesics, and exercises to improve strength, flexibility, and proprioception.[26] Prolotherapy using dextrose for treatment of OSS has been evaluated, and 1 small study reported good results, with a dextrose-treated group more likely to be pain-free and participating in full activities than groups treated with lidocaine injections or physical therapy only. However, prolotherapy currently is not considered part of the standard of care for OSS.[27]

Another common traction apophysitis of the knee is Sinding-Larsen-Johansson syndrome, a traction apophysitis of the inferior pole of the patella. It usually occurs at a slightly younger age than OSS and responds to a similar treatment regimen.

Other Traction Apophysitides

Traction apophysitides are also common in the pelvis and foot. The sartorius attaches to the anterior superior iliac spine (ASIS), the rectus femoris to the anterior inferior iliac spine (AIIS), the hamstring to the ischial tuberosity, and the abdominal muscles to the iliac crest (Figure 6 and Table 1). Repetitive microtrauma related to traction from any of these muscle groups on the corresponding apophysis can lead to pain. As with the knee and foot, conservative management with activity modification, as needed, analgesics, ice, and physical therapy typically lead to resolution of symptoms. The ASIS and AIIS apophysitides are common in running athletes, whereas ischial tuberosity apophysitis frequently occurs in jumping athletes and athletes who perform splits, such as gymnasts, dancers, and cheerleaders. Iliac crest apophysitis is often seen in sports requiring repetitive trunk rotation, such as soccer.

Calcaneal apophysitis is a common diagnosis in children and adolescents. It is bilateral in 60% of patients.[28] Physical examination typically reveals pain with palpation or squeezing of the calcaneal apophysis and decreased dorsiflexion.[28] It is a self-limiting condition, and most patients improve with stretching, strengthening, use of heel cups, and analgesics.[28] A radiograph is not needed for the diagnosis, and the amount of fragmentation of the apophysis is not necessarily related to the

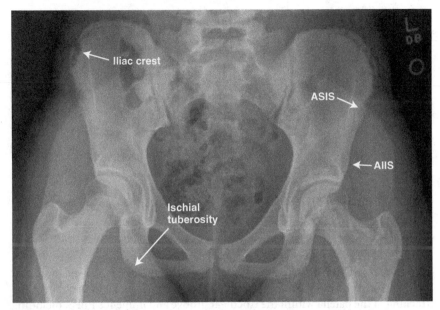

Fig 6. Normal pelvic apophyses.

Table 1
Pelvic apophyses

Muscle	Apophyseal attachment
Sartorius	Anterior superior iliac spine (ASIS)
Rectus femoris	Anterior inferior iliac spine (AIIS)
Hamstring	Ischial tuberosity
Abdominal muscles	Iliac crest

amount of pain the athlete experiences but can be used to rule out other conditions (Figure 7). Occasionally, nighttime splinting or immobilization with a walking boot is needed, but that is uncommon.

Case 6: Knee Pain in a Runner
A 14-year-old, 9th-grade cross-country runner presents with 8 weeks of gradual onset of bilateral anterior knee pain. This is her first year running with the high school team, and her weekly running mileage is almost twice what it was during middle school. Her pain began about 4 weeks into the season and has increased such that it is affecting her speed. She denies acute injury, swelling, locking, or instability.

Physical examination shows no swelling. She has tenderness with palpation of the patellar facets, both medially and laterally. She has decreased hip abductor, hip flexor, and gluteus medius strength. She has a significant valgus moment and pain with single leg squat. Knee radiographs are normal.

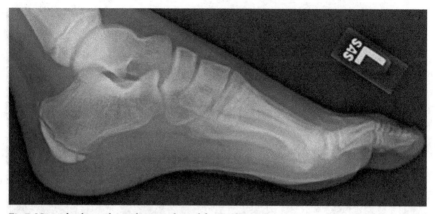

Fig 7. Normal calcaneal apophysis on lateral foot radiograph.

She was diagnosed with patellofemoral pain syndrome (PFPS), caused by abnormal patellar tracking.[29] Multiple static and dynamic stabilizers may affect the tracking of the patella within the trochlear groove and influence PFPS, including Q-angle, genu varum or valgum, quadriceps, hip abductor and hip external rotator strength, and iliotibial band and quadriceps flexibility.[29-31]

Patellofemoral pain syndrome is a common diagnosis, accounting for 16% to 25% of running injuries.[29,32,33] Patients usually report gradual onset of pain around or underneath the patella. Running, sitting for long periods of time ("theater sign"), and going up and down steps usually exacerbate pain. Occasionally, patients report their knee "giving way", which is related to quadriceps inhibition secondary to pain.[34] Often, a history of recent change in activity level can be elicited, as in the case described.

Typically, there is no evidence of swelling on examination, and range of motion is full and pain-free. J-tracking of the patella, an indication of patellar maltracking, may be noted with lateral deviation of the patella during terminal extension of the knee. Palpation elicits pain of the patellar facets and retinaculum. Evaluation of patella mobility may reveal restricted (<1 quadrant of motion) or excessive patellar glide (>2 quadrants of motion). Patellar grind test/inhibition usually recreates pain in PFPS. Weakness of the hip external rotators, which can contribute to lateral patellar tracking, is indicated by internal rotation of the knee during single leg squat.[30] Inadequate flexibility of both the iliotibial band and the quadriceps have been identified as risk factors for PFPS.[29]

Radiographs of the knee can eliminate other possible causes of knee pain, including osteochondritis dissecans, fracture, and tumor. A sunrise, or axial, view may demonstrate lateral tilting of the patella (Figure 8).

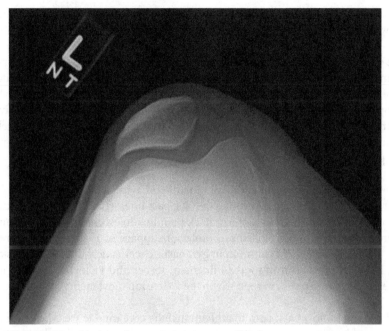

Fig 8. Sunrise view of the knee demonstrating excess patellar tilt.

Treatment should be tailored to address any strength or flexibility deficits in the hip, quadriceps, or hamstring musculature noted on physical examination.[35] Training errors, such as abrupt increases in mileage, pace, or training volume, should be corrected. Analgesics can be used to manage pain until symptoms improve with rest and physical therapy. Taping and bracing may help some patients; however, these methods have not been found to add benefit in controlled trials.[29]

Case 7: Back Pain in a Gymnast
A 13-year-old level 7 (intermediate level) gymnast presents with complaints of low back pain. She has experienced intermittent pain for about a year but for the last 6 weeks she has felt more persistent pain of greater intensity. She has recently been working on a back handspring series on the beam. She notes that her pain is worse with activities requiring back extension. She also has pain when she sits for long periods of time in school. She denies radicular pain, bowel or bladder problems, weakness, numbness, or tingling.

On physical examination, she has limited extension of the back secondary to pain. She has a positive stork test (single leg extension) and pain with palpation of the spinous processes and paraspinous musculature of the lumbar spine from L3-L5.

Radiographs (anteroposterior, lateral, and oblique) demonstrated a spondylolysis with a grade I spondylolisthesis in the lateral view (Figure 9).

She was removed from all extension-based activities but was permitted to perform light, low-impact, pain-free, physical activity. Physical therapy to maintain core strength and flexibility was prescribed. A functional brace alleviated her symptoms during the school day. She was pain-free after 9 weeks of activity restriction and physical therapy. A gradual return to gymnastics (over 8 weeks) with addition of extension-based activities last allowed for a successful return to her previous level of competition.

Low back pain is a frequent complaint in athletes, with about 10% of all adolescent athletes being affected.[36] Spondylolysis, pars interarticularis stress fracture, accounts for as much as 47% of low back pain in adolescent athletes. Although spondylolysis and spondylolisthesis (anterior slippage of 1 vertebral body relative to another) are most common in gymnasts, cheerleaders, dancers, and skaters, it also is often seen in football linemen, soccer and volleyball players, and other athletes who perform repetitive hyperextension movements of the back.[37,38]

Risk factors for low back pain in athletes include core muscle weakness and hip flexor and hamstring inflexibility.[37] Training volume and intensity also contribute to the risk for low back pain.

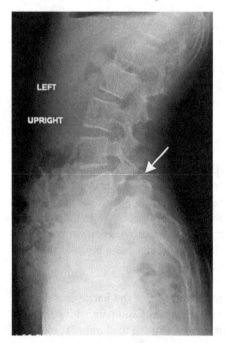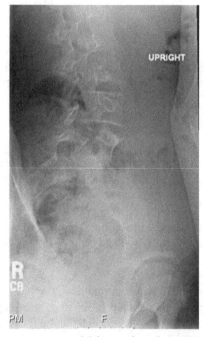

Fig 9. **A:** Lateral radiograph of the lumbar spine demonstrating spondylolysis with grade I spondylolisthesis. **B:** Oblique (Scottie dog) view of the lumbar spine demonstrating spondylolysis.

In spondylolysis, physical examination usually reveals pain with extension and the stork test. Decreased hamstring or hip flexor flexibility may be present. Pain with palpation of the spinous processes or paraspinous musculature also may be present.

Radiographs can be used to evaluate for the presence of fracture, neoplasm, and spondylolysis or spondylolisthesis. Oblique views best demonstrate spondylolysis. However, normal radiographs do not rule out the diagnosis of spondylolysis, so advanced imaging such as single photon emission computed tomography (SPECT) or MRI may be needed to diagnose spondylolysis.

Treatment includes rest from all painful activities. Physical therapy to strengthen the core musculature and to improve posture and hamstring and hip flexor flexibility should be prescribed. Bracing is controversial. Some authors recommend rigid, thoracolumbar orthoses to limit extension and rotation, others recommend functional braces to provide support, and still others restrict activity without bracing.[37]

Other causes of chronic back pain in athletes include mechanical back pain, facet syndrome, and sacroiliac (SI) joint dysfunction. Mechanical low back pain can be caused by muscle, ligament, facet joint, or joint capsule pain.[37] These athletes often have pain with flexion and/or extension and tenderness to palpation of the paraspinous musculature. Radiographs and advanced imaging studies will be normal, thus ruling out spondylolysis. Treatment involves activity modification, analgesics, and physical therapy similar to that for spondylolysis. Sacroiliac joint dysfunction may also cause pain with extension, but pain is more localized to the buttocks region on examination with both extension and palpation. The FABER (flexion, abduction, external rotation) test may be positive. Specific SI tests (eg, March test, ASIS compression test, ASIS malrotation) may be positive. Radiographs typically are negative. If infection of the SI joint or spondyloarthropathy is suspected, laboratory workup and MRI may be needed for further evaluation. Treatment includes analgesics for pain, activity modification, and physical therapy. In recalcitrant cases, guided injection of the SI joint may be needed.

OVERTRAINING ISSUES

Overtraining and Burnout

Case 8: Fatigue in a Swimmer
A 15-year-old male elite swimmer who trains year-round and competes internationally presents with a chief complaint of fatigue and muscle soreness. He participates in 3 practices per day, 6 to 7 days per week, starting at 0400 until 2100. He has been swimming since he was 6 years old. Physical examination is completely normal. Results of all his previous laboratory studies performed by a previous provider were normal.

This case illustrates important points seen in overtraining and burnout in young athletes. Currently there is little research in young athletes because most of the focus has been on college-age athletes and adults. There is a spectrum of conditions that include overreaching at one end and overtraining at the other extreme, which can lead to burnout. Overreaching has been defined as intense training that leads to decreased performance and psychological symptoms.[39-41] A full recovery is possible after a short period of rest. Overtraining syndrome has been defined as an extreme of overreaching that causes decreases in performance for more than 2 months and symptoms that are more severe, have a maladaptive physiology, and are not explained by other diseases.[39-41] Burnout in children and adolescents is unique because there is often more of a psychological component than in adults.

Burnout was defined by R. E. Smith as a " response to chronic stress in which a young athlete ceases to participate in a previously enjoyable activity."[42] The exact epidemiology of burnout in young athletes is not known because the current literature lacks standard terminology. However, it has been reported that 30% to 35% of adolescent athletes have experienced overreaching at some point in their lives.[40,41,43-45]

Smith described 4 stages of burnout in young athletes: (1) the athlete is placed in a situation with varying demands; (2) the demands are perceived by the athlete as being excessive; (3) the athlete experiences varying physiologic responses; and (4) burnout consequences develop, such as withdrawal from a sport.[40-42]

A variety of risk factors are related to the development of burnout in young athletes. They can be divided into environmental factors and personal characteristics, and are outlined in Table 2.[40,41,45-47]

The symptoms of overtraining and burnout are varied, often are nonspecific, and are commonly found in the healthy adolescent population (Table 3).[39-41,45,47] In order to make the diagnosis of overtraining and burnout, the physician must first include it as a possibility in the differential diagnosis. A comprehensive history that includes questions regarding an extensive training history and any decreases in performance is essential. Other specific historical items include investigating for the presence of other potential triggers and instituting very limited and focused testing. Table 4 outlines the specifics related to making the diagnosis.[39-41,48]

The treatment of overtraining and burnout is varied depending on the etiology. Any specific organic disease that is present should be treated appropriately. An extended period of rest, or relative rest, is the key intervention to allow recovery of the body and mind. This is a paradigm shift from the young athlete's typical behavior and can be difficult for the athlete to understand or follow. It is important to work with mental health experts because of the high incidence of a psychological component in young athletes. Any anxiety, depression, or sleep

Table 2
Factors related to burnout in young athletes

Environmental factors
  Extremely high training volumes
  Extremely high time demands
  Demanding performance expectations (imposed by self or significant other)
  Frequent intense competition
  Inconsistent coaching practices
  Little personal control in sport decision-making
  Negative performance evaluations (critical instead of supportive)
Personal characteristics
  Perfectionism
  Need to please others
  Nonassertiveness
  Unidimensional self-conceptualization (focusing only on one's athletic involvement)
  Low self-esteem
  High perception of stress (high anxiety)

From DiFiori JP, Benjamin HJ, Brenner J, et al. Overuse injuries and burnout in youth sports: a position statement from the American Medical Society for Sports Medicine. *Clin J Sport Med.* 2014;24(1)3-20, with permission.

Table 3
Symptoms of overtraining syndrome/burnout

Fatigue	Insomnia	Loss of appetite
Depression	Irritability	Weight loss
Bradycardia or tachycardia	Agitation	Lack of mental concentration
Loss of motivation or interest	Decreased self-confidence	Heavy, sore, stiff muscles
Hypertension	Anxiety	Restlessness
Sleep disturbances	Nausea	Frequent illness

From DiFiori JP, Benjamin HJ, Brenner J, et al. Overuse injuries and burnout in youth sports: a position statement from the American Medical Society for Sports Medicine. *Clin J Sport Med.* 2014;24(1)3-20, with permission.

disturbances should be treated with counseling and medication when indicated. Once the athlete is ready to return to training, it is crucial that the athlete's expectations be more realistic and any adult-controlled factors corrected in order to prevent burnout from reoccurring.

Prevention of overtraining and burnout can be accomplished by avoiding over-scheduling and excessive time commitment to training, as described in this case of the competitive swimmer.[40,41] A health care professional could consider using a Profile of Mood States (POMS) to monitor the athlete's mental health. The POMS is a psychological rating scale used to measure distinct moods states. In addition, athletes, parents, and physicians need to keep alert for signs and symptoms of burnout.

Table 4
Diagnosis of overtraining syndrome/burnout

History
  Decreased performance persisting despite weeks to month of recovery
  Disturbances in mood
  Lack of signs/symptoms or diagnosis of other possible causes of underperformance
  Lack of enjoyment participating in sport
  Inadequate nutritional and hydration intake
Presence of potential triggers
  Increased training load with adequate recovery
  Monotony of training
  Excessive number of competitions
  Sleep disturbance
  Stressors in family life (parental pressure)
  Stressors in sporting life (coaching pressure and travel demands)
  Previous illness
Testing (if indicated by history)
  Consider laboratory studies: complete blood count, comprehensive metabolic panel, erythrocyte
  sedimentation rate, C-reactive protein, iron studies, creatine kinase, thyroid studies, cytomegalovirus
  and Epstein-Barr virus titers
  Profile of Mood States (POMS): A psychometric tool for global measurement of mood, tension,
  depression, anger, vigor, fatigue, and confusion

From DiFiori JP, Benjamin HJ, Brenner J, et al. Overuse injuries and burnout in youth sports: a
position statement from the American Medical Society for Sports Medicine. *Clin J Sport Med.*
2014;24(1)3-20, with permission.

Tournaments and Year-Round Training

Young athletes who compete in tournaments in which they participate in multiple games during a short period of time (eg, a weekend), are at increased risk for multiple problems. These include heat illness, nutritional deficiencies, overtraining injuries, and burnout.[49]

Year-round training in a single sport has become more common for young athletes. Often the motivation is financial, with parents and athletes hoping to capture a piece of the very small "pie," leading to college scholarships and, potentially, a professional career. It has been documented that only 3.3% to 11.3% of high school athletes compete at the National Collegiate Athletic Association (NCAA) level (does not signify scholarships).[50] In addition, only 0.03% to 0.5% of high school athletes make it to the professional level.[50] It has been documented that athletes who participate in a variety sports have fewer injuries and play sports longer than those who specialize before puberty.[40,41,47,49,51,52]

GENERAL PREVENTION RECOMMENDATIONS

In order to help prevent overuse and overtraining injuries, the following recommendations should be encouraged[4,40,41,49]:

- Young athletes should be encouraged to have 1 to 2 days per week off from competitive sports to allow recovery and adaptation of their bodies and minds. During this time off they should be encouraged to do other recreational activities that they enjoy.
- Young athletes should be encouraged to take 2 to 3 months off from their sport throughout the year. The time off does not have to be consecutive, and they can remain active doing other activities or recreational sports.
- Young athletes should be encouraged to participate on only 1 team at a time. If they do participate with multiple teams during the same season, the prevention guidelines previously described or sports-specific guidelines (eg, pitch count limits) should be incorporated into that time.[16]
- Athletes should gradually increase their weekly training time, number of repetitions, or total distance using the 10% rule as a general guideline (only increase by 10% each week).
- Parents and athletes should be cautioned about participation in weekend tournaments in which playing time can exceed 6 hours per day.
- Most young athletes should avoid early specialization in a single sport.[47,52]

The primary goal for all young athletes should be to have fun while participating in sports that they enjoy and learning lifelong physical activity and healthy competition skills. Young athletes should be taught how to recognize signals of overtraining and then alter their training as needed.[49,53]

References

1. National Council of Youth Sports. Report on trends and participation in organized youth sports. Available at: www.ncys.org/pdfs/2008/2008-ncys-market-research-report.pdf. Accessed October 25, 2014
2. National Federation of State High School Association. 2013-14 High School Athletics Participation Survey. Available at: www.nfhs.org/ParticipationStatics/PDF/2013-14_Participation_Survey_PDF.pdf. Accessed October 25, 2014
3. Luke A, Lazaro RM, Bergeron MF, et al. Sports-related injuries in youth athletes: is overscheduling a risk factor? Clin J Sport Med. 2011;21(4):307-314
4. Valovich McLeod TC, Decoster LC, et al. National Athletic Trainers' Association position statement: prevention of pediatric overuse injuries. J Athl Train. 2011;46:206-220
5. Lyman S, Fleisig GS, Waterbor JW, et al. Longitudinal study of elbow and shoulder pain in youth baseball pitchers. Med Sci Sports Exerc. 2001;33(11):1803-1810
6. Hang DW, Chao CM, Hang Y-S. A clinical and roentgenographic study of Little League elbow. Am J Sports Med. 2004;32(1):79-84
7. Wilk KE, Macrina LC, Cain EL, Dugas JR, Andrews JR. Rehabilitation of the overhead athlete's elbow. Sports Health. 2012;4(5):404-414
8. Benjamin HJ, Briner WW. Little League elbow. Clin J Sport Med. 2005;15(1):37-40
9. Olsen SJ. Risk factors for shoulder and elbow injuries in adolescent baseball pitchers. Am J Sports Med. 2006;34(6):905-912
10. Fleisig GS, Andrews JR, Cutter GR, et al. Risk of serious injury for young baseball pitchers: a 10-year prospective study. Am J Sports Med. 2011;39(2):253-257
11. Anloague PA, Spees V, Smith J, Herbenick MA, Rubino LJ. Glenohumeral range of motion and lower extremity flexibility in collegiate-level baseball players. Sports Health. 2012;4(1):25-30

12. Johnson JN, Houchin G. Adolescent athlete's shoulder: a case series of proximal humeral epiphysiolysis in nonthrowing athletes. *Clin J Sport Med.* 2006;16(1):84-86

13. Osbahr DC, Kim HJ, Dugas JR. Little League shoulder. *Curr Opin Pediatr.* 2010;22(1):35-40

14. Lyman S, Fleisig GS, Andrews JR, Osinski ED. Effect of pitch type, pitch count, and pitching mechanics on risk of elbow and shoulder pain in youth baseball pitchers. *Am J Sports Med.* 2002;30(4):463-468

15. Yang J, Mann BJ, Guettler JH, Dugas JR. Risk-prone pitching activities and injuries in youth baseball findings from a national sample. *Am J Sports Med.* 2014;42(6):1456-1463

16. American Sports Medicine Institute. American Sports Medicine Institute: position statement for youth baseball pitchers. 2014:1-2. Available at: www.asmi.org/research.php?page=research&section=positionStatement. Accessed October 4, 2014

17. Bak K, Faunø P. Clinical findings in competitive swimmers with shoulder pain. *Am J Sports Med.* 1997;25(2):254-260

18. McMaster WC, Troup J. A survey of interfering shoulder pain in United States competitive swimmers. *Am J Sports Med.* 1993;21(1):67-70

19. Rupp S, Berninger K, Hopf T. Shoulder problems in high level swimmers—impingement, anterior instability, muscular imbalance? *Int J Sports Med.* 1995;16(8):557-562

20. Sein ML, Walton J, Linklater J, et al. Shoulder pain in elite swimmers: primarily due to swim-volume-induced supraspinatus tendinopathy. *Br J Sports Med.* 2010;44(2):105-113

21. Bak K. The practical management of swimmer's painful shoulder: etiology, diagnosis, and treatment. *Clin J Sport Med.* 2010;20(5):386-390

22. DiFiori JP. Wrist pain, distal radial physeal injury, and ulnar variance in the young gymnast. *Am J Sports Med.* 2005;34(5):840-849

23. DiFiori JP, Puffer JC, Mandelbaum BR, Mar S. Factors associated with wrist pain in the young gymnast. *Am J Sports Med.* 1996;24(1):9-14

24. Gholve PA, Scher DM, Khakharia S, Widmann RF, Green DW. Osgood Schlatter syndrome. *Curr Opin Pediatr.* 2007;19(1):44-50

25. Kujala UM, Kvist M, Heinonen O. Osgood-Schlatter disease in adolescent athletes. Retrospective study of incidence and duration. *Am J Sports Med.* 1985;13(4):236-241

26. Frush TJ, Lindenfeld TN. Peri-epiphyseal and overuse injuries in adolescent athletes. *Sports Health.* 2009;1(3):201-211

27. Topol GA, Podesta LA, Reeves KD, et al. Hyperosmolar dextrose injection for recalcitrant Osgood-Schlatter disease. *Pediatrics.* 2011;128(5):e1121-e1128

28. Micheli LJ, Ireland ML. Prevention and management of calcaneal apophysitis in children: an overuse syndrome. *J Pediatr Orthop.* 1987;7(1):34-38

29. Dixit S, DiFiori JP, Burton M, Mines B. Management of patellofemoral pain syndrome. *Am Fam Physician.* 2007;75(2):194-202

30. Fulkerson JP. Diagnosis and treatment of patients with patellofemoral pain. *Am J Sports Med.* 2002;30(3):447-456

31. Meira EP, Brumitt J. Influence of the hip on patients with patellofemoral pain syndrome: a systematic review. *Sports Health.* 2011;3(5):455-465

32. Taunton JE. A retrospective case-control analysis of 2002 running injuries. *Br J Sports Med.* 2002;36(2):95-101

33. Clement DB, Taunton JE, Smart GW, McNicol KL. A survey of overuse running injuries. *Phys Sportsmed.* 1981;9:47-58

34. Post WR. Clinical evaluation of patients with patellofemoral disorders. *Arthroscopy.* 1999;15(8):841-851

35. Frye JL, Ramey LN, Hart JM. The effects of exercise on decreasing pain and increasing function in patients with patellofemoral pain syndrome: a systematic review. *Sports Health.* 2012;4(3):205-210

36. d'Hemecourt PA, Gerbino PG, Micheli LJ. Back injuries in the young athlete. *Clin Sports Med.* 2000;19(4):663-679

37. Purcell L, Micheli L. Low back pain in young athletes. *Sports Health.* 2009;1(3):212-222

38. Rassi El G, Takemitsu M, Woratanarat P, Shah SA. Lumbar spondylolysis in pediatric and adolescent soccer players. *Am J Sports Med.* 2005;33(11):1688-1693

39. Meeusen R, Duclos M, Gleeson M, et al. Prevention, diagnosis and treatment of the Overtraining syndrome. *Eur J Sport Sci.* 2006;6(1):1-14

40. DiFiori JP, Benjamin HJ, Brenner JS, et al. Overuse injuries and burnout in youth sports: a position statement from the American Medical Society for Sports Medicine. *Clin J Sport Med.* 2014;24(1):3-20

41. DiFiori JP, Benjamin HJ, Brenner JS, et al. Overuse injuries and burnout in youth sports: a position statement from the American Medical Society for Sports Medicine. *Br J Sports Med.* 2014;48(4):287-288

42. Smith RE. Sport psychology toward a cognitive-affective model of athletic burnout. *J Sport Exerc Psychol.* 1986;8(1):36-50

43. Matos NF, Winsley RJ, Williams CA. Prevalence of nonfunctional overreaching/overtraining in young English athletes. *Med Sci Sports Exerc.* 2011;43(7):1287-1294

44. Raglin J, Sawamura S, Alexiou S, Hassmén P. Training practices and staleness in 13 to 18-year-old swimmers: a cross-cultural study. *Pediatr Exerc Sci.* 2000;12(1):61-70

45. Winsley R, Matos N. Overtraining and elite young athletes. *Med Sport Sci.* 2011;56:97-105

46. Gould D. Intensive sport participation and the prepubescent athlete: competitive stress and burnout. In: Cahill BR, Pearl AJ, eds. *Intensive Participation in Children's Sports.* Champaign, IL: Human Kinetics; 1993:19-38

47. Malina RM. Early sport specialization: roots, effectiveness, risks. *Curr Sports Med Rep.* 2010;9(6):364-371

48. Morgan WP, Brown DR. Psychological monitoring of overtraining and staleness. *Br J Sports Med.* 1987;21:107-114

49. Brenner JS; American Academy of Pediatrics Council on Sports Medicine and Fitness. Overuse injuries, overtraining, and burnout in child and adolescent athletes. *Pediatrics.* 2007;119(6):1242-1245

50. National Collegiate Athletic Association. Estimated probability of competing in athletics beyond the high school interscholastic level. Available at: www.ncaa.org/sites/default/files/Probability-of-going-pro-methodology_Update2013.pdf. Accessed October 25, 2014

51. American Academy of Pediatrics Committee on Sports Medicine and Fitness. Intensive training and sports specialization in young athletes. *Pediatrics.* 2000;106(1):154-157

52. Jayanthi N, Pinkham C, Dugas L, Patrick B, LaBella C. Sports specialization in young athletes: evidence-based recommendations. *Sports Health.* 2013;5(3):251-257

53. Small E. Chronic musculoskeletal pain in young athletes. *Pediatr Clin North Am.* 2002;49(3):655-662, vii

Adolesc Med 026 (2015) 100–115

Rehabilitation of Musculoskeletal Injuries in Young Athletes

Gabriel Brooks, PT, DPT, MTC, SCS[a]*;
Jon Almquist, ATC, VATL, ITAT[b]

[a]Baylor College of Medicine, Texas Children's Hospital, Department of Pediatrics,
Section of Adolescent Medicine and Sports Medicine, Houston, Texas;
[b]Fairfax Family Practice Comprehensive Concussion Center, Fairfax, Virginia

INTRODUCTION

Musculoskeletal disorders and diseases are the leading causes of pain, physical disability, and physician visits throughout the world, representing as much as 30% of primary care visits in North America.[1-4] During the school year from 2012 to 2013, there were 2.5 million sports injury-related emergency department (ED) visits for patients aged 6 to 18 years, which comprised 23% of all ED injury-related visits.[5] The leading diagnoses for sports-injury related visits to the ED were fractures, dislocations, sprains and strains, open wounds, and contusions. Fourteen percent of medical visits to ambulatory care centers in the United States cited musculoskeletal signs and symptoms as the primary reason for the visit. Although musculoskeletal injury is common, there is a disparity in the preparedness of physicians to care for these injuries. As recently as 2003, only 40% of US medical schools had a required preclinical musculoskeletal course, and just 20% had a required clinical clerkship.[6] The lack of musculoskeletal training in medical school curricula has been well documented,[7-11] and subsequent surveys of students, residents, and practicing physicians have consistently demonstrated a lack of confidence in diagnosing and managing musculoskeletal problems.[1,7,10,11] This information is not new, yet it is noteworthy because the physician is most frequently the practitioner who determines an athlete's return to play status after injury. The objectives of this article are to review the key concepts of management for musculoskeletal injuries, rehabilitation, and assessment of readiness to return to play.

---

*Corresponding author
E-mail address: gpbrooks@texaschildrens.org

It is sound practice to place efforts toward primary prevention of injury so that athletes can reach their full potential for the season and reduce the likelihood of time loss injury.[12-18] Toward that end, it is the authors' recommendation that a specific risk assessment for musculoskeletal injury be included in the preseason physical examination.

PRIMARY PREVENTION

Screening efforts are one method of primary prevention that seeks to identify risk factors predictive of injury within the athletic population. In addition to the objective criteria, functional sports-specific testing provides insight into the athlete's ability to progressively return to sports practice conditions after the summer break or time off from injury. Sports-specific functional testing under fatigued conditions provides a more comprehensive assessment of an athlete's readiness to return to competition. Young, motivated athletes, as well as their parents, may not admit to limitations if the desire to return to sport overrides the perceived importance of the problem. Given space and time constraints, decisions for final return to practice or competition can be referred to the physical therapist or athletic trainer. Examples of screening efforts that may be used include the general musculoskeletal preseason examination, the group preparticipation physical examination (PPE), and the specialty PPE. Although screening examinations typically take place in groups and by nature are general, they may uncover functional deficits indicating the need for a more focused examination. The pediatrician should then perform a differential examination or refer the athlete for a more comprehensive evaluation. The rehabilitation process subsequently can be initiated.

Abnormalities noted on the musculoskeletal screening should be referred to the physical therapist or athletic trainer for focused remediation of the impairments before the athlete begins the season. A few examples of findings from the PPE that are predictive risk factors include the following:

- Prior sports injury.[19]
- Asymmetry of the shoulder total arc of motion (external to internal) in which the rotation range of motion arc differs by ≥5 degrees on the dominant side compared to the nondominant side[20] (Figure 1).
- A single leg squat that demonstrates functional knee valgus in which the hip internally rotates to place the knee medial to the ankle.[21] The clinical presentation of this risk factor is shown in Figure 2.
- A Beighton scale score of >2 points.[22] Examples are shown in Figures 3 to 6.

The physician may wish to include a more robust movement screening system in addition to the standard PPE to ensure that the patient's balance and ease of movement have been adequately tested.[23] One example of this type of assessment is the Functional Movement Screen (FMS).[24] In the FMS there are 7 movement tests each with a possible 3 points making a total of 21 possible points. Of

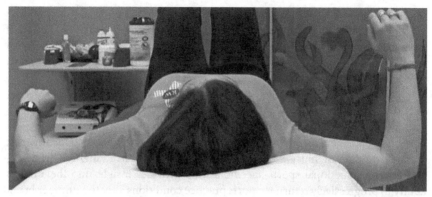

Fig 1. With the patient in supine, a difference between the total arc of shoulder rotation motion on the athlete's throwing side (R) compared to the non-throwing side (L) >5 degrees is a risk factor for injury.

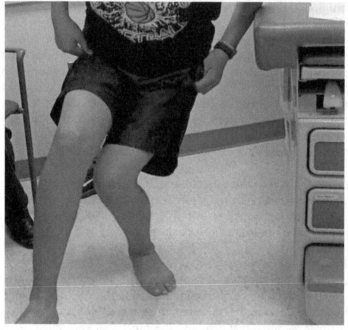

Fig 2. The patient performs a single leg squat and deviates into functional valgus on the load bearing side. This is a positive predictor of numerous sports injuries to the leg.

the 7 movement tests, 5 are tested bilaterally and 2 movements, the deep squat and the trunk stability push up, are tested as 1 full body, symmetrical movement. Each test is scored on a point scale from 0 to 3 as follows:

0 = patient reports pain during the movement
1 = patient demonstrates failure to complete the movement or loss of balance during the movement

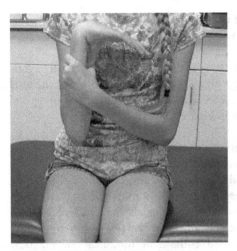

Fig 3. In the Beighton hypermobility screening test 1 point of a maximum 9 points is assigned for each thumb that can be brought to the volar side of the wrist in wrist flexion.

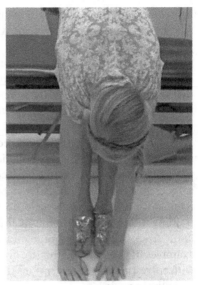

Fig 4. In the Beighton hypermobility screening test 1 point of a maximum 9 points is assigned for the ability to place the palms flat on the floor from standing with the knees straight.

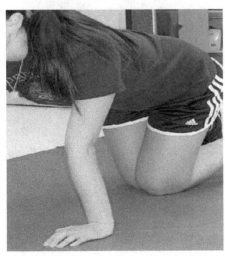

Fig 5. In the Beighton hypermobility screening test 1 point of a maximum 9 points is assigned for each elbow that hyperextends.

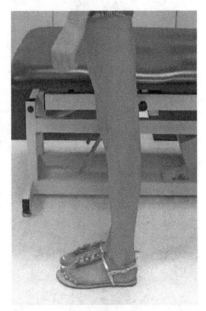

Fig 6. In the Beighton hypermobility screening test 1 point of a maximum 9 points is assigned for each knee that hyperextends.

2 = patient completes the movement with compensation
3 = patient performs the movement without any compensation

For each movement, the highest score from 3 trials is recorded and used to generate an overall composite FMS score with a maximum score of 21. For the tests that are assessed bilaterally, the lowest score is used. Examples of the movements from this screening system are shown in Figures 7 to 10.

Whatever methods are used for screening, when athletes are identified as *at risk* for injury in the PPE, a rehabilitation plan should be developed between the physician, patient and family, physical therapist, and athletic trainer. The physical therapist will then proceed with targeted interventions to address the impairments. The treatments used to accomplish these goals may include balance training to improve neuromuscular performance, muscular strengthening, flexibility training, joint manipulation, and equipment modification. Practical examples of these treatments are given in Table 1. The treatment goals are listed with corresponding interventions that are commonly used in physical therapy to meet those goals.

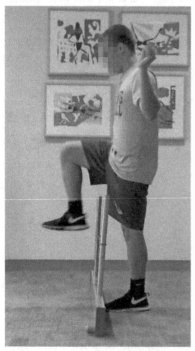 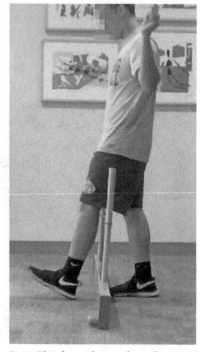

Fig 7. This figure depicts the mid-point of the FMS screen movement test called "Hurdle Step".

Fig 8. This figure depicts the end point of the FMS test movement called "Hurdle Step".

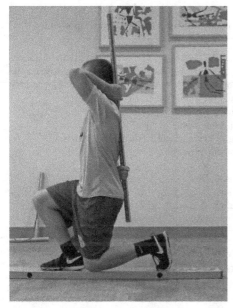

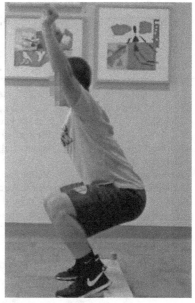

Fig 9. This figure depicts the FMS test movement called "In line lunge."

Fig 10. This figure depicts the end point of the FMS test movement called "Deep Squat."

IMPROVING MUSCLE STRENGTH

Muscular strength and endurance training in sport are implicitly important, but there is widespread misunderstanding in community-based sports programs about proper dosing of the exercise variables. The American Academy of Pediatrics (AAP) recommends that strength training in children be adequately supervised with an instructor to athlete ratio of ≤1:10.[25] Supervision may be provided by an athletic trainer with pediatric sports specialization or physical therapist with sports specialization and experience in pediatrics. A strength training professional with a pediatric-specific credential, such as American College of Sports Medicine (ACSM) certification, may also supervise strength training sessions.

The AAP does not address coaching in their statement on strength training, nor have recommendations been established for coaches' credentials to supervise strength training. It is important that coaches have the specific knowledge and skills appropriate for this population to ensure proper management of the athlete and optimal skill acquisition. The primary author routinely sees the consequences of inappropriate weight lifting regimens performed by young athletes manifest as lumbar spondylolysis, joint sprains, and varied muscle strains. Olympic lifts are frequently the reported mechanism of injury. Because children acquire the neuromotor skills that they will use for sports throughout their lifetime between 5 years of age and 8 years of age, it is critical to have well-qualified professionals instruct-

Table 1

Treatment methods for physical impairments identified in the preparticipation exam.

Goals	Treatment
Regain and improve strength	Progressive resistive exercise. The format of resistive exercise may be isometric or isotonic and each may be used in an Open kinetic chain (OKC) context or the Closed kinetic chain (CKC) context.
Normalize joint accessory mobility	Manipulate joint if hypomobile Stabilize joint if hypermobile Bracing, taping, or neuromuscular re-education exercises
Improve proprioception, kinesthesia	Balance and stability exercises
Improve neuromuscular control, elegance	Motion analysis studies Athlete education Multimodal cuing Motor control retraining

ing practices and consulting with sports programs to ensure that skill development activities result in motor patterns that are safe and sustainable for the long term.

Neuromuscular training in rehabilitation is designed to improve an athlete's afferent-efferent communications to minimize potentially injurious movements during a task and to improve economy, lessen strain, and ensure optimal function before return to sport. Treatment efforts aimed at improving proprioception, kinesthesia, balance, agility, and reaction time are examples of neuromuscular training modalities. An example of this type of training is an athlete performing balance board activities to improve proprioception and thus reduce the risk of future ankle sprain (Figure 11).

REHABILITATION PROFESSIONALS IN SECONDARY CARE CENTERS

There is a need for primary care physicians to possess the knowledge and skills to diagnose and treat musculoskeletal injuries, including referral to qualified physical therapists or certified athletic trainers for rehabilitation. However, of all medical visits for musculoskeletal injuries in ambulatory care centers in the United States, physical therapy was prescribed for only 2.3% of the cases.[26]

The reasons for the low number of referrals made to physical therapy is not known. Clarifying the role of rehabilitation specialists in the continuum of care may assist the primary care physician in making the needed referral. Physical therapists are licensed by each state and may obtain board certification under the American Board of Physical Therapy Specialties. Musculoskeletal injuries are most typically managed by the sports clinical specialist (SCS) or the orthopedic clinical specialist (OCS).

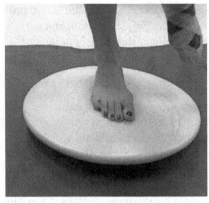
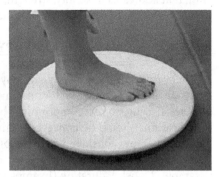

Fig 11. The athlete performs balance board activities to challenge ankle stability and improve proprioception thus reducing the risk of future ankle sprain.

Physical therapists frequently collaborate with certified athletic trainers along the care continuum. Athletic trainers are most commonly employed by schools, sports organizations, and clinics, where they provide emergency and acute injury care, as well as coordination of care for injured players, equipment maintenance, and rehabilitation services.[27] The pattern of collaboration varies among regions and facilities, and sometimes there is substantial overlap between the 2 professions. High school athletes may have access to a certified athletic trainer in the school who can provide a more seamless continuum of care throughout the athlete's recovery.

COMPREHENSIVE INJURY REHABILITATION

Rest alone is insufficient to effect recovery from injury and does not reduce the risk of reinjury, yet physical therapy is prescribed in only 2.3% of musculoskeletal injury cases.[28] With the low frequency of referral to physical therapy, many conditions are not fully rehabilitated when the athlete resumes activity. Given the frequency of reinjury upon return to sport, it should be emphasized that complete rehabilitation is essential.

When a physician makes the decision to return an athlete to competition after injury, it is often without using objective criteria to determine readiness.[28-30] Therefore, it would be helpful to review the known risk factors for injury and the rehabilitation for those impairments. Only when the risk factors have been eliminated should the athlete return to play.

In contrast to rest as the treatment regimen, a comprehensive rehabilitation program that addresses flexibility, strength, endurance, proprioception, and correction of faulty movement patterns significantly reduces the risk of reinjury.[14-19]

PRESCRIBING PHYSICAL THERAPY

It is important for the primary care physician to inform the rehabilitation professional of any medical factor that influences exercise prescription, such as diabetes, dysautonomia, compromised bone health, or coagulopathy.[25] Any contraindications should be conveyed to the therapist. To facilitate the referral to physical therapy, consider writing a prescription that includes the following information: diagnosis, other relevant disease (Example: diabetes), frequency (Example: 2×/wk.), duration (Example: 8 weeks), special precautions (Example: Ehlers-Danlos syndrome), and specific impairments that you want to highlight (Example: scapular dyskinesis in shoulder elevation or Trendelenburg gait deviation in the hip).

An example of how the physician might generate a referral to rehabilitation is given in Table 2. It begins with the examination findings, progresses to how the physician might request treatment, and concludes with what is commonly done in response to that request. The physician's findings on examination are listed with corresponding referral options for the impairments and the most common treatment resulting from those referrals.

METHODS OF TREATMENT USED IN REHABILITATION

Cryotherapy

Cryotherapy is used in primary and secondary centers and is recommended for acute injuries to mitigate the inflammatory response and reduce pain.[31] The cold pack should be applied to the injured body part on a 10-minute on and 10-minute off schedule. The body part then should be allowed to rewarm for 1 hour before the ice is reapplied. Cryotherapy is known to limit perfusion and nerve conduction velocity, which can be helpful in the management of swelling and pain. However, after icing, the athlete's proprioception and kinesthesia are impaired,[31] so the athlete's protective responses also are impaired under these circumstances. If the athlete is allowed to play immediately after icing, the sensory impairment may prevent the athlete from adequately protecting the injury. Therefore, ice should be used after activity or when 30 minutes for rewarming can be assured before the athlete begins activity.

Manual Therapy

Manual therapy is the manipulative treatment of joint movement restrictions.[32] It is a skilled treatment that allows the physical therapist to restore the joint's

Table 2
Writing a referral to rehabilitation services.

Examination finding	Writing the prescription	Corresponding treatments
Loss of joint range of motion	If restriction is muscular: "Stretching/flexibility training" (PT, AT)	Low-load, long-duration stretching (30s to 2 min each) +/− active lengthening exercises "Contract-relax" (aka reciprocal or autogenic inhibition)
	If restriction is in the joint capsule or a soft tissue adhesion is present: "Manual therapy" (PT)	Manual manipulation of the joint +/− surrounding soft tissues to restore normal joint dynamics
Muscle weakness	If impairment is in endurance: "Muscle strengthening–endurance" (PT, AT)	15-30 repetitions using lower weight
	If impairment is a loss of strength: "Muscle strengthening (PT, AT)	3 sets of repetitions to failure at 30-60% Estimated 1RM
	If impairment is in power: "Muscle power training" (PT, AT)	Low no. of repetitions of explosive muscle actions (Examples:, jumping, sprinting, throwing)
Ill-fitting equipment	Equipment fitting consultation (PT, AT)	Review of proper sports equipment to mitigate risk of injury and maximize performance (Examples: make adjustments to an ill-fitting helmet, discard improper running shoes or orthoses and receive recommendations based on patient anatomy and function)

Note: Where a treatment may be provided by either a physical therapist (PT) or an athletic trainer (AT) both initials appear. Where the treatment skill is more specialized and requires advanced clinical skill, only the physical therapist designation (PT) appears. PT is a standard abbreviation for Physical Therapist and AT is a standard abbreviation for Athletic Trainer.

normal mechanical movement when it has been altered by injury or immobilization. The concept of joint dysfunction refers to a state of altered mechanics in which there is an increase or a decrease from the expected normal or the presence of an aberrant motion. Where hypomobility exists, the treatment of choice is joint manipulation, stretching, and activity that promotes movement. When hypermobility exists, treatment of the joint in question is not manipulation but stabilization by exercise, passive supports, or correction of movement impairments. When making a referral to physical therapy, the physician requesting "manual therapy" need only indicate the region (Example: shoulder). However, if any specialty needs exist, such as postoperative precautions, the physician may wish to communicate them along with the request.

Stretching

If the range of motion about a joint is limited in quality or quantity, that impairment should be corrected in order to prevent further injury and improve performance.[33] Stretching is more effective when it is performed with low intensity and long durations after, rather than before, activity. In contrast, warm ups are performed before activity. They are an important part of the athlete's regimen, but they do not contribute toward actual lengthening of the muscle and its associated connective tissue. Examples include high kicks, toe touches/reverse dead lifts, skipping, and crossover steps.

Strengthening

For children and adolescents, the recommended frequency of strength training is 2 to 3 times per week, for a duration of at least 8 weeks, and an exercise intensity that allows for 2 to 3 sets of repetitions to volitional failure for each exercise. Use of 1-repetition maximum lifts is discouraged, especially for skeletally immature athletes. Training with 10-repetition maximums and predicted maximums are recommended in place of 1RM loads for young athletes.[25] The specific tasks involved in Olympic weight lifting maneuvers (dead lift, squat, snatch and clean) have poor transfer to other sports and are not predictive of athletic performance in sports outside of performing the identical task under powerlifting competition conditions. Powerlifting and bodybuilding are discouraged for pediatric athletes.

In rehabilitation contexts, specific strength impairments are targeted and corrected; however, as the patient improves, a more general strengthening program can be engaged. This type of program should address all the major muscle groups, including the core stabilizing musculature, and it should include exercises that move through the complete range of motion. More sports-specific areas can be addressed later when strength and stability have been achieved.[25] One such example is seen in soccer players who are known to have a high incidence of hamstring injuries and a high rate of recurrence.[34] The risk of hamstring strain can be reduced by performing long-arc, eccentric phase hamstring strengthening exercises.[35,36]

Balance and Neuromuscular Control

Retraining of balance and neuromuscular control is an important part of rehabilitation that is used to improve efficiency of motion and reduce the risk of injury. It is of great importance that neuromotor control and proprioceptive sense be restored after injury because a previously unrehabilitated injury is an excellent predictor of future sports injury.[19] Any program aimed at reducing the risk of injury should recognize the presence or absence of validated predictors of injury during an athlete's functional testing.[37] This identification of risk factors should be made at several points along the continuum of care and again before returning to sport. These validated predictors of injury are essentially movement impairments that can be corrected with training, and they can be used as outcome measures for rehabilitation or injury prevention programs.

Sports injuries are understood to be multifactorial in cause, and injuries generally cannot be prevented by addressing a single risk factor in isolation. Comprehensive preventive programs reduce injury risk by addressing multiple risk factors within a formal season-long program.[12,13,15-18,37-39] Proprioceptive and neuromuscular training have demonstrated significant reductions in the number of risk factors and the number of injuries during an athletic season.[12,13,15-18,40-42] Primary care physicians should feel comfortable recommending such programs for athletes when the programs are composed of evidence-based interventions.

Bracing and Taping for Athletics

Bracing and taping are commonly used to stabilize injuries in athletes. Use of ankle lace-up braces is recommended for athletes who have a history of ankle injury within the last year.[40,41,43] Ankle lace-up braces are more effective at reducing reinjury than ankle taping, and each is more effective than no support.[42] The athlete should not be dependent on the brace but should also engage in an ankle functional retraining program for recovery of strength, flexibility, balance, and proprioception. Objective criteria should be used to assess functional ankle stability before and after a training program is implemented to determine whether the desired improvement has taken place.[28]

Knee braces are more controversial than ankle braces. The evidence is mixed regarding the effect of bracing the knee to prevent injury, and data recommending prophylactic knee bracing to decrease the rate and severity of knee ligament injury in athletes are not available.[44,45] However, bracing after injury may protect the affected tissue from further damage, and the physician should make an individual determination of need.

CLEARING THE ATHLETE FOR SPORT PARTICIPATION

Once rehabilitation has been completed, the athlete must be formally cleared to participate in sport. Judging an athlete's readiness to return to sport can be complex. Making that judgment without objective criteria may allow an athlete to return to sport prematurely and may result in sub-optimal athletic performance or reinjury.[29] The decision to return an athlete to sport can be improved with use of objective criteria. Two methods for obtaining the athlete's readiness to return to play are functional outcome questionnaires and more objective criteria-based testing.

Functional Outcomes Questionnaires

One method of determining an athlete's readiness to return to play is to have the patient complete a validated functional outcome questionnaire. Examples of these questionnaires include the Kerlan-Jobe Orthopedic Clinic (KJOC) shoulder and elbow questionnaire,[46] the Penn shoulder scale,[47] and the Lower Limb Functional Index.[48] These functional outcome measures can be administered and scored in less than 3 minutes and can be used at regular intervals during the episode of care to demonstrate improvement. Objective documentation of function scores can help the physician make return to sport decisions.

Criteria-Based Testing

Use of additional testing methods to determine an athlete's readiness to return to competitive play is recommended. Two types of criteria-based testing can be performed: (1) a functional test that is based on movement quality (for example the Y balance test for upper the quarter or lower quarter[49,50]); and (2) the FMS or dynamic movement assessment.

Technical tests seek to quantify impairments for comparison to normative values. Examples are isokinetic dynamometry or motion analysis studies, including motion capture software. Intensive studies can be performed using high-speed cameras, global positioning system (GPS)-derived kinetic data, or infrared cameras, which read biomarkers to measure critical elements of performance.

Objective testing is an important part of the decision-making process to determine an athlete's sport-specific readiness. The objective data may be used together with the physician's understanding of the athlete's specific physical demands and the overall impression of the patient. Determination of the athlete's readiness to return to sport can made by the physician or may be referred to the physical therapist or athletic trainer. Some questions that physicians may use to help determine an athlete's readiness to compete include:

- Is the athlete's strength consistent with normative values?
- Is the joint range of motion full and easily accessed?
- Has the athlete successfully completed a sport-specific functional skills progression without provocation of symptoms?
- What are the demands of this athlete's position in this sport, and can this athlete meet those demands safely?
- To what level of competition is the athlete returning? (The speeds and forces will be higher in higher levels of competition.)

Asking these types of questions may help the physician to assess the degree to which the athlete has been rehabilitated or the degree of readiness that the athlete possesses for return to play.

SUMMARY

Caring for young athletes challenges the physician to use primary preventive measures to prevent injury and to respond with secondary measures when injuries do occur. An enhanced knowledge of the rehabilitation process will assist the physician in making the appropriate referrals and in evaluating the patient's condition before clearing that athlete. Use of criteria-based testing may aid the primary care physician in determining an athlete's readiness for sport.

References

1. Monrad SU, Zeller JL, Craig CL, DiPonio LA. Musculoskeletal education in US medical schools: lessons from the past and suggestions for the future. *Curr Rev Musculoskelet Med.* 2011;4:91-98
2. Musculoskeletal diseases: leading cause of disability and health care cost. Available at: www.usbjd. org/about/index.cfm?pg=fast.cfm. Accessed August 28, 2014
3. Pinney SJ, Regan WD. Educating medical students about musculoskeletal problems: are community needs reflected in the curricula of Canadian medical schools? *J Bone Joint Surg Am.* 2001;83A:1317-1320
4. National high school sports-related injury surveillance study. Available at: www.ucdenver.edu/academics/colleges/PublicHealth/research/ResearchProjects/piper/projects/RIO/Pages/StudyReports.aspx. Accessed August 28, 2014
5. Simon TD, Bublitz C, Hambidge SJ. Emergency department visits among pediatric patients for sports-related injury: basic epidemiology and effect of race/ethnicity and insurance status. *Pediatr Emerg Care.* 2006;22:309-315
6. DiCaprio MR, Covey A, Bernstein J. Curricular requirements for musculoskeletal medicine in American medical schools. *J Bone Joint Surg Am.* 2003;85A:565-567
7. Clawson DK, Jackson DW, Ostergaard DJ. It's past time to reform the musculoskeletal curriculum. *Acad Med.* 2001;76:709-710
8. Freedman KB, Bernstein J. The adequacy of medical school education in musculoskeletal medicine. *J Bone Joint Surg Am.* 1998;80:1421-1427
9. Freedman KB, Bernstein J. Educational deficiencies in musculoskeletal medicine. *J Bone Joint Surg Am.* 2002;84A:604-608
10. Day CS, Yeh AC, Franko O, et al. Musculoskeletal medicine: an assessment of the attitudes and knowledge of medical students at Harvard Medical School. *Acad Med.* 2007;82:452-457

11. Lynch JR, Gardner GC, Parsons RR. Musculoskeletal workload versus musculoskeletal clinical confidence among primary care physicians in rural practice. *Am J Orthop (Belle Mead NJ)*. 2005;34:487-491

12. Noyes FR, Barber-Westin SD. Neuromuscular retraining intervention programs: do they reduce noncontact anterior cruciate ligament injury rates in adolescent female athletes? *Arthroscopy*. 2014;30:245-255

13. McHugh MP, Tyler TF, Miravella MR, Mullaney MJ, Nicholas SJ. The effectiveness of a balance training intervention in reducing the incidence of non-contact ankle sprains in high school football players. *Am J Sports Med*. 2007;35:1289-1294

14. Hupperets MD, Verhagen EA, Heymans MW, et al. Potential savings of a program to prevent ankle sprain recurrence. *Am J Sports Med*. 2010;38:2194-2200

15. Emery CA, Meeuwisse WH. The effectiveness of a neuromuscular prevention strategy to reduce injuries in youth soccer: a cluster-randomized controlled trial. *Br J Sports Med*. 2010;44:555-562

16. Verhagen E, Van der Veek A, Twisk J, Bouter L, Bahr R. The effect of a proprioceptive balance board training program for the prevention of ankle sprains. *Am J Sports Med*. 2004;32:1385-1393

17. Beynnon BD, Murphy DF, Alosa DM. Predictive factors for lateral ankle sprains: a literature review. *J Athl Train*. 2002;37:376-380

18. Mohammadi F. Comparison of 3 preventive methods to reduce the recurrence of ankle inversion sprains in male soccer players. *Am J Sports Med*. 2007;35:922-926

19. Ryan J, DeBurca N, McCreesh K. Risk factors for groin/hip injuries in field-based sports: a systematic review. *Br J Sports Med*. 2014;48:1089-1096

20. Manske, R, Wilk, K, Davies, G, Ellenbecker, T, Reinold, M. Glenohumeral motion deficits: friend or foe? *Int J Sports Phys Ther*. 2013;8:537-553

21. Loudon JK, Reiman MP. Lower extremity kinematics in running athletes with and without a history of medial shin pain. *Int J Sports Phys Ther*. 2012;7:356-364

22. Cameron KL, Duffey ML, DeBerardino TM, et al. Association of generalized joint hypermobility with a history of glenohumeral joint instability. *J Athl Train*. 2010;45:253-258

23. Lisman P, O'Connor FG, Deuster PA, Knapik JJ. Functional movement screen and aerobic fitness predict injuries in military training. *Med Sci Sports Exerc*. 2013;45:636-643

24. Schneiders AG, Davidsson A, Hörman E, Sullivan SJ. Functional movement screen normative values in a young, active population. *Int J Sports Phys Ther*. 2011;6:75-82

25. Council on Sports Medicine and Fitness. Strength training by children and adolescents. Available at: pediatrics.aappublications.org/content/121/4/835.full. Accessed August 28, 2014

26. NAMCS. National Hospital Ambulatory Medical Care Survey: 2010 outpatient department summary tables. Available at: www.cdc.gov/nchs/ahcd/web_tables.htm#2010. Accessed August 28, 2014

27. National Athletic Trainers' Association. Profile of athletic trainer. Available at: www.NATA.org/public. Accessed August 28, 2014

28. Clanton TO, Matheny LM, Jarvis HC, Anastasia B, Jeronimus AB. Return to play in athletes following ankle injuries. *Sports Health*. 2012;4:471-474

29. Myer GD, Martin L Jr, Ford KR, et al. No association of time from surgery with functional deficits in athletes after anterior cruciate ligament reconstruction: evidence for objective return-to-sport criteria. *Am J Sports Med*. 2012;40:2256-2263

30. Hewett TE, Di Stasi SL, Myer GD. Current concepts for injury prevention in athletes after anterior cruciate ligament reconstruction. *Am J Sports Med*. 2013;41:216-224

31. Brooks GP, Cline J, Fitzgerald D, Hergenroeder AC. Musculoskeletal injury in the young athlete: overview of rehabilitation for non-operative injuries. In: Basow BD, ed. *UpToDate*. Wellesley, MA: UpToDate; 2011

32. Cleland JA, Mintken PE, McDevitt A, et al. Manual physical therapy and exercise versus supervised home exercise in the management of patients with inversion ankle sprain: a multicenter randomized clinical trial. *Orthop Sports Phys Ther*. 2013;43:443-455

33. Woods K, Bishop P, Jones E. Warm-up and stretching in the prevention of muscular injury. *Sports Med.* 2007;37:1089-1099

34. Schache A. Eccentric hamstring muscle training can prevent hamstring injuries in soccer players. *J Physiother.* 2012;58:58

35. Brunker P, Nealon A, Morgan C, Burgess D, Dunn A. Recurrent hamstring muscle injury: applying the limited evidence in the professional football setting with a 7-point programme. *Br J Sports Med.* 2014;48:929-938

36. Petersen J, Thorborg K, Nielsen MB, Budtz-Jørgensen E, Hölmich P. Preventive effect of eccentric training on acute hamstring injuries in men's soccer: a cluster-randomized controlled trial. *Am J Sports Med.* 2011;39:2296-2303

37. Hewett TE, Myer GD, Ford KR, et al. Biomechanical measures of neuromuscular control and valgus loading of the knee predict anterior cruciate ligament injury risk in female athletes: a prospective study. *Am J Sports Med.* 2005;33:492-501

38. Gilchrist J, Mandelbaum BR, Melancon H, et al. A randomized controlled trial to prevent noncontact anterior cruciate ligament injury in female collegiate soccer players. *Am J Sports Med.* 2008;36:1476-1483

39. Mandelbaum BR, Silvers HJ, Watanable DS, et al. Effectiveness of a neuromuscular and proprioceptive training program in preventing anterior cruciate ligament injuries in female athletes: 2-year follow up. *Am J Sports Med.* 2005;33:1003-1010

40. McGuine T, Brooks A, Hetzel S. The effect of lace-up ankle braces on injury rates in high school basketball players. *Am J Sports Med.* 2011;9:1840-1848

41. Frey C, Feder KS, Sleight J. Prophylactic ankle brace use in high school volleyball players: a prospective study. *Foot Ankle Int.* 2010;31:296-300

42. Seah R, Mani-Babu S. Managing ankle sprains in primary care: what is best practice? A systematic review of the last 10 years of evidence. *Br Med Bull.* 2011;97:105-135

43. Surve I, Schwellnus MP, Noakes T, Lombard C. A 5-fold reduction in the incidence of recurrent ankle sprains in soccer players using the Sport-Stirrup orthosis. *Am J Sports Med.* 1994;22:601-606

44. Rishiraj N, Taunton J, Lloyd-Smith R, et al. The potential role of prophylactic/functional knee bracing in preventing knee ligament injury. *Sports Med.* 2009;39:937-960

45. Pietrosimone BG, Grindstaff TL, Linens SW, Uczekaj E, Hertel J. A systematic review of prophylactic braces in the prevention of knee ligament injuries in collegiate football players. *J Athl Train.* 2008;43:409-415

46. Franz JO, McCulloch PC, Kneip CJ, Noble PC, Lintner DM. The utility of the KJOC score in professional baseball in the United States. *Am J Sports Med.* 2013;41:2167-2173

47. Leggin BG, Michener LA, Shaffer MA, et al. The Penn shoulder score: reliability and validity. *J Orthop Sports Phys Ther.* 2006;36:138-151

48. Gabel CP, Melloh M, Burkett B, Michener LA. Lower limb functional index: development and clinometric properties. *Phys Ther.* 2012;92:98-110

49. Gorman PP, Butler RJ, Plisky PJ, Kiesel KB. Upper quarter Y balance test: reliability and performance comparison between genders in active adults. *J Strength Cond Res.* 2012;26:3043-3048

50. Faigenbaum AD, Myer GD, Fernandez IP, et al. Feasibility and reliability of dynamic postural control measures in children in first through fifth grades. *Int J Sports Phys Ther.* 2014;9:140-148

Adolesc Med 026 (2015) 116–142

The Female Athlete Triad: Energy Deficiency, Physiologic Consequences, and Treatment

Albert C. Hergenroeder, MD[a]*; Mary Jane De Souza, PhD[b], Roberta H. Anding, MS, RD/LD, CDE, CSSD[a]

[a]*Baylor College of Medicine, Texas Children's Hospital, Department of Pediatrics, Section of Adolescent Medicine and Sports Medicine, Houston, Texas;*
[b]*The Pennsylvania State University, University Park, Pennsylvania*

INTRODUCTION

Historically, opportunities for women to engage in physical activity increased dramatically with the passing of Title IX. The increased participation of young girls and women in sport and exercise has been associated with recognition of the benefits of exercise for cardiovascular, nutritional, bone, and mental health.[1] However, in some young athletes the energy cost of exercise exceeds their energy intake, resulting in an energy deficit. This chronic energy deficit can have adverse health consequences. This article describes how chronic energy deficiency manifests as menstrual dysfunction and low bone mass, referred to as the *female athlete triad*. After reading this article, the reader should be able to describe the physiology of the female athlete triad, recognize its clinical manifestations, and recommend a treatment plan to address it.

DEFINITION OF THE FEMALE ATHLETE TRIAD

Numerous studies in the late 1970s and early 1980s confirmed the health consequences of chronic energy deficiency, ie, low bone mass and stress fractures in some female athletes.[2-4] Those reports focused primarily on the observance of amenorrhea and delayed menarche in long-distance runners[4] and ballet dancers.[5,6] An authoritative review by Loucks and Horvath[7] in 1985 helped highlight the importance of exercise-associated menstrual disturbances as a focal area of research and synthesized the available information on the potential causes of

---

*Corresponding author
E-mail address:* alberth@bcm.edu

reproductive disturbances in exercising women. Researchers focused attention on the potential contributions of body composition, eating habits and behaviors, training regimens, diet, and physical and psychological issues as causative factors of these exercise-associated menstrual disturbances. Shortly thereafter, a group of researchers brought together by the American College of Sports Medicine (ACSM) in 1992 named and defined the female athlete triad as a condition comprising disordered eating (DE), amenorrhea, and low bone mass.[8]

The first Position Stand on the Female Athlete Triad was published in 1997 by the ACSM.[9] In that original presentation, the triad was defined as proposed by Yeager et al[8] in 1993; that is, the triad was defined as a medical condition consisting of clinical endpoints of DE, amenorrhea, and osteoporosis. In 2007, the development of a new model for understanding the female athlete triad emerged as result of many lessons learned from several decades of research that greatly advanced our understanding of the condition.[10] The new triad model published in 2007 established that the components of the female athlete triad were known to be interrelated because energy deficiency associated with DE played a causal role in the development of menstrual disturbances[11-13] and that both energy deficiency and a low estrogen environment associated with amenorrhea played a causal role in initiating bone loss in these athletes.[14-16]

In the new triad model, these interrelationships were reaffirmed.[10] However, each component of the female athlete triad is represented along a health continuum of severity ranging from a healthy status to an unhealthy clinically significant status. At the *healthy* end of the continuum of the triad, the components include optimal energy availability, the presence of normal ovulatory menstrual cycles, and optimal bone health.[10] At the *unhealthy* clinically significant end of the continuum of the triad, each component is defined by clinically significant outcomes, including low energy availability with or without DE, functional hypothalamic amenorrhea (FHA), and osteoporosis.[10]

Important new features of the 2007 triad model highlight the fact that many athletes may not present with the severe clinically significant outcomes of the triad.[10] Indeed, athletes may display intermediate, or subclinical, presentations of 1 or more of the conditions of the triad, and, most importantly, progression along the 3 continuums can occur at different rates. The subclinical conditions include mild to moderate degrees of low energy availability with or without DE, subtle menstrual disturbances such as luteal phase defects and anovulatory menstrual cycles, and mild to moderate degrees of bone loss. For example, an athlete may show signs of restrictive eating but may not meet the clinical criteria for an eating disorder. She also may display subtle menstrual disturbances, such as a change in menstrual cycle length, anovulation, or luteal phase defects, but may not yet have developed amenorrhea. Likewise, she may be losing bone mass but may not yet have dropped below her age-matched normal range for bone mineral density (BMD). Although the conditions represented by each continuum can present independent of the other 2, it is more likely that, because of the clear associations among the 3 conditions, an athlete suffering from 1 element of the female athlete triad is also suffering from the others, even if only in a subclinical manner. Thus, it is important to understand that an athlete may present at different stages on each continuum and has the capacity to change stages on each continuum at varying rates. For example, changes can occur daily when considering energy status, monthly when considering the time course necessary for energetic changes to affect menstrual function, and annually when considering the time course necessary for energetic and menstrual changes to affect bone health.[10]

EPIDEMIOLOGY

The highest prevalence of amenorrhea in athletes is observed in sports that emphasize leanness, such as figure skating, ballet, long-distance running, and gymnastics, but investigators have observed menstrual abnormalities in a wide variety of other sports.[3,4,7,17-19] The prevalence of amenorrhea has been reported to range from 6% to 43% in runners[3,4,17,20-22] and as high as 69% in ballet dancers.[23]

Based on a recent systematic review of observational studies and cross-sectional studies that included 10,498 participants with a mean age of 21.8 ± 3.5 year and a mean body mass index of 20.8 ± 2.6 kg/m², the presence of all 3 components of the Triad ranged from 0% to 16% in primarily older adolescent and young adult athletes.[24] The prevalence of having any 2 of the components was estimated to range from 2.7% to 27% and of having 1 of the components ranged from 16% to 60%.[24] When the athletes were grouped as lean sport athletes, a higher prevalence of the combination of menstrual disturbances and low BMD (3.3% vs 1.0%), menstrual disturbances and DE (6.8%-57.8% vs 5.4%-13.5%), and low BMD and DE (5.6% vs 1.0%) was observed when compared to the non-lean sport athletes.[24]

In high school female athletes, the full triad, which is the simultaneous observance of all 3 components, occurs at a rate of 1% to 1.2%.[25,26] However, when individual components are evaluated, higher prevalence rates are observed. For example, bone loss was reported at a rate of 16% to 21%, menstrual disturbance 24% to 54%, and DE 4% to 18%.[26] Twenty-three percent had none of the components of the triad.[25] Consequently, the problems discussed in this article will be commonly encountered by pediatricians who care for high school female athletes.

PHYSIOLOGY OF ENERGY DEFICIENCY AND THE HYPOTHALAMIC-PITUITARY-OVARIAN AXIS

Research to date has established that the primary etiology of triad-related clinical sequelae is chronic energy deficiency.[12,13,27] The energy deficiency is a product of the athlete failing to consume an adequate volume of calories to meet the total cost of energy expenditure, which, of course, includes exercise energy expenditure.[10] In the triad position stand, the concept of low energy availability is presented as a causal factor for triad clinical outcomes and is represented by energy intake minus the amount of calories used for all energetic processes except exercise energy expenditure.[10]

In all mammals during conditions of low energy availability, the body repartitions energy away from reproduction and growth and toward other life-sustaining processes such as thermoregulation, cell maintenance, immunity, and locomotion to meet total energy demands.[28] Thus, in female athletes who fail to consume adequate volumes of energy to support their total expenditure needs, a repartitioning of energetic fuels is observed.[10] This repartitioning of energy away from growth and reproduction is associated with menstrual disturbances and bone loss.[10,15] Notably, the reliance of reproductive function on energy availability is also observed in nonathletic, non-Westernized women who experience seasonal food availability and high energy expenditures during harvesting of food and in whom reproductive suppression is also observed.[29-31] Energy deficiency in these cases occurs because of low energy availability, which results from limited food resources, and high energy expenditure because of work in the fields or travel between remote locations.[29,30] Irrespective of the cause of the energy deficiency, a low energy availability persists and a relative chronic energy drain is observed. The concept of a chronic energy drain was first reported by Michelle Warren[6] in 1980, and its relationship to menstrual disturbances has been noted since then.

Low energy availability and energy deficiency are associated with a series of metabolic adjustments that help to support the conservation of energy (ie, energetic fuel). The metabolic adjustments to low energy availability and energy conservation include decreased resting energy expenditure (REE); suppressed triiodothyronine (TT_3), insulinlike growth factor-1 (IGF-1) and leptin concentrations; and elevated reverse TT_3, ghrelin, peptide YY, and cortisol concentrations.[32-37] Suppression of REE and TT_3 has been well documented in amenorrheic, exercising women with low energy availability and energy deficiency.[14,34,38,39] In a series of well-controlled experiments, Dr Anne Loucks[12,16,40,41] documented that low energy availability is associated with suppressed TT_3 and IGF-1, and with decreased luteinizing hormone (LH) pulsatility, used as a proxy marker of reproductive function. The experiments by Dr Loucks also demonstrated that markers of bone formation were suppressed, and that increased bone resorption was observed when estradiol was suppressed by low energy availability.[16]

A causal relationship between low energy availability and menstrual cyclicity was convincingly provided by the exercise training studies of Dr Nancy Williams et al.[13,42] Those investigators demonstrated that amenorrhea could be induced in monkeys during exercise training when energy intake was restricted, and that amenorrhea could be reversed by increasing food intake without any moderation of daily exercise training. The work by Dr Williams highlights the finding that resumption of ovulatory cycles in monkeys was dose dependent such that the monkeys that increased food intake the most, recovered ovulatory function in the shortest period of time.[13] A key marker of energy balance, total TT_3, was significantly related to both the induction and the reversal of amenorrhea, thus providing additional evidence supporting the energy availability hypothesis.[13,42]

Additional evidence for the relationship between energy deficiency and energy-related menstrual disturbances comes from the results of cross-sectional studies in exercising women with subtle menstrual disturbances. De Souza et al[34,35,43] provided evidence that subtle menstrual disturbances such as luteal phase defects and anovulation in exercising women are associated with similar metabolic adjustments that are observed in amenorrheic exercising women, albeit less severe but, nonetheless, similar.

Chronic energy deficiency often is not reliably indicated by low body weight, nor is energy balance indicated by stable body weight.[44] Energy-conserving metabolic adaptations that act to reduce energy expenditure and body weight can, in some cases, result in maintenance of weight, although at a lower weight, thus presenting as restoration of energy balance despite ongoing underlying chronic alterations that indicate a metabolic and endocrine environment characteristic of energy conservation.[44] In our laboratory, we have successfully used the ratio of REE (as measured in the laboratory) to the Harris-Benedict[45] predicted REE (measured REE/predicted REE) to predict the presence of an energy deficiency[11,14,34] The Harris-Benedict equation[45] has been used to predict REE in many published reports[46-48] of REE in underweight women; therefore, we decided that this equation was likely to be useful for our purposes. Furthermore, a reduced ratio of measured REE to predicted REE by the Harris-Benedict equation[45] is often in the range from 60% to 80% in clinical models of starvation, such as anorexia nervosa (AN).[46-48] Consequently, among exercising women, we operationally defined energy deficiency as a ratio of measured REE to predicted REE that is less than 90%; on the other hand, energy replete was defined as a ratio of measured REE to predicted REE that is greater than 90%.[11,14,34] This strategy not only has been used in several published articles but also has been corroborated by alterations in concentrations of metabolic hormones (TT_3 and ghrelin) that are indicative of an energy deficiency state.[11,14,34]

BONE ACCUMULATION AND LOSS ACROSS THE LIFESPAN

The skeleton consists of 2 types of bone: cortical and trabecular (or cancellous) bone. Vertebral bodies (the femoral neck and the distal radius), which are common sites of osteoporotic fracture, are composed primarily of cancellous bone.[49] The accumulation of cortical bone occurs from conception through the third decade of life, with a marked rise during puberty.[50] The peak in trabecular mass may be achieved during the second decade, especially in the femoral neck, with some later accrual in the lumbar spine.[50-52] Between the ages of 12 and 16 years, women may accrue 40% of their adult skeleton or bone mass.[53] The percentiles of individuals' femoral neck volume and bone mineral content (BMC) in the 5%, 50%, or 95% of the population distribution during adulthood are established at some time during pubertal growth. Periosteal apposition during growth is the main determinant of bone size throughout life and an important determinant of bone mass and volumetric BMD in old age.[54]

That most bone mass is acquired by the end of the second decade of life underscores the importance of maximizing those environmental factors (eg, exercise, nutrition, and hormonal status) that will facilitate achievement of a woman's genetically endowed peak bone mass.

As healthy women age beyond the third decade, osteoblastic activity, or bone formation, begins to lag behind osteoclastic activity, or bone resorption, and net bone loss occurs.[55] Cross-sectional measurements of lumbar spine BMD of women aged 20 to 90 years showed a 1% loss of BMD per year of age starting early in the third decade. Because some women may not achieve their genetically endowed bone mass potential during adolescence as a consequence of inadequate exercise, energy availability, or estrogen status, osteoporosis has its origins in adolescence. Osteoporosis is a disease characterized by reduced bone mass and increased bone fragility.[56,57] Of the 25 million Americans who are at high risk for osteoporosis, an estimated 85% are women.[58] On average, post-hip fracture women died 4 years earlier than expected.[59] Estimated medical expenditures for treatment of osteoporosis in the United States were $13.8 billion in 1995 and are expected to be $25 billion by 2025.[60-63] The attendant mortality, morbidity, and financial effect of osteoporosis make this disease a major public health problem that will increase in significance as the number of Americans older than 85 years is expected to be 20 million by 2040.[64]

Peak bone mass is determined by genetics, puberty, nutritional factors, exercise, and hormonal status. Each of these determinants will be discussed here, with a focus on the role of estrogen in bone health.

Genetics

Genetics accounts for the largest variance in peak bone mass. Estimates of the genetic contributions to bone mass vary by axial and appendicular skeleton sites and the measurement being reported, and have been reported to account for 34% to 75% of the variance in bone mass.[65-71]

Puberty

Bone mass increases during childhood and adolescence through a combination of increases in bone length, bone diameter, and thickness and density of cortical bone.[72] Cortical bone constitutes approximately 80% of the skeletal mass and trabecular bone approximately 20%.[73] Bone turnover and remodeling are accelerated during the premenarchal years,[74] and accelerated bone mineralization, especially of trabecular bone in the lumbar spine and femoral neck, occurs during puberty. Furthermore, there is regionalization of bone development, such that the growth velocity of the femur peaks around 21 months before menarche, the humerus and tibia peak 18 months before menarche, and the radius and trunk attain peak growth velocity at 17 months and 12 months before menarche, respectively. Attainment of peak bone mass occurs postpuberty, as demonstrated in the femoral neck, which reaches peak bone mass by age 16 years.

Minimal increase of BMD occurs beyond 2 years postmenarche.[75] Most bone mass is acquired by the end of the second decade; however, most of the increase in bone size and density occurs relatively early in puberty.[50,75,76] A small fraction of bone mass accretion occurs in the third decade, and maximum cortical width may not be reached until the end of the third decade.[76-79] The total increase in whole-body bone mineral and half the increase in spine mineral during puberty are related to changes in bone size rather than to an increase in bone mineral per unit volume.[51]

Is Delayed Menarche a Factor in Bone Mass Acquisition that Carries into Adulthood?

The American Society of Reproductive Medicine defines a late age of menarche as menarche that occurs at age 15 years or later.[80] A later age of menarche at age 14 years versus menarche at age 12 years was associated with a detrimental effect on distal tibial microarchitecture in healthy 20-year-old women and premenopausal middle-aged women.[81] Age of menarche (mean 13.2 vs 12.2 years) was significantly related to lower lumbar spine BMD in a cross-section of exercising women (mean age 22 ± 0.5-years), 37 of whom were ovulatory and 45 amenorrheic.[82] Later menarche is a risk factor for stress fractures in military cadets and 17- to 26-year-old track and field athletes.[83,84] The age of menarche was inversely related to stiffness and failure load at the distal tibia and radius in female adolescents.[85] During puberty, the rise in estrogen concentration that accompanies menarche inhibits periosteal apposition of long bones and stimulates endosteal apposition.[81] Regarding the mechanism accounting for the association between later menarche, bone strength, and bone mass, later menarcheal age has been associated with a greater bone diameter leading to greater cross-sectional area but smaller cortical thickness.[86] However, it has been proposed that the effect of later menarche may differ in sedentary and exercising women because of the osteogenic nature of habitual weight-bearing physical activity.[82] Late menarche is reported to affect BMD independent of DE and menstrual irregularity.[87]

Nutritional Factors

Body Weight

Body weight is the single best predictor of BMD in populations of children and adolescents.[88] Body weight and pubertal stage are positively associated with BMD in adolescent females.[51,88-91] The effect of weight as a determinant of BMD may be tempered in mid to late puberty compared to early puberty.[51,91,92] Yet the association between body weight and bone mass is complicated and affected by body composition and sex steroid exposure. For example, total body and lumbar spine BMD are associated with lean body mass and estradiol concentrations in exercising women.[93,94] Weight as a marker of nutrition is a covariate in understanding the association of amenorrhea and reduced BMD.[95,96] The extremes of weight are harmful for bone health, that is, excessive leanness is a risk factor for osteoporosis,[97] and obesity may be a detriment for bone health development.[98]

Calcium and Vitamin D

ineralization requires optimal calcium intake through child-
e, and adulthood. Between 5% and 10% of the variance in peak
counted for by calcium intake. Therefore, girls and women
aged to consume the dietary reference intake of calcium.

mended daily intake of elemental calcium is 1300 mg, and the
y intake of vitamin D is 600 IU for 9- to 18-year-old girls and
ase in calcium intake to 1500 mg/day has been proposed for
and young adults with amenorrhea.[89,100-102] However, in adolescent girls with AN, increased calcium intake without increased body weight may not improve BMD because of increased excretion and decreased absorption of calcium.[97] Most adolescent girls and women consume less than the recommended daily requirement for calcium.[102,103]

Exercise

As physical activity in children and adolescents increases, so does bone strength.[1] The converse also holds true: low levels of physical activity are associated with poor bone strength.[104] In the Iowa Bone Development Study, 185 boys and 148 girls had 3 BMC measurements at 5, 8, and 11 years of age and wore activity monitors for 4 days. Adjusting for age, height, weight, somatic maturity, and moderate to vigorous physical activity (MVPA), MVPA at age 5 years predicted BMC at ages 8 and 11 years.[105] Leisure time sports was associated with bone accrual in children older than 2 years, with a greater effect seen in boys.[106] Mechanical loading increases bone accretion.[107-109]

Weight-bearing exercise favors bone formation.[110] The impact load on bone with walking and running is 2 to 5 times body weight and is up to 12 times body weight in jumping and landing, as occurs in gymnastics.[111] Gymnasts tend to have higher BMD than non-gymnasts, with the greatest difference seen in the upper extremities.[112] However, exercise to the point at which menstrual disturbances occur, such as amenorrhea, anovulation, or luteal phase inadequacy, reverses the beneficial effect of exercise on BMD, and bone loss may result.[85,95,113-116]

Bone mass and size of retired gymnasts were greater than in age-matched controls unless the former had amenorrhea, in which case there was no difference compared with controls.[117] The problem is not the exercise per se but the inability to compensate for the high energy expenditure with adequate calories, thereby resulting in low energy availability, therein the genesis of the female athlete triad.

Does Exercise During Adolescence and Early Adulthood Provide Lasting Benefit?

Elite runners and tennis players from 1950 to 1977, currently 40 to 65 years of age, had higher spine and hip BMD compared to an inactive control group, controlling for age, height, weight, and smoking status.[118] What is unknown about this study is the prevalence of menstrual disturbances related to training requirements during their training years. In 105 retired dancers in the Australian Ballet (mean age 51 ± 14 years), there was no overall difference between the hip and spine compared to controls matched for age, menopausal status, height, and weight.[119] Cigarette smoking, associated with lower BMD, was more common in the dancers. Those dancers with a history of 5 or fewer periods per year during dance had a lower spine (8%) and radius (10%) BMD but not at the hip. Retired elite ballet dancers (mean age 51 years) had similar BMD at weight-bearing sites compared to aged-matched controls, even though they continued to exercise twice as much as the controls. However, those with a history of 5 or fewer menstrual cycles per year during the dance years had lower radial (10%) and spinal (8%) BMD compared to matched controls.[119] It seems that the benefits of improved bone mass with weight-bearing exercise are trumped by the hypoestrogenemia associated with chronic energy drain and the associated amenorrhea/oligomenorrhea.

Bone Strength

Bone strength is related to bone geometry, that is, the size of bone plays an important role in the strength of bone such that a larger bone typically is a stronger bone.[70] Although BMD accounts for a significant proportion of bone strength, changes in material composition and geometry can offset the effects of low bone mass.[73] Bone mineral density, represented in the units gm/cm^2 obtained from dual energy x-ray absorptiometry (DXA) measurements, is a 2-dimensional estimate of BMD based on the projected area in the coronal plane of the bone being measured, but it does not account for bone depth. Bone mineral density is a surrogate for, but not necessarily a measure of, bone strength.[120] This is reflected in the 2014 Consensus Statement for Return to Play for the Female Athlete Triad,[121] which states that the decision to treat or not treat with pharmacologic therapies does not depend on BMD Z-scores alone but also on additional risk factors such as fracture history, genetics, cumulative triad risk factors, which have been associated with an increased risk for low BMD and bone stress injury, and the rate of bone loss with non-pharmacologic treatment.[121] Black women have greater and Asian women lower or comparable BMD compared with non-Hispanic white women, yet the former 2 groups have osteoporotic hip fracture rates that are one-half to one-third that of the latter.[69] Bone strength in female runners is related to bone size more than BMD, as the bending strength of bone increases exponentially with bone surface area and distance from the center.[122]

Most clinical fractures are a result of compression, bending, and torsion. In the latter 2, the cross-sectional area of a structure is more important in resisting loads than is its mass or density.[64] As the diameter of bone is increased, less material (ie, density) is needed for the same bending stiffness. At weight-bearing sites, female athletes tend to have larger bone diameters compared to sedentary controls, and greater bone strength as a result of increased trabecular area and lower cortical bone density because of delayed mineralization of expanding bone.[123]

What Are the Short-Term Injury Implications of Menstrual Disorders on Bone Health?

Odds ratios for low BMD in young girls with fractures of the femur, radius, and spine range were 2.0, 2.2, and 2.6, respectively, compared to age-matched girls who had no fractures in these bones.[124] Bone mass density is reduced and stress fractures are increased in athletes with secondary amenorrhea.[125] The relationship between excess exercise, amenorrhea, and injury has been confirmed in adolescent females. Menstrual status is an important marker of BMD in patients with and without identified eating disorders, and those with amenorrhea and oligomenorrhea have risk of lower BMD.[93,96,121,126-130]

In a prospective study of high school female athletes, musculoskeletal injury, including stress fractures, was associated with the female athlete triad.[26] The population at risk increases when considering not just those young women with the full female athlete triad but also women with components of the triad. One report suggests that most young athletes have at least 1 component of the triad.[25] High school athletes with DE were twice as likely to sustain an injury, and those with menstrual irregularity had more severe injuries.[87]

Stress fractures among preadolescent and adolescent girls are associated with leanness sports (eg, gymnastics, running track, and cheerleading) and menstrual dysfunction.[131] Fractures have been correlated with decreased bone mass gain during puberty in girls. In a prospective study of female runners, a previous stress fracture was associated with a 6-fold increase in the risk of a stress fracture over 1 year.[132] In that report, menarche at age older than 15 years, BMI less than 19, and previous participation in dance or gymnastics each increased the risk of a stress fracture between 2 to 3 times compared to those without a stress fracture. However, when all 4 factors (BMI <19, menarche >15 years, previous participation in dance or gymnastics, and previous stress fracture) were present, the risk of stress fracture increased 100-fold.

Medium-Term Bone Mass Outcomes and Menstrual Disturbance

Former gymnasts who were amenorrheic and oligomenorrheic during their athletic careers had lumbar spine BMD values that were 84% and 94% of the lumbar spine BMD of gymnasts who had always been eumenorrheic.[61] This was despite several years of oral contraceptive use or regular menses during baseline (age 31 years) or at follow-up 8 years later. Eighty-seven percent of female runners (mean age 18.7 years at 3-year follow-up) who had low bone mass for chronologic age at 15 years still had it at 3-year follow up. Thus, short-term bone losses persist for those with the female athlete triad. Those likely to improve reduced their training volume and increased their fat and lean mass.[133]

Long-Term Bone Health and the Female Athlete Triad

In healthy young adults, bone formation and bone resorption are tightly coupled in bone forming units or bone metabolic units.[73,134] When they are uncoupled and bone formation lags behind bone resorption, bone loss occurs.[55] Bone loss results from disturbances of bone remodeling, which is a continuous process of maintaining the integrity of the boney skeleton.[135] The annual rates of cancellous and cortical bone turnover are estimated to be 25% and 2% to 3%, respectively, in adults. Estrogen deficiency is associated with the uncoupling of bone resorption and formation within a bone remodeling unit. When bone resorption exceeds bone formation, as in estrogen deficiency, the cavities created by bone osteoclasts are not replaced, resulting in thinning of more widely spaced trabeculae, and eventually can lead to perforation of trabeculae.[135] The resultant bone microarchitecture impairment has been recognized in amenorrheic adolescent athletes.[85,123]

Most bone mass is accumulated by the end of adolescence. Disordered eating and eating disorders result in low energy availability and interfere with normal bone acquisition, which can lead to permanent deficits.[87] Cognitive dietary restraint (CDR) refers to the chronic effort to achieve or sustain a desired body weight by consciously restricting food intake and is described as DE.[136] Mean BMD and Z-scores were significantly lower for the total body and the lumbar spine in the 18- to 35-year-old females with high CDR than in those with normal CDR scores. Oligomenorrhea was higher in the women with high CDR compared to those with normal CDR scores. Adolescents with DE are greater risk for the development of osteopenia and osteoporosis. DE was associated with a fracture risk in adulthood that is 2 to 7 times higher than that in adolescents without an eating disorder, especially for non-spine fractures. We are aware that eating disorders and DE are not synonymous, however, there is a continuum between the components of the female athlete triad and diagnosable eating disorders, and much of the literature regarding poor outcomes for bone health refer to patients with identified eating disorders.

In the context of bone health and the female athlete triad, a problem is that within 1 year of the diagnosis of AN it is reported that half of anorexia nervosa patients with osteopenia had been diagnosed with AN within the past year, suggesting that either the onset of bone loss occurs early in the disease process or the disease had existed undetected for some time.[129]

Bone fragility is a function of growth- and age-related factors that influence skeletal size, architecture, and mass.[137] Peak bone mass, most of which is acquired by the end of the second decade, is a major determinant of osteoporosis.[50,75] The risk of osteoporosis in the postmenopausal period is related to the peak bone mass achieved and the rate of postmenopausal bone loss. The disease may have its onset in adolescence if the genetic potential of peak bone mass is not achieved during the second decade.[50,62,75] Conditions that interfere with the pubertal process of bone accrual, such as prolonged energy deficiency and the associated menstrual abnormalities, are likely to increase the risk of osteoporosis in adulthood. These conditions may manifest either as a clinical eating disorder or as the less severe subclinical DE; however, both of these may be observed in female athletes and are associated with low bone mass and hypoestrogenia.[87,127,133,138] Notably, these unhealthy eating behaviors and reduced bone mass may persist long term.

TREATMENT

The treatment approach that we endorse assumes that other primary medical causes of menstrual disturbances and chronic energy deficiency have been ruled out. Such an evaluation is not discussed in this article. The treatment approach is crucial here and is consistent with the Female Athlete Triad Coalition Consensus Paper published in 2014.[121] It is directed toward restoring positive energy balance by reducing energy expenditure and increasing energy intake, and in doing so reproductive function can be restored and bone mass improved. This approach is supported by more than 30 years of research.[14,121,127,139-142] For example, reduced training, increased caloric intake, and weight gain are associated with return of spontaneous menses in runners, and spontaneous return of menses is associated with improved BMD.[127] Female runners who did not reduce their running mileage showed no significant change in estrogen levels or BMD, whereas those who reduced their weekly mileage by 43% increased their body weight 5%, resumed their menses, increased their estrogen levels, and increased their BMD.[140] Catch-up in bone mass in adolescent female runners was associated with reducing training volume and increasing lean and fat mass.[133] Recovery of BMD in patients with AN is most significantly related to weight gain and resumption of menses.[126]

In our experience, at the time of presentation to the physician, some patients with female athlete triad have a diagnosable eating disorder; however, many do not meet all the criteria for an eating disorder and present with other components of the female athlete triad that place them at risk for bone loss. Disordered eating, for example, is associated with low BMD even in the absence of menstrual irregularity in young female runners.[20] The physician will also often be confronted with the patient with 1 or more components of the female athlete triad. Using screening tools to identify athletes with eating disorders versus DE may have a role in research projects, yet considering the heterogeneity of eating disorders and DE, clinical expertise is required to rule in or out an eating disorder in individual patients. For example, it was reported that body weight was higher in a group of older adolescent/young adult runners with higher eating disorder scores (indicating more eating disorder pathology) than in a group of patients with normal eating disorder scores.[20] Yet patients with bulimia nervosa often have normal weight, so lumping all eating disorders together is simplistic. The diagnosis of an eating disorder may take several clinic visits.

It is in this context that a team approach is necessary in the diagnosis and management of the female athlete triad. The members of the multidisciplinary team should include a primary care or sports medicine physician, a sports dietitian, and mental health practitioner.[121] Depending on the individual patient's needs, other members of the team may include a consultation from an adolescent medicine specialist, endocrinologist, orthopedic surgeon, psychiatrist, exercise physiologist, certified athletic trainer, family members who provide feedback, or a coach.[121] We begin with medical nutritional therapy.

Medical Nutritional Therapy

Central to the development of the female athlete triad is low energy availability or underfueling. Although menstrual dysfunction and bone stress injuries are the identifiable endpoints, it is the low energy availability relative to exercise and training that is the central etiology. It is important to identify high-risk sports, the energy consumed, the amount used in physical activity, and the determination of energy and protein needs. The physician may not have the time or the availability of an experienced sports dietitian to conduct a comprehensive nutrition assessment. Therefore, this section is intended to be a practical guide to assist in identifying the high-risk female athlete and provide the athlete with practical strategies for improving her health and performance.

The identification of high-risk athletes can be considered an initial screening. In a study by Torstveit and Sundogt-Borgen,[143] 669 athletes were screened for the female athlete triad, and more than 70% were in sports that emphasized leanness. Leanness is emphasized in distance running, dance, cheerleading, and gymnastics, but energy drain can occur in any sport. Other warning signs include recent restrictive dietary patterns, fatigue during performance, recent weight loss, and declining performance.

Diets that have become exclusive or limiting may indicate a restrictive eating pattern. This includes gluten restriction in the absence of celiac disease or gluten sensitivity, recent vegetarianism or veganism, fat-free diet, or even popular restrictive diet plans such as a detoxification diet or the Paleo diet. In addition to reducing total calories, restrictive dietary patterns may contribute to the development of stress fractures. Although not all studies support the role of calcium in the prevention of stress fractures, low-fat dairy products rich in calcium, potassium, and vitamin D have been linked with an improvement in BMD in female distance runners.[144] Vegan diets by definition eliminate dairy products, and vegans are at risk for low intake of calcium and vitamin D.[145]

It is important to determine meal frequency, barriers to consuming adequate amounts of food, such as an early morning practice, finances, and religious, traditional, and acceptable solutions to the energy deficits. Diet histories are deceptive because the athlete often seems to be making healthy choices but the amount of energy is insufficient to support normal physiologic function or athletic performance. Athletes may complain of declining performance with their healthy diet choices despite increases in training. Orthorexia is often considered a form of DE. It often manifests as an athlete who wants to eat perfectly and often is fearful of eating foods away from home because of unknown food preparation techniques. It also is possible that the athlete is not forthright about her dietary intake or patterns.[146]

Estimates of Energy Needs

Adequate energy availability to support sport and normal physiologic function is 45 kcal/kg fat-free mass (FFM).[147] Inadequate intake is considered to be less than 30 kcal/kg FFM. In order to use this formula, 2 key elements must be determined: FFM and calorie intake. An accurate accounting of usual intake using 3-day food records must be obtained and energy intake calculated. Athletes must be instructed on portion sizes and strategies to estimate intake. Food models can be useful in this assessment. In addition, use of the metabolic costs of certain exercise (METS) can be used to estimate the calories expended in physical activity. Ainsworth et al[148] have reported such activities and MET values.

Determination of FFM can be calculated by DXA while obtaining BMD, or by air displacement plethysmography, calipers, or bioelectrical impedance in a well-hydrated athlete.[149] These methods are the standards for determining body composition and energy need. Body mass index (body weight/height <17.5 kg/m^2 or weight $<85\%$ of estimated ideal body weight [IBW], see estimate of IBW following)[150] or rapid recent weight loss in the absence of injury or illness in an adolescent can be used to alert the physician to the likelihood of under-fueling. However, neither of these calculations is predictive of under-fueling in the female athlete who is also engaged in a regular moderate-intensity strength training program. Conversely, the under-fueled athlete will often experience a down regulation of metabolic rate to compensate for chronic/acute reduction in calories. In a clinical setting this can be manifest by bradycardia, hypothermia, and postural orthostatic tachycardia syndrome. Although the magnitude of energy reduction is difficult to determine for an individual, a 10% reduction in weight is consistent with excess weight loss in a previously healthy athlete.[151]

The end or slowing of growth and development can be determined by a number of methods, including review of the height and weight growth charts and assessment of the stage of pubertal maturation or Tanner stage.[152] Female athletes who are Tanner stage 5 have completed their growth and development regardless of chronologic age. As such, adult prediction estimates of energy need can be used. The Hamwi equation is the best known, using an estimate of IBW.[150] Estimated IBW is calculated by allowing 100 pounds for the first 5 feet of height and an additional 5 pounds for each inch in height above 5 feet. Using this method, the estimated IBW for a female who is 5 feet 4 inches is 100 pounds + (5 pounds/inch × 4 inches) = 120 pounds. The IBW in pounds is multiplied by 10 to give an estimate of calories for that person's basal metabolic rate. The basal metabolic rate is what an individual needs just to accommodate basal needs (eg, lying in bed with no activity). If the athlete is in season and is working out daily, using IBW × 20 will give an estimate of total daily calorie needs for an active individual. Therefore, the same athlete discussed earlier would need 2400 calories per day as a reference point (120 × 20 = 2400) This is a simple equation designed to provide a quick estimate and is not as accurate as using energy availability by FFM measurement, but it is inherently more practical.

For younger athletes (ie, still in puberty), prediction equations of energy need are available for adolescents. Although they are not specifically designed for athletes, they can be adjusted based on current level of activity. Most female athletes need an activity factor of active or very active. The benefit of using this formula is the online version of this equation available at http://fnic.nal.usda.gov/fnic/interactiveDRI/. Using the calorie calculation in Table 1 for an active athlete who is 5 feet 4 inches, weighs 125 pounds, and is 15 years old, the estimate of daily energy needs is 2437. Given the complexity of this equation, the Hamwi equation is a close approximation for physicians regardless of the age of the athlete.[150]

Table 1
Institute of Medicine, Food and Nutrition Board, and National Academy of Sciences Daily Reference Intakes for Energy for Children and Adolescents

Females	
Age 9-18 years	$EER^{(1)} = 135.3 - (30.8 \times age \, [years]) + PA \times [(10.0 \times weight \, [kg]) + (934 \times height \, [m])] + 25$
	$PA^{(2)} = 1.00 = Sedentary$
	$1.16 = Low \, active$
	$1.31 = Active$
	$1.56 = Very \, active$

[1] Estimated Energy Requirement
[2] Physical Activity

From *Dietary Reference Intakes for Energy, Carbohydrate, Fiber, Fat, Fatty Acids, Cholesterol, Protein, and Amino Acids (Macronutrients).* Washington, DC: The National Academies Press; 2005: 182. Available at: fnic.nal.usda.gov/dietary-guidance/dri-nutrient-reports/energy-carbohydrate-fiber-fat-fatty-acids-cholesterol-protein. Accessed March 13, 2015.

Protein Needs

In the absence of adequate calories, protein can become a source of energy via gluconeogenesis. The energy restrictive female athlete may have lost lean muscle weight in addition to body fat, which can contribute to a decline in performance.[153] Sports nutrition guidelines indicate that adolescent athletes need more protein than their nonathletic counterparts.[154] Adult protein needs for athletes are estimated to be 1.2 to 1.7 g/kg body weight across all sports. Although estimates of protein needs in the adolescent female are lacking in the literature, an average of 1.5 g/kg is a reasonable goal.[155] Others have estimated the protein need of the energy restricted athlete to be 1.6 to 2 g/kg.[156] Although this estimate is for the adult population, it is practical to estimate a protein need between 1.5 and 2 g/kg for rebuilding lean mass lost. In the past 5 years there has an increased interest in branch chain amino acids, specifically leucine and its unique ability to stimulate muscle protein synthesis.[156] Animal proteins, particularly whey protein, are rich in leucine, whereas plant-based proteins can have significantly less leucine.[156] The increased amount of protein needed and the need for adequate leucine may pose a dilemma for vegetarian or vegan athletes.[157] These diets are best planned by a dietitian with experience in vegetarian diets for sports, such as a Certified Specialist in Sports Dietetics (CSSD).

Case Example

The following case demonstrates how a treatment plan could be initiated in the primary care physician's office if a multidisciplinary team is not immediately available.

Kelly is an 18-year-old elite female distance runner. She is 5 foot 4 inches tall and weighs 98 pounds. She presents with hypothermia, bradycardia, and postural orthostatic tachycardia syndrome. She is Tanner stage 5. She is vegetarian and eats "very well," consuming lots of fruits and vegetable and all organic foods. Menarche began at age 15 years, and her last menstrual period was 12 months ago. Other causes of her secondary amenorrhea have been ruled out. Her estimated daily calorie intake is approximately 1500 calories.

Calculation of Estimated IBW
Because Kelly is an adult, her calorie needs can be estimated by multiplying her estimated IBW × 20, where IBW = 100 pounds for the first 5 feet of height and 5 pounds for each inch afterward. For Kelly, IBW = 100 + (5 × 4) = 100 + 20 = 120 pounds. Her estimated % IBW is 98/120 = 82%.

Because Kelly is physically active, her estimated daily calorie needs are 120 × 20 = 2400 calories. She is hypothermic and bradycardic, which represent a hypometabolic state as a result of under-fueling. This condition will need to be considered as her weight is being monitored.

We would suggest that Kelly add between 200 to 600 calories to her daily intake, which is consistent with the 2014 consensus statement.[121] A gradual increase in energy intake also is recommended to prevent overfeeding, which can lead to physical and psychological problems with the increased energy intake prescription. Simple approximately 500-calorie additions include ¾ cup of nuts, 12 ounces of juice, and an energy bar (sports bar such as Powerbar, Gatorade bar), or a peanut butter and jelly sandwich and 8 ounces of soy milk. Energy-dense, low-volume foods, such as nuts, dried fruit, and shelf-stable fortified milk products, can be used to reduce intestinal discomfort and provide portable snacks that are convenient to bring to practice or to carry throughout the day for a student athlete. If intestinal discomfort limits intake, spreading intake throughout the day via frequent meals and snacks is advisable. Gradual increase in energy intake is also recommended to prevent overfeeding.

In addition, we would recommend that Kelly reduce her training volume by 25%, for example, reduce her running mileage from 60 to 45 miles per week.

We would see her again in 1 to 2 weeks. If her weight and vital signs were improved, we would consider allowing her to increase her mileage incrementally while adding in the necessary calories to account for the increase mileage (100 calories/mile). Any measurable increase in weight (eg, 100 g) is deemed successful, and calories are adjusted to promote gradual consistent weight gain. We would then follow her every 1 to 2 weeks until her weight reached closer to 85% of estimated IBW and her vital signs continued to improve. If Kelly was unable to improve her weight and vital signs after the first visit or subsequently reversed progress after improvement, we would progressively increase the recommended daily calorie intake and reduce the calorie expenditure to the point of stopping running if necessary.

When to Involve a Mental Health Professional

A mental health professional is not required to be part of the initial treatment team if an eating disorder is not diagnosed. However, one should be consulted if an eating disorder is diagnosed or if the patient's medical condition does not progress, specifically, if weight and vital signs do not improve, suggesting that an eating disorder may be present. These initial follow-up visits should occur at 1- to 2-week intervals.

Beyond Exercise Restriction and Increased Energy Intake

The Female Athlete Triad Coalition 2014 Consensus Panel on the Female Athlete Triad emphasizes that non-pharmacologic treatment strategies should be prioritized, particularly focusing on achieving resumption of menses, given the importance of menses and normal estrogen status to bone health.[121] The improvement in menstrual function with strategies to improve energy availability can occur within several months but may take longer than 1 year.

This 2014 consensus statement also included the following qualifications. Weight gain alone will promote BMD improvement; however, normalization of BMD is unlikely to occur with weight gain alone, as reported by others, suggesting the need to address energy and estrogen-related mechanisms together.[14,127] Nutritional and hormonal recovery is recommended to improve mineralization of trabecular bone and growth of cortical bone, including that in women with the female athlete triad and eating disorders.[123,126,158]

Some expert opinions support a role for estrogen supplementation, which had demonstrated improved BMD in women with severe AN or with FHA.[141,159-161] The 2014 Consensus Statement on the Female Athlete Triad supports a role for treatment of athletes with a history of multiple fractures if there is a lack of response to non-pharmacologic therapy for at least 1 year and if new fractures occur during the non-pharmacologic management.[121] Lack of response to therapy was defined as a clinically significant (not defined) reduction in BMD Z-scores after 1 year of non-pharmacologic therapy or the occurrence of a clinically significant fracture during that year.[121] The consensus statement goes on to state "that prolonged non-pharmacologic therapy despite lack of response is of concern in younger athletes who are in the process of accruing peak bone mass because the adolescent and young adult years are critical windows in time during which they optimize bone accrual, and deficits incurred during this time may be irreversible. Furthermore, the threshold for pharmacologic treatment in the young athlete with low BMD, stress fractures, or impaired bone accrual is less clear." In the 2014 consensus statement and in the 2007 ACSM Triad Position Stand,[10] increases in BMD are associated with increases in weight and resumption of menses more so than administration of combined oral contraceptive (COC) to athletes with FHA. As such, non-pharmacologic treatments likely need to be implemented to optimize the effectiveness of treatment as the first step in a treatment plan.[139]

Mechanical loading contributes to the development of bone mass and geometry, and this adaptive response of bone to mechanical loading requires a functional estrogen receptor ER-α.[162] The relative contribution of ER-α polymorphism and physical activity to BMC depends on the level of physical activity and the region of the skeleton being studied, thus highlighting the complicated relationship between exercise, nutritional status, estrogen status, and genetics. Estrogen concentration is a strong predictor of lumbar spine BMD, as 70% of the lumbar spine is trabecular bone.[126] The presence of both energy deficiency and estrogen deficiency exacerbates alterations of bone metabolism in exercising women.[14] Estrogen modulates osteoclast resorptive activity so that the effect of estrogen deficiency is increased bone resorption.[163,164] Women with FHA experience increased bone resorption related to estrogen deficiency.[93]

The bulk of the evidence suggests that COC pill use alone does not improve BMD in patients with AN and in patients with FHA compared to subjects not treated with COC.[141,165-168] It has been suggested that the failure of oral contraceptive therapy to improve BMD may be related to the suppression of hepatic production of IGF-1 with oral estrogen administration.[126] Alternatively, the nutrition factors that are associated with return of menses are likely to be accompanied by an increase in bone-trophic hormones, such as IGF-1.

Estrogen supplementation in young females with FHA and eating disorders remains controversial, however. Estrogen/progestin supplementation is not recommended as a first-line treatment, yet its role as a later intervention is endorsed by expert opinion.[121,169] One consensus statement says that COC pills do not increase BMD in those with the female athlete triad, yet they endorse a role for estrogen as a later treatment. Others suggest that estrogen and progesterone therapy may be considered in women with AN who have low bone density and a clinically significant fracture history if weight gain strategies are not effective despite best efforts.[142] In addition, transdermal estrogen and cyclic progesterone may be considered when bone Z-scores are low and are decreasing over time (no interval given; however, the convention is to measure BMD annually) despite all efforts at weight gain, given the limited time during adolescence during which to optimize bone accrual and prevent irreversible bone deficits.

The guidelines regarding duration and mechanism of delivery (eg, oral or transdermal) are not provided. There have been and remain methodologic limitations to studies designed to determine the role of estrogen replacement in women with FHA, including high dropout rates. Those with the highest risk factors (ie, lowest weight and highest rate of menstrual irregularity) were the most likely to discontinue the oral contraceptives, making it difficult to conduct randomized controlled trials.[141] There are few data supporting guidelines for those younger than 18 years.

It is reported that contraceptive therapy creates an exogenous ovarian steroid environment that often provides a false sense of security for patients with amenorrhea when induced withdrawal bleeding occurs.[170] However, there is no evidence indicating that allowing these women to remain amenorrheic speeds the return of eventual spontaneous menses, and amenorrhea has been removed as a criterion for AN.[171] The 2014 Female Athlete Consensus Statement indicates that estrogen replacement therapy be considered if the BMD Z-scores are less than or equal to –2.0 with clinically significant fractures and a lack of response to non-pharmacologic therapy for more than 1 year, or a clinically significant reduction (not defined) in BMD Z-scores after non-pharmacologic therapy for more than 1 year or the occurrence of new clinically significant fractures during the year of non-pharmacologic therapy.[121] Two of the authors have a practice in which it is not uncommon to receive referrals from primary care providers for patients with components of the female athlete triad, with or without a diagnosed eating disorder, who have been not responsive to non-pharmacologic therapy, including dietary and/or psychological treatment for more than 1 year. Often these patients did not have a baseline DXA measurement, so assessing a reduction in

BMD over 1 year is not possible. In this context, considering estrogen replacement is consistent with the consensus guidelines.[121] We have been using a transdermal estrogen patch with cyclic progestin most recently for eating disorder patients, and we have discussed its use with those who do not have a diagnosed eating disorder but have prolonged amenorrhea.[172]

CONCLUSION

Patients with the female athlete triad can be challenging to treat, with or without an identified eating disorder or DE. Implementation of the treatment plan, especially for (but not limited to) adolescents, focusses on reversing the chronic energy deficiency, which requires implementing increased energy intake and reduced energy expenditure. This requires support from coaches and parents. It is a shared responsibility. If the physician recommends reduction of exercise, then the parents and coaches need to reinforce this recommendation. To not do so is to abrogate their responsibility.

References

1. Strong WB, Malina RM, Blimkie CJ, et al. Evidence based physical activity for school-age youth. *J Pediatr*. 2005;146:732-737
2. Baker ER, Mathur RS, Kirk RF, Williamson HO. Female runners and secondary amenorrhea: correlation with age, parity, mileage, and plasma hormonal and sex-hormone-binding globulin concentrations. *Fertil Steril*. 1981;36:183-187
3. Dale E, Gerlach DH, Wilhite AL. Menstrual dysfunction in distance runners. *Obstet Gynecol*. 1979;54:47-53
4. Feicht CB, Johnson TS, Martin BJ, Sparkes KE, Wagner WW Jr. Secondary amenorrhoea in athletes. *Lancet*. 1978;2:1145-1146
5. Frisch RE, Wyshak G, Vincent L. Delayed menarche and amenorrhea in ballet dancers. *N Engl J Med*. 1980;303:17-19
6. Warren MP. The effects of exercise on pubertal progression and reproductive function in girls. *J Clin Endocrinol Metab*. 1980;51:1150-1157
7. Loucks AB, Horvath SM. Athletic amenorrhea: a review. *Med Sci Sports Exerc*. 1985;17:56-72
8. Yeager KK, Agostini R, Nattiv A, Drinkwater B. The female athlete triad: disordered eating, amenorrhea, osteoporosis. *Med Sci Sports Exerc*. 1993;25:775-777
9. Otis CL, Drinkwater B, Johnson M, Loucks A, Wilmore J. American College of Sports Medicine position stand. The female athlete triad. *Med Sci Sports Exerc*. 1997;29:i-ix
10. Nattiv A, Loucks AB, Manore MM, et al. American College of Sports Medicine position stand. The female athlete triad. *Med Sci Sports Exerc*. 2007;39:1867-1882
11. De Souza MJ, Hontscharuk R, Olmsted M, Kerr G, Williams NI. Drive for thinness score is a proxy indicator of energy deficiency in exercising women. *Appetite*. 2007;48:359-367
12. Loucks AB, Thuma JR. Luteinizing hormone pulsatility is disrupted at a threshold of energy availability in regularly menstruating women. *J Clin Endocrinol Metab*. 2003;88:297-311
13. Williams NI, Caston-Balderrama AL, Helmreich DL, et al. Longitudinal changes in reproductive hormones and menstrual cyclicity in cynomolgus monkeys during strenuous exercise training: abrupt transition to exercise-induced amenorrhea. *Endocrinology*. 2001;142:2381-2389
14. De Souza MJ, West SL, Jamal SA, et al. The presence of both an energy deficiency and estrogen deficiency exacerbate alterations of bone metabolism in exercising women. *Bone*. 2008;43:140-148
15. De Souza MJ, Williams NI. Beyond hypoestrogenism in amenorrheic athletes: energy deficiency as a contributing factor for bone loss. *Curr Sports Med Rep*. 2005;4:38-44

16. Ihle R, Loucks AB. Dose-response relationships between energy availability and bone turnover in young exercising women. *J Bone Miner Res.* 2004;19:1231-1240
17. Sanborn CF, Martin BJ, Wagner WW Jr. Is athletic amenorrhea specific to runners? *Am J Obstet Gynecol.* 1982;143:859-861
18. Carlberg KA, Buckman MT, Peake GT, Riedesel ML. Body composition of oligo/amenorrheic athletes. *Med Sci Sports Exerc.* 1983;15:215-217
19. Schwartz B, Cumming DC, Riordan E, et al. Exercise-associated amenorrhea: a distinct entity? *Am J Obstet Gynecol.* 1981;141:662-670
20. Cobb KL, Bachrach LK, Greendale G, et al. Disordered eating, menstrual irregularity, and bone mineral density in female runners. *Med Sci Sports Exerc.* 2003;35:711-719
21. Glass AR, Deuster PA, Kyle SB, et al. Amenorrhea in Olympic marathon runners. *Fertil Steril.* 1987;48:740-745
22. Shangold MM, Levine HS. The effect of marathon training upon menstrual function. *Am J Obstet Gynecol.* 1982;143:862-869
23. Abraham SF, Beumont PJ, Fraser IS, Llewellyn-Jones D. Body weight, exercise and menstrual status among ballet dancers in training. *Br J Obstet Gynaecol.* 1982;89:507-510
24. Gibbs JC, Williams NI, De Souza MJ. Prevalence of individual and combined components of the female athlete triad. *Med Sci Sports Exerc.* 2013;45:985-996
25. Hoch AZ, Pajewski NM, Moraski L, et al. Prevalence of the female athlete triad in high school athletes and sedentary students. *Clin J Sport Med.* 2009;19:421-428
26. Nichols JF, Rauh MJ, Lawson MJ, Ji M, Barkai HS. Prevalence of the female athlete triad syndrome among high school athletes. *Arch Pediatr Adolesc Med.* 2006;160:137-142
27. De Souza MJ, Williams NI. Physiological aspects and clinical sequelae of energy deficiency and hypoestrogenism in exercising women. *Hum Reprod Update.* 2004;10:433-448
28. Wade GN, Schneider JE, Li HY. Control of fertility by metabolic cues. *Am J Physiol.* 1996;270:E1-E19
29. Jasienska G, Ellison PT. Physical work causes suppression of ovarian function in women. *Proc Biol Sci.* 1998;265:1847-1851
30. Ellison PT. Advances in human reproductive ecology. *Annu Rev Anthropol.* 1994;23:255-275
31. Ellison PT. Energetics and reproductive effort. *Am J Hum Biol.* 2003;15:342-351
32. Danforth E Jr, Burger A. The role of thyroid hormones in the control of energy expenditure. *Clin Endocrinol Metab.* 1984;13:581-595
33. Danforth E Jr, Burger AG. The impact of nutrition on thyroid hormone physiology and action. *Annu Rev Nutr.* 1989;9:201-227
34. De Souza MJ, Lee DK, VanHeest JL, et al. Severity of energy-related menstrual disturbances increases in proportion to indices of energy conservation in exercising women. *Fertil Steril.* 2007;88:971-975
35. De Souza MJ, Leidy HJ, O'Donnell E, Lasley B, Williams NI. Fasting ghrelin levels in physically active women: relationship with menstrual disturbances and metabolic hormones. *J Clin Endocrinol Metab.* 2004;89:3536-3542
36. Laughlin GA, Yen SS. Nutritional and endocrine-metabolic aberrations in amenorrheic athletes. *J Clin Endocrinol Metab.* 1996;81:4301-4309
37. Scheid JL, Williams NI, West SL, VanHeest JL, De Souza MJ. Elevated PYY is associated with energy deficiency and indices of subclinical disordered eating in exercising women with hypothalamic amenorrhea. *Appetite.* 2009;52:184-192
38. Kaufman BA, Warren MP, Dominguez JE, et al. Bone density and amenorrhea in ballet dancers are related to a decreased resting metabolic rate and lower leptin levels. *J Clin Endocrinol Metab.* 2002;87:2777-2783
39. Myerson M, Gutin B, Warren MP, et al. Resting metabolic rate and energy balance in amenorrheic and eumenorrheic runners. *Med Sci Sports Exerc.* 1991;23:15-22
40. Loucks AB, Heath EM. Induction of low-T3 syndrome in exercising women occurs at a threshold of energy availability. *Am J Physiol.* 1994;266:R817-R823

41. Loucks AB, Verdun M, Heath EM. Low energy availability, not stress of exercise, alters LH pulsatility in exercising women. *J Appl Physiol.* 1998;84:37-46

42. Williams NI, Helmreich DL, Parfitt DB, Caston-Balderrama A, Cameron JL. Evidence for a causal role of low energy availability in the induction of menstrual cycle disturbances during strenuous exercise training. *J Clin Endocrinol Metab.* 2001;86:5184-5193

43. De Souza MJ, Van Heest J, Demers LM, Lasley BL. Luteal phase deficiency in recreational runners: evidence for a hypometabolic state. *J Clin Endocrinol Metab.* 2003;88:337-346

44. Leibel RL, Rosenbaum M, Hirsch J. Changes in energy expenditure resulting from altered body weight. *N Engl J Med.* 1995;332:621-628

45. Harris JA, Benedict FG. *A Biometric Study of the Basal Metabolism in Man.* Publication No. 279. Washington, DC: Carnegie Institution of Washington, DC; 1919

46. Marra M, Polito A, De Filippo E, et al. Are the general equations to predict BMR applicable to patients with anorexia nervosa? *Eat Weight Disord.* 2002;7:53-59

47. Melchior JC, Rigaud D, Rozen R, Malon D, Apfelbaum M. Energy expenditure economy induced by decrease in lean body mass in anorexia nervosa. *Eur J Clin Nutr.* 1989;43:793-799

48. Polito A, Fabbri A, Ferro-Luzzi A, et al. Basal metabolic rate in anorexia nervosa: relation to body composition and leptin concentrations. *Am J Clin Nutr.* 2000;71:1495-1502

49. Eastell R, Mosekilde L, Hodgson SF, Riggs BL. Proportion of human vertebral body bone that is cancellous. *J Bone Miner Res.* 1990;5:1237-1241

50. Gilsanz V, Gibbens DT, Roe TF, et al. Vertebral bone density in children: effect of puberty. *Radiology.* 1988;166:847-850

51. Katzman DK, Bachrach LK, Carter DR, Marcus R. Clinical and anthropometric correlates of bone mineral acquisition in healthy adolescent girls. *J Clin Endocrinol Metab.* 1991;73:1332-1339

52. Volgyi E, Tylavsky FA, Xu L, et al. Bone and body segment lengthening and widening: a 7-year follow-up study in pubertal girls. *Bone.* 2010;47:773-782

53. Lloyd T, Petit MA, Lin HM, Beck TJ. Lifestyle factors and the development of bone mass and bone strength in young women. *J Pediatr.* 2004;144:776-782

54. Zebaze RM, Jones A, Knackstedt M, Maalouf G, Seeman E. Construction of the femoral neck during growth determines its strength in old age. *J Bone Miner Res.* 2007;22:1055-1061

55. Riggs BL, Melton LJ 3rd. Involutional osteoporosis. *N Engl J Med.* 1986;314:1676-1686

56. Bronner F. Calcium and osteoporosis. *Am J Clin Nutr.* 1994;60:831-836

57. Johnston CC Jr, Slemenda CW. Pathogenesis of osteoporosis. *Bone.* 1995;17:19S-22S

58. McBean LD, Forgac T, Finn SC. Osteoporosis: visions for care and prevention: a conference report. *J Am Diet Assoc.* 1994;94:668-671

59. Frost SA, Nguyen ND, Center JR, Eisman JA, Nguyen TV. Excess mortality attributable to hip-fracture: a relative survival analysis. *Bone.* 2013;56:23-29

60. Ray NF, Chan JK, Thamer M, Melton LJ 3rd. Medical expenditures for the treatment of osteoporotic fractures in the United States in. 1995: report from the National Osteoporosis Foundation. *J Bone Miner Res.* 1997;12:24-35

61. Keen AD, Drinkwater BL. Irreversible bone loss in former amenorrheic athletes. *Osteoporos Int.* 1997;7:311-315

62. National Osteoporosis Foundation. *Clinician's Guide to Prevention and Treatment of Osteoporosis.* Washington, DC: National Osteoporosis Foundation; 2014

63. Burge R, Dawson-Hughes B, Solomon DH, et al. Incidence and economic burden of osteoporosis-related fractures in the United States, 2005-2025. *J Bone Miner Res.* 2007;22:465-475

64. Melton L, Chao E, Lamne J. Osteoporosis: etiology, diagnosis and management. In: Riggs B, Melton JF, eds. *Biomechanical Aspects of Fractures.* New York: Raven Press; 1988:111

65. Danielson ME, Cauley JA, Baker CE, et al. Familial resemblance of bone mineral density (BMD) and calcaneal ultrasound attenuation: the BMD in mothers and daughters study. *J Bone Miner Res.* 1999;14:102-110

66. Pocock NA, Eisman JA, Hopper JL, et al. Genetic determinants of bone mass in adults: a twin study. *J Clin Invest.* 1987;80:706-710

67. Wosje KS, Binkley TL, Fahrenwald NL, Specker BL. High bone mass in a female Hutterite population. *J Bone Miner Res.* 2000;15:1429-1436
68. Krall EA, Dawson-Hughes B. Heritable and life-style determinants of bone mineral density. *J Bone Miner Res.* 1993;8:1-9
69. Villa ML, Marcus R, Ramirez Delay R, Kelsey JL. Factors contributing to skeletal health of postmenopausal Mexican-American women. *J Bone Miner Res.* 1995;10:1233-1242
70. Tabensky A, Duan Y, Edmonds J, Seeman E. The contribution of reduced peak accrual of bone and age-related bone loss to osteoporosis at the spine and hip: insights from the daughters of women with vertebral or hip fractures. *J Bone Miner Res.* 2001;16:1101-1107
71. Flicker L, Hopper JL, Rodgers L, et al. Bone density determinants in elderly women: a twin study. *J Bone Miner Res.* 1995;10:1607-1613
72. Kalkwarf HJ, Zemel BS, Gilsanz V, et al. The bone mineral density in childhood study: bone mineral content and density according to age, sex, and race. *J Clin Endocrinol Metab.* 2007;92:2087-2099
73. Marcus R, Feldman D. Osteoporosis. In: Marcus R, Feldman D, Kelsey J, eds. *Osteoporosis.* San Diego, CA: Academic Press; 1996:15
74. Forbes GB. Body size and composition of perimenarchal girls. *Am J Dis Child.* 1992;146:63-66
75. Theintz G, Buchs B, Rizzoli R, et al. Longitudinal monitoring of bone mass accumulation in healthy adolescents: evidence for a marked reduction after 16 years of age at the levels of lumbar spine and femoral neck in female subjects. *J Clin Endocrinol Metab.* 1992;75:1060-1065
76. Harel Z, Gold M, Cromer B, et al. Bone mineral density in postmenarchal adolescent girls in the United States: associated biopsychosocial variables and bone turnover markers. *J Adolesc Health.* 2007;40:44-53
77. Recker RR, Davies KM, Hinders SM, et al. Bone gain in young adult women. *JAMA.* 1992;268:2403-2408
78. Wastney ME, Ng J, Smith D, et al. Differences in calcium kinetics between adolescent girls and young women. *Am J Physiol.* 1996;271:R208-R216
79. Bonjour J, Theintz G, Buchs B, Slosman D, Rizzoli R. Critical years and stages of puberty for spinal and femoral bone mass accumulation during adolescence. *J Clin Endocrinol Metab.* 1991;73:55-63
80. Practice Committee of American Society for Reproductive Medicine. Current evaluation of amenorrhea. *Fertil Steril.* 2008;90:S219-S225
81. Chevalley T, Bonjour JP, Ferrari S, Rizzoli R. Deleterious effect of late menarche on distal tibia microstructure in healthy. 20-year-old and premenopausal middle-aged women. *J Bone Miner Res.* 2009;24:144-152
82. Mallinson RJ, Williams NI, Hill BR, De Souza MJ. Body composition and reproductive function exert unique influences on indices of bone health in exercising women. *Bone.* 2013;56:91-100
83. Bennell KL, Malcolm SA, Thomas SA, et al. Risk factors for stress fractures in track and field athletes. A twelve-month prospective study. *Am J Sports Med.* 1996;24:810-818
84. Cosman F, Ruffing J, Zion M, et al. Determinants of stress fracture risk in United States Military Academy cadets. *Bone.* 2013;55:359-366
85. Ackerman KE, Putman M, Guereca G, et al. Cortical microstructure and estimated bone strength in young amenorrheic athletes, eumenorrheic athletes and non-athletes. *Bone.* 2012;51:680-687
86. Seselj M, Nahhas RW, Sherwood RJ, et al. The influence of age at menarche on cross-sectional geometry of bone in young adulthood. *Bone.* 2012;51:38-45
87. Thein-Nissenbaum J. Long term consequences of the female athlete triad. *Maturitas.* 2013;75:107-112
88. Ponder SW, McCormick DP, Fawcett HD, et al. Spinal bone mineral density in children aged 5.00 through 11.99 years. *Am J Dis Child.* 1990;144:1346-1348
89. Slemenda CW, Reister TK, Hui SL, et al. Influences on skeletal mineralization in children and adolescents: evidence for varying effects of sexual maturation and physical activity. *J Pediatr.* 1994;125:201-207
90. Chan GM. Dietary calcium and bone mineral status of children and adolescents. *Am J Dis Child.* 1991;145:631-634
91. Lloyd T, Rollings N, Andon MB, et al. Determinants of bone density in young women. I. Relationships among pubertal development, total body bone mass, and total body bone density in premenarchal females. *J Clin Endocrinol Metab.* 1992;75:383-387

92. Rubin K, Schirduan V, Gendreau P, et al. Predictors of axial and peripheral bone mineral density in healthy children and adolescents, with special attention to the role of puberty. *J Pediatr.* 1993;123:863-870
93. Scheid JL, Toombs RJ, Ducher G, et al. Estrogen and peptide YY are associated with bone mineral density in premenopausal exercising women. *Bone.* 2011;49:194-201
94. Petit MA, Beck TJ, Lin HM, et al. Femoral bone structural geometry adapts to mechanical loading and is influenced by sex steroids: the Penn State Young Women's Health Study. *Bone.* 2004;35:750-759
95. Warren MP, Brooks-Gunn J, Fox RP, et al. Lack of bone accretion and amenorrhea: evidence for a relative osteopenia in weight-bearing bones. *J Clin Endocrinol Metab.* 1991;72:847-853
96. White CM, Hergenroeder AC, Klish WJ. Bone mineral density in 15- to 21-year-old eumenorrheic and amenorrheic subjects. *Am J Dis Child.* 1992;146:31-35
97. Abrams SA, Stuff JE. Calcium metabolism in girls: current dietary intakes lead to low rates of calcium absorption and retention during puberty. *Am J Clin Nutr.* 1994;60:739-743
98. Mughal MZ, Khadilkar AV. The accrual of bone mass during childhood and puberty. *Curr Opin Endocrinol Diabetes Obes.* 2011;18:28-32
99. Ross AC, Manson JE, Abrams SA, et al. The 2011 report on dietary reference intakes for calcium and vitamin D from the Institute of Medicine: what clinicians need to know. *J Clin Endocrinol Metab.* 2011;96:53-58
100. Johnston CC Jr, Miller JZ, Slemenda CW, et al. Calcium supplementation and increases in bone mineral density in children. *N Engl J Med.* 1992;327:82-87
101. Shangold M, Rebar RW, Wentz AC, Schiff I. Evaluation and management of menstrual dysfunction in athletes. *JAMA.* 1990;263:1665-1669
102. Matkovic V, Ilich JZ. Calcium requirements for growth: are current recommendations adequate? *Nutr Rev.* 1993;51:171-180
103. Institute of Medicine. Dietary reference intakes for calcium and vitamin D. November 2010 report brief. National Academy of Sciences. www.iom.edu/Reports/2010/Dietary-Reference-Intakes-for-Calcium-and-Vitamin-D/Report-Brief.aspx Accessed February 11, 2015
104. Farr JN, Blew RM, Lee VR, Lohman TG, Going SB. Associations of physical activity duration, frequency, and load with volumetric BMD, geometry, and bone strength in young girls. *Osteoporos Int.* 2011;22:1419-1430
105. Janz KF, Letuchy EM, Eichenberger Gilmore JM, et al. Early physical activity provides sustained bone health benefits later in childhood. *Med Sci Sports Exerc.* 2010;42:1072-1078
106. Heidemann M, Jespersen E, Holst R, et al. The impact on children's bone health of a school-based physical education program and participation in leisure time sports: the Childhood Health, Activity and Motor Performance School (the CHAMPS) study, Denmark. *Prev Med.* 2013;57:87-91
107. Hind K, Burrows M. Weight-bearing exercise and bone mineral accrual in children and adolescents: a review of controlled trials. *Bone.* 2007;40:14-27
108. Carter DR. Mechanical loading history and skeletal biology. *J Biomech.* 1987;20:1095-1109
109. Grimston SK, Willows ND, Hanley DA. Mechanical loading regime and its relationship to bone mineral density in children. *Med Sci Sports Exerc.* 1993;25:1203-1210
110. Aloia JF, Cohn SH, Ostuni JA, Cane R, Ellis K. Prevention of involutional bone loss by exercise. *Ann Intern Med.* 1978;89:356-358
111. McNitt-Gray JL. Kinetics of the lower extremities during drop landings from three heights. *J Biomech.* 1993;26:1037-1046
112. Burt LA, Greene DA, Ducher G, Naughton GA. Skeletal adaptations associated with pre-pubertal gymnastics participation as determined by DXA and pQCT: a systematic review and meta-analysis. *J Sci Med Sport.* 2013;16:231-239
113. Drinkwater BL, Nilson K, Chesnut CH 3rd, et al. Bone mineral content of amenorrheic and eumenorrheic athletes. *N Engl J Med.* 1984;311:277-281
114. Christo K, Prabhakaran R, Lamparello B, et al. Bone metabolism in adolescent athletes with amenorrhea, athletes with eumenorrhea, and control subjects. *Pediatrics.* 2008;121:1127-1136

115. Prior JC, Vigna YM, Schechter MT, Burgess AE. Spinal bone loss and ovulatory disturbances. N Engl J Med. 1990;323:1221-1227

116. Cann CE, Martin MC, Genant HK, Jaffe RB. Decreased spinal mineral content in amenorrheic women. JAMA. 1984;251:626-629

117. Ducher G, Eser P, Hill B, Bass S. History of amenorrhoea compromises some of the exercise-induced benefits in cortical and trabecular bone in the peripheral and axial skeleton: a study in retired elite gymnasts. Bone. 2009;45:760-767

118. Etherington J, Harris PA, Nandra D, et al. The effect of weight-bearing exercise on bone mineral density: a study of female ex-elite athletes and the general population. J Bone Miner Res. 1996;11:1333-1338

119. Khan KM, Green RM, Saul A, et al. Retired elite female ballet dancers and nonathletic controls have similar bone mineral density at weightbearing sites. J Bone Miner Res. 1996;11:1566-1574

120. Nelson DA, Koo WW. Interpretation of absorptiometric bone mass measurements in the growing skeleton: issues and limitations. Calcif Tissue Int. 1999;65:1-3

121. De Souza MJ, Nattiv A, Joy E, et al. 2014 Female Athlete Triad Coalition Consensus Statement on Treatment and Return to Play of the Female Athlete Triad:1st International Conference held in San Francisco, California, May 2012, and 2nd International Conference held in Indianapolis, Indiana, May 2013. Br J Sports Med. 2014;48:289

122. Smock AJ, Hughes JM, Popp KL, et al. Bone volumetric density, geometry, and strength in female and male collegiate runners. Med Sci Sports Exerc. 2009;41:2026-2032

123. Ackerman KE, Nazem T, Chapko D, et al. Bone microarchitecture is impaired in adolescent amenorrheic athletes compared with eumenorrheic athletes and nonathletic controls. J Clin Endocrinol Metab. 2011;96:3123-3133

124. Goulding A, Cannan R, Williams SM, et al. Bone mineral density in girls with forearm fractures. J Bone Miner Res. 1998;13:143-148

125. Lindberg JS, Fears WB, Hunt MM, et al. Exercise-induced amenorrhea and bone density. Ann Intern Med. 1984;101:647-648

126. Miller KK, Lee EE, Lawson EA, et al. Determinants of skeletal loss and recovery in anorexia nervosa. J Clin Endocrinol Metab. 2006;91:2931-2937

127. Drinkwater BL, Nilson K, Ott S, Chesnut CH 3rd. Bone mineral density after resumption of menses in amenorrheic athletes. JAMA. 1986;256:380-382

128. Castro J, Lazaro L, Pons F, Halperin I, Toro J. Predictors of bone mineral density reduction in adolescents with anorexia nervosa. J Am Acad Child Adolesc Psychiatry. 2000;39:1365-1370

129. Bachrach LK, Guido D, Katzman D, Litt IF, Marcus R. Decreased bone density in adolescent girls with anorexia nervosa. Pediatrics. 1990;86:440-447

130. Grinspoon S, Miller K, Coyle C, et al. Severity of osteopenia in estrogen-deficient women with anorexia nervosa and hypothalamic amenorrhea. J Clin Endocrinol Metab. 1999;84:2049-2055

131. Loud KJ, Gordon CM, Micheli LJ, Field AE. Correlates of stress fractures among preadolescent and adolescent girls. Pediatrics. 2005;115:e399-e406

132. Tenforde AS, Sayres LC, McCurdy ML, Sainani KL, Fredericson M. Identifying sex-specific risk factors for stress fractures in adolescent runners. Med Sci Sports Exerc. 2013;45:1843-1851

133. Barrack MT, Van Loan MD, Rauh MJ, Nichols JF. Body mass, training, menses, and bone in adolescent runners: a 3-yr follow-up. Med Sci Sports Exerc. 2011;43:959-966

134. Parfitt AM. Quantum concept of bone remodeling and turnover: implications for the pathogenesis of osteoporosis. Calcif Tissue Int. 1979;28:1-5

135. Dempster DW, Lindsay R. Pathogenesis of osteoporosis. Lancet. 1993;341:797-801

136. Neimeyer GJ, Khouzam N. A repertory grid study of restrained eaters. Br J Med Psychol. 1985;58(Pt 4):365-367

137. Seeman E, Karlsson MK, Duan Y. On exposure to anorexia nervosa, the temporal variation in axial and appendicular skeletal development predisposes to site-specific deficits in bone size and density: a cross-sectional study. J Bone Miner Res. 2000;15:2259-2265

138. Wiksten-Almstromer M, Hirschberg AL, Hagenfeldt K. Reduced bone mineral density in adult women diagnosed with menstrual disorders during adolescence. Acta Obstet Gynecol Scand. 2009;88:543-549

139. Joy E, De Souza MJ, Nattiv A, et al. 2014 female athlete triad coalition consensus statement on treatment and return to play of the female athlete triad. *Curr Sports Med Rep.* 2014;13:219-232

140. Lindberg JS, Powell MR, Hunt MM, Ducey DE, Wade CE. Increased vertebral bone mineral in response to reduced exercise in amenorrheic runners. *West J Med.* 1987;146:39-42

141. Cobb KL, Bachrach LK, Sowers M, et al. The effect of oral contraceptives on bone mass and stress fractures in female runners. *Med Sci Sports Exerc.* 2007;39:1464-1473

142. Misra M, Klibanski A. Anorexia nervosa and bone. *J Endocrinol.* 2014;221: R163-R176

143. Torstveit MK, Sundgot-Borgen J. Participation in leanness sports but not training volume is associated with menstrual dysfunction: a national survey of 1276 elite athletes and controls. *Br J Sports Med.* 2005;39:141-147

144. Nieves JW, Melsop K, Curtis M, et al. Nutritional factors that influence change in bone density and stress fracture risk among young female cross-country runners. *PM R.* 2010;2:740-750

145. Craig WJ. Health effects of vegan diets. *Am J Clin Nutr.* 2009;89:1627S-1633S

146. Segura-Garcia C, Papaianni MC, Caglioti F, et al. Orthorexia nervosa: a frequent eating disordered behavior in athletes. *Eat Weight Disord.* 2012;17:e226-e233

147. Loucks AB, Kiens B, Wright HH. Energy availability in athletes. *J Sports Sci.* 2011;29(Suppl 1):S7-S15

148. Ainsworth BE, Haskell WL, Whitt MC, et al. Compendium of physical activities: an update of activity codes and MET intensities. *Med Sci Sports Exerc.* 2000;32:S498-S504

149. Fogelholm M, van Marken Lichtenbelt W. Comparison of body composition methods: a literature analysis. *Eur J Clin Nutr.* 1997;51:495-503

150. Hamwi G. Changing dietary concepts. In: Danowski TS, ed. *Diabetes Mellitus: Diagnosis and Treatment.* New York: American Diabetes Association; 1964;73-78

151. Cahill GF Jr. Fuel metabolism in starvation. *Annu Rev Nutr.* 2006;26:1-22

152. Abbassi V. Growth and normal puberty. *Pediatrics.* 1998;102:507-511

153. Stiegler P, Cunliffe A. The role of diet and exercise for the maintenance of fat-free mass and resting metabolic rate during weight loss. *Sports Med.* 2006;36:239-262

154. Rodriguez NR, DiMarco NM, Langley S. Position of the American Dietetic Association, Dietitians of Canada, and the American College of Sports Medicine: Nutrition and athletic performance. *J Am Diet Assoc.* 2009;109:509-527

155. Aerenhouts D, Van Cauwenberg J, Poortmans JR, Hauspie R, Clarys P. Influence of growth rate on nitrogen balance in adolescent sprint athletes. *Int J Sport Nutr Exerc Metab.* 2013;23:409-417

156. Phillips SM, Van Loon LJ. Dietary protein for athletes: from requirements to optimum adaptation. *J Sports Sci.* 2011;29(Suppl 1):S29-S38

157. Venderley AM, Campbell WW. Vegetarian diets: nutritional considerations for athletes. *Sports Med.* 2006;36:293-305

158. Misra M, Prabhakaran R, Miller KK, et al. Weight gain and restoration of menses as predictors of bone mineral density change in adolescent girls with anorexia nervosa-1. *J Clin Endocrinol Metab.* 2008;93:1231-1237

159. Warren MP, Miller KK, Olson WH, Grinspoon SK, Friedman AJ. Effects of an oral contraceptive (norgestimate/ethinyl estradiol) on bone mineral density in women with hypothalamic amenorrhea and osteopenia: an open-label extension of a double-blind, placebo-controlled study. *Contraception.* 2005;72:206-211

160. Klibanski A, Biller BM, Schoenfeld DA, Herzog DB, Saxe VC. The effects of estrogen administration on trabecular bone loss in young women with anorexia nervosa. *J Clin Endocrinol Metab.* 1995;80:898-904

161. Hergenroeder AC, Smith EO, Shypailo R, et al. Bone mineral changes in young women with hypothalamic amenorrhea treated with oral contraceptives, medroxyprogesterone, or placebo over 12 months. *Am J Obstet Gynecol.* 1997;176:1017-1025

162. Zaman G, Jessop HL, Muzylak M, et al. Osteocytes use estrogen receptor alpha to respond to strain but their ERalpha content is regulated by estrogen. *J Bone Miner Res.* 2006;21:1297-1306

163. Oursler MJ, Pederson L, Fitzpatrick L, Riggs BL, Spelsberg T. Human giant cell tumors of the bone (osteoclastomas) are estrogen target cells. *Proc Natl Acad Sci U S A.* 1994;91:5227-5231

164. Oursler MJ, Osdoby P, Pyfferoen J, Riggs BL, Spelsberg TC. Avian osteoclasts as estrogen target cells. *Proc Natl Acad Sci U S A.* 1991;88:6613-6617
165. Grinspoon S, Thomas E, Pitts S, et al. Prevalence and predictive factors for regional osteopenia in women with anorexia nervosa. *Ann Intern Med.* 2000;133:790-794
166. Gibson JH, Mitchell A, Reeve J, Harries MG. Treatment of reduced bone mineral density in athletic amenorrhea: a pilot study. *Osteoporos Int.* 1999;10:284-289
167. Golden NH, Lanzkowsky L, Schebendach J, et al. The effect of estrogen-progestin treatment on bone mineral density in anorexia nervosa. *J Pediatr Adolesc Gynecol.* 2002;15:135-143
168. Warren MP, Brooks-Gunn J, Fox RP, et al. Persistent osteopenia in ballet dancers with amenorrhea and delayed menarche despite hormone therapy: a longitudinal study. *Fertil Steril.* 2003;80:398-404
169. Seifert-Klauss V, Prior JC. Progesterone and bone: actions promoting bone health in women. *J Osteoporos.* 2010;2010:845180
170. Bergstrom I, Crisby M, Engstrom AM, et al. Women with anorexia nervosa should not be treated with estrogen or birth control pills in a bone-sparing effect. *Acta Obstet Gynecol Scand.* 2013;92:877-880
171. Beck TJ, Ruff CB, Warden KE, Scott WW Jr, Rao GU. Predicting femoral neck strength from bone mineral data: a structural approach. *Invest Radiol.* 1990;25:6-18
172. Misra M, Katzman D, Miller KK, et al. Physiologic estrogen replacement increases bone density in adolescent girls with anorexia nervosa. *J Bone Miner Res.* 2011;26:2430-2438

Adolesc Med 026 (2015) 143–162

The Adolescent Dancer: Common Medical Concerns and Relevant Anticipatory Guidance

Kathleen A. Linzmeier, MD[a]; Chris G. Koutures, MD[b]*

[a]Pediatric Resident, University of California-Irvine, Children's Hospital
of Orange County Pediatric Residency Program, Orange, California;
[b]Pediatric and Sports Medicine Specialist, Private Practice, Anaheim Hills, California

With recent trends indicating growing injury rates in both classical and competitive dance disciplines, adolescent medicine specialists will be more apt to encounter dedicated young dancers and thus become part of the dance medicine team.[1] By the early adolescent years, many young performers have decided to eschew other forms of organized sport or physical activity and solely specialize in dance. This increased focus frequently translates into several hours of dance activity per day, often with only 1 to 2 days off per week from organized dance activities.

A fear of being told to "just stop dancing" often makes dancers and other performers hesitant to seek medical care.[1] Many medical professionals initially may profess a lack of familiarity and comfort with medical care of dancers and other performing artists. Adolescent medicine physicians who take the time to learn some basic dance terms and use evidence-based anticipatory guidance skills along with knowledge of adolescent growth and development can become ideal resources for dancers and their families.

This article opens by defining the nature of dance, including key terms for the medical professional. Review of concerns regarding overuse, effect of dance on adolescent development, and common injuries seen in particular forms of dance are addressed. The article concludes with important prevention recommendations.

*Corresponding author
E-mail address: chris@dockoutures.com

DEFINING KEY DANCE TERMS

Being comfortable discussing the dance studio environment and types of dance will greatly enhance rapport between medical care professionals, dancers, families, and instructors.

Most dancers prefer "sprung" wooden *floors* to concrete or other harder surfaces that do not have ample cushioning to reduce the cumulative impact of repetitive jumps and leaps.[1] *Mirrors* are often placed on side walls to allow review of technique by participants and instructors, although they also invite the inevitable comparisons of body image and skills with other dancers. Alongside at least 1 wall is the *barre*, which is a wooden rail about 3 feet high that dancers hold for balance. Dancers working to hone basic skills or who are recovering from injury can use the mirrors and barre to focus on proper technique and for physical support. The middle of the dance floor is known as *center stage* and is used for more advanced skills, including leaps, turns, and throws. *Blocking* or *marking steps* allow dancers to walk or move in unison with the rest of the troop without jumping, leaping, turning, or lifts, and are a sensible modification for partial participation while dancers are recovering from injury.

TYPES OF DANCE CLASSES

- *Technique* or *"tech"* courses: Basics of movements are emphasized in these courses. They often are held earlier in the day and may include use of mirrors and the barre for balance.
- *Choreography courses:* The whole troupe uses the entire dance floor to rehearse pieces. These courses often include *partnering* in which dancers pair off in lifting and turning with each other. The courses are more commonly held later in the day and more frequently scheduled closer to a show or competition.
- *Summer intensives:* These weeks- or months-long courses focus on particular types of dance, often on a try-out or audition basis. They regularly take place at prominent dance studios, academies, or theater company locations. Participants must balance the high-level experience with dance commitments before and after the intensive while they also try to ensure appropriate nutrition and rest while eating in cafeterias and living in a dormitory (ie, they often are away from home for the first time).

COMMON FORMS OF DANCE

- *Ballet:* Classical form focusing on 5 basic positions (Figure 1) that emphasize *plié* (knee flexion and ankle dorsiflexion) (Figure 2), *relevé* (ankle and first toe plantarflexion), *turnout* (hip external rotation) (Figure 3A) and ultimately *en pointe* (Figure 3B) in which the entire body weight is balanced in the tips of the toes with the ankle in full plantarflexion. Dancers en pointe use firm

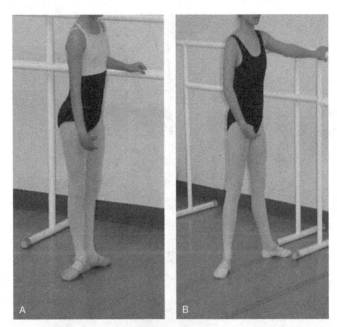

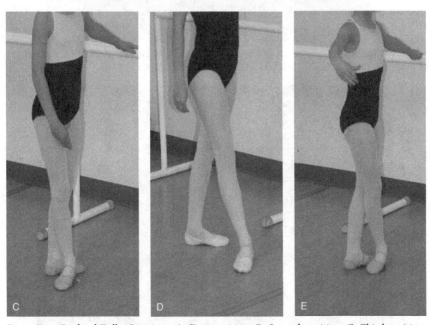

Fig 1. Five Cardinal Ballet Positions. A, First position; B, Second position; C, Third position; D, Fourth position; E, Fifth position. Note the extent of hip external rotation in each position.

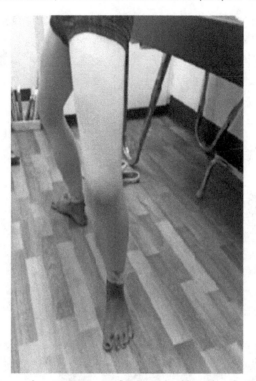

Fig 2. Plié in ballet second position. Knee in flexion and ankle in dorsiflexion. Ideal alignment has hip lined up with mid-patella and second metatarsal head.

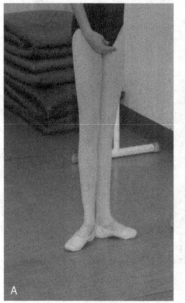
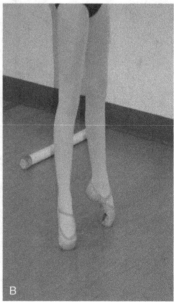

Fig 3. A, Ballet turnout; B, Ballet pointe position.

wooden pointe shoes, often with lamb's wool toe covers for comfort and protection that enables the ankle plantarflexion and toe extension. All other forms of ballet are done either barefoot or with very thin ballet slippers.

- *Modern:* Less hip external rotation and faster than classical ballet.
- *Jazz:* Involves sharp, precise, angular high kicks, slides, and splits on the floor without hip external rotation. Performers can use more supportive footwear.
- *Lyrical:* Fusion of ballet and jazz that focuses on individualized expression.
- *Tap:* Repetitive dorsiflexion/plantarflexion of the feet to strike toes against the dance floor. Performers use specialized tap shoes with metal tips.
- *Hip-hop:* Very physical form of dance that uses more upright, upper body emphasis (*new-school hip-hop style*) or a floor-based, total body emphasis (*old-school hip-hop style*).
- *Cultural or ethnic dance:* Often includes partnering, use of dance lines, high leg kicks, and large groups of participants.
- *Competitive dance:* Often involves team-based routines, but all team members may not be at the same skill level, leaving less prepared performers at higher risk for injury. Emerging interest in competitive dance with emphasis on scoring high marks from judges creates particular concerns for overuse and injury in adolescent dancers. Rehearsing and training for competitive events may place less emphasis on progressive skill acquisition and more on immediate readiness to perform advanced routines and movements that could overwhelm underprepared dancers.

PRINCIPLES OF DANCE MEDICINE

Physicians who profess understanding of the nature and demands of dance can more readily develop rapport with performers, who often are reluctant to seek medical attention.

- Physicians can frame recommendations for dance modifications, rest, and adequate nutrition in a positive, performance-enhancing manner, which tends to be better received by dancers, parents, and instructors.[1]
- The presence of previous injury significantly increases risk for future new injury or reinjury, often because of inadequate recovery.[2] Physicians should emphasize the need for appropriate rehabilitation plans to reduce the risk of ongoing injury concerns.[1]
- Complete removal from the dance environment can be emotionally difficult for the adolescent dancer and may not be absolutely necessary, and such advice from the physician may be routinely disregarded by the committed dancer.
- The physician should emphasize what performers can do rather than what they can't do in order to enhance adherence by dancers. Suggested modifications can include increased barre work, use of blocking steps, working the upper body only, or limited jumps, leaps, turns, and lifts.

- Working on rehabilitation exercises during dance periods will allow dancers to remain active among their peers and have appropriate time to complete necessary commitments. Favored cross-training choices include yoga and Pilates, which are nonimpact activities that help build flexibility and core strength.
- A multidisciplinary approach, including offers to communicate with instructors to provide collaborative care, can build more positive relationships.

DANCE AND ADOLESCENT DEVELOPMENT

Female performance artists, including dancers, gymnasts, and figure skaters, may experience delayed pubertal onset, growth spurt, and age of menarche compared to age-matched females not participating in these activities.[3] This delay may result from the athlete's attempts to avoid selection bias because growth spurts are not favored developments by many coaches/instructors and from reduced energy availability and caloric intake. In many cases, maturation is accelerated once the performer retires from or reduces the amount of activity. Performers, such as gymnasts, eventually can attain predicted adult height levels but again, later than their peers.[4]

Even with this potential for delayed growth, many female dancers attain their growth spurt ahead of age-matched male dancers, which can create unique issues on the dance floor. These issues are most notable with partnering, in which the male dancer lifts his female counterpart. Proper lifting technique calls for the male to place his hands on the lateral chest wall of the female, and many adolescent boys may not appropriately lift now taller and more developed females because of inadequate strength or hesitancy to place their hands near the emerging breast area. This often results in the male dancer placing his hands lower on the female's rib cage, which increases the injury risk for both partners.

The adolescent growth spurt may cause rapid changes in the length of extremities. This may predispose to relative deficiencies in shoulder, hip, and buttock strength and coordination, such as increased knee valgus, tibial internal rotation, and foot hyperpronation with landing and turning.[5] Increased body weight along with scoliosis and decreased hip external rotation in particular can lead to back injuries.[5] Injuries to the physeal plates at the end of long bones and apophyseal attachment sites of tendon to bone are encountered more frequently during the adolescent growth spurt (females in Tanner 3 and males in Tanner 4).[2] Focal pain in these regions requires radiographic evaluation and often reduction of activity to allow appropriate healing.

Dancers are not immune from the multitude of environmental and cognitive changes that occur during adolescence and can frequently affect dance participation. Concerns about emerging sense of identity combined with challenges about sexuality, alcohol and drug use, and peer and family relationships need to be openly addressed to optimize the emotional health of young dancers.

Although many adolescent dancers opt to increase frequency and complexity of dance commitments during growth periods, a more sensible recommendation might be to reduce overall time commitment and focus on "relearning" basic movement skills and patterns.[2]

NUTRITIONAL CONCERNS IN THE ADOLESCENT DANCER

Body image issues are common among many adolescents but can be more glaringly apparent in the dance environment.[1,3] Relative energy deficiency in sports (RED-S) because of inadequate caloric intake combined with significant energy expenditure are common findings in the adolescent dance community and can result in both immediate and longer-term adverse physical and emotional issues.[6] The female athlete triad of abnormal menstrual function, disordered eating patterns, and low bone density is a common consequence of insufficient energy availability.[7] (See *The Female Athlete Triad: Energy Deficiency, Physiologic Consequences, and Treatment,* pp. 116-142 in this issue.) Both male and female dancers with poor energy availability are at higher risk for musculoskeletal injuries with complicated or delayed recoveries, increased risk of acute respiratory illness, and psychological and physical burnout.[6]

Insufficient caloric and nutrient intake may be caused by several factors. (1) Dancers often are unaware that they may expend several thousand calories over many hours of dance on a daily basis. (2) Many dancers have suboptimal intake of dairy and meat because they lack time to purchase/prepare/consume these foods, they are under financial constraints, or they follow diets that may select against the intake of animal products. This leads to concerns over adequate micronutrient intake of calcium, vitamin D, and iron.[8] (3) During training, dancers may pay inadequate attention to fluid and carbohydrate intake, which leads to difficulties in maintaining optimal cognition, motivation, and motor skill performance.[8]

Direct comparisons with other dancers, use of mirrors, the favoring of tighter-fitting or revealing garments, and even particular comments from instructors or peers about weight all can heighten a dancer's potential for development of restrictive eating patterns.

Because many performers will not present for medical care with direct complaints about these issues, the astute adolescent specialist should make detailed inquiries about the type and amount of food intake, specific amounts and intensity of dance participation, age of menarche and frequency of menstrual cycles, and self-directed or outside pressures to control weight.[6,7] Sequential monitoring of height, weight, and body mass index (BMI) on age-appropriate growth curves can identify at-risk individuals. In particular, evidence suggests that adolescent females with BMI less than the 28% percentile have a higher rate of menstrual dysfunction.[9] Aggressive intervention, including nutritional and sports/dance medicine specialist consultation, laboratory evaluation, mental health support, and modifications of dance and other physical activity, may be indicated in dancers who exhibit signs or symptoms suggestive of RED-S or female athlete triad.[6,7]

ADOLESCENT DANCER AND BONE HEALTH

Bone health is optimized by sufficient caloric, vitamin D, and calcium intake combined with appropriate levels of weight-bearing physical activity. Adolescence is a key period for bone development, with most females accruing their peak bone density by late adolescence,[10] so any process that interferes with bone strength can have both short- and long-term adverse consequences.

Although dance is a solid impact loading activity for bone development, excessive amounts of dance can overload the bone and lead to fatigue. Dance is also mainly an indoor activity that reduces cumulative sunlight exposure, leading to potential vitamin D insufficiency. These 2 factors combined with inadequate intake of calcium and total calories confer a higher potential for bone stress injuries, namely, in lower extremity bones such as the metatarsals, sesamoids, tibia, fibula and femur, in adolescent dancers.[1]

DANCE COMMITMENT AND SCHEDULES

Adolescent dancers commonly have both technical and choreography classes in multiple disciplines on a weekly basis, often taught by a variety of instructors and at a multitude of dance venues or studios. Many classical dance studios have featured productions in early winter and again in late spring or early summer, with the summer months often free from organized commitments. However, the emergence of competitive dance has shifted the performance calendar to a more year-round commitment.

Properly crafted training programs that maximize performance while minimizing injury risk follow the concepts of *periodization*, in which blocks of higher-intensity activity are combined with periods of lower-intensity training, absolute rest, and appropriate alternate forms of physical activity in efforts to reduce injury.[11] In the dance community with its multiple classes, locations, and instructors, a lack of communication often dooms any sense of a coordinated training program and places the adolescent dancer at high risk for physical and emotional overload during a particularly vulnerable period.

Unless dancers have a primary instructor who can help monitor for signs of overload and impending injury, the direct coordinating and communicating onus unfortunately falls on individual dancers and families who commonly are unaware and unable to fully execute this important role.

INJURIES IN DANCE

Dancers are susceptible to multiple types of injury because of microtrauma from the repetitive nature of their activities, improper technique, and underlying aberrant anatomy, making it more difficult for them to carry out proper dance positions. From 60% to 90% of dancers are injured during their careers, with most injuries affecting the lower extremities and back.[12-14] Dance-specific movements, such as repetitive lifting, leaping, jumping, turning, externally rotating, plantar flexing, and landing, can lead to particular injury patterns, such as shoulder and back pain, spondylolysis, sacroiliac dysfunction, knee pain, and a variety of ankle and foot injuries.

LIFTING AND PARTNERING: BACK AND SHOULDER PAIN

The lifting requirements of dance highlight the important interaction between technique, muscle strength, and postural alignment.[13] Lifting is not isolated to male dancers; female dancers are also encouraged to use aggressive upper extremity movements that can place stress on the shoulder girdle and back. Proper alignment allows for musculoskeletal balance and enables dancers to move efficiently. It is important to assess alignment in all dancers, including the evaluation of posture in common dance positions in order to identify their effect on function.

Standard posture is evaluated using a plumb line that, when evaluated from a lateral view, should fall through the external auditory meatus and bodies of the cervical vertebrae, bisect the trunk, and fall slightly posterior to the center hip joint through the greater trochanter with the pelvis in neutral position. Misalignment can contribute to pain, resulting in compensatory movements, muscle imbalance, and injury.

Particular poor postures that contribute to muscle imbalance and a vicious cycle of pain include forward head posture, rounded shoulders, and kyphosis. Underlying weakness of the scapular muscles combined with tight pectoral muscles pull the shoulders forward. This leads to the rounded shoulders and kyphotic posture of the upper back (Figure 4) and resultant scapular abduction, which results in decreased cervical range of motion.[13] Surrounding muscles then develop compensatory movement patterns that can predispose dancers to further injury. Muscle imbalances may be exacerbated during periods of rapid growth when soft tissue and muscle are unable to keep pace with the rate of bone growth, which overall can contribute to decreased flexibility and compensatory mechanisms.[15]

This forward posture is often exacerbated by the "slouching posture" exhibited by many adolescents and their preponderance to lean forward when they are reading or using electronic devices. Addressing more appropriate positions both on and off the dance floor is crucial to correcting these injury patterns.

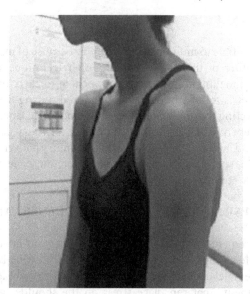

Fig 4. Forward position of chin, neck and both shoulders.

Common injuries resulting from this imbalance include subacromial impinge-ment and bursitis, rotator cuff tendinitis, acromioclavicular joints synovitis and sprains, and shoulder instability. Rehabilitation of these injuries should aim to restore proper alignment, biomechanics, and muscle balance.

LEAPS, FLIPS, AND TURNS: LOWER BACK AND SACROILIAC PAIN

Back pain has been estimated to occur in 60% to 80% of ballet and modern dancers in whom it most often is localized to the lumbar spine.[13] Hyperlordosis is a major risk factor contributing to back pain. Hyperlordosis usually is an acquired posture in dancers resulting from anatomic misalignment, muscle imbalance, and poor technique.[13] The muscle imbalance involves relatively weak abdominal muscles with tight soft tissue fascia connections in the thoracolum-bar region leading to increased prominence and tightness of the both the middle and lower back regions.

Structural imbalance is more significant during the adolescent growth spurt, when lumbar fascia elongation may not be able to keep up with bony growth, thus leading to tethering and subsequent lordosis.[15,16] Some dancers compensate for this structural imbalance by developing a mild round-back kyphotic posture in an attempt to rebalance the torso forward over the pelvis. It is important to not attribute any back pain in such athletes to their kyphotic posture alone but also to address the need for increased flexibility of tight lumbodorsal fascia. This can be achieved with stretches of the flexed lower back and hip flexor muscles along with improved strengthening of weak anterior abdominal muscles.

Dancers also may adopt hyperlordosis of the lower back as a compensatory mechanism for limited hip external range of motion in an attempt to achieve more perfect turnout.[17,18] Increased lordosis at the lumbo-pelvic junction creates flexion at the hip joint, which leads to increased external rotation. However, this trick for increasing turnout should be avoided because it encourages poor technique. Continued hyperlordosis requires contraction of the gluteals and hamstrings in addition to hyperextension of the knees in order to maintain pelvic stability. Such compensatory mechanisms ultimately will lead to injuries such as spondylolysis and iliopsoas tendinitis.[19]

Tightness of the anterior chest leading to limitations in active shoulder flexion can predispose a young dancer to hyperlordosis and resultant lumbosacral injuries. A dancer who cannot attain full shoulder flexion (reaching up) often "cheats" by forcing the lower back into greater degrees of hyperextension. This only exacerbates the cumulative overload on the lumbosacral region. Evaluating shoulder range of motion and correcting deficits in shoulder flexion both are essential aspects of a complete assessment and rehabilitation plan for lumbosacral pain in the dancer.

Dancers are particularly vulnerable to posterior lumbar vertebral stress injuries given the extreme hyperextension and hyperlordosis required in many elements of dance.[13,16] Spondylolysis involves an abnormality in the pars interarticularis of the vertebral arch.[20] It represents a stress or fatigue fracture most commonly described as an overuse injury as a result of repetitive microtrauma from extension, flexion, and rotation of the spine. The injury can involve any vertebra of the lumbar spine but most often is localized to the middle and lower segments.

Physical examination reveals pain with provocative hyperextension. Pain often is exaggerated on the ipsilateral side of the pathologic defect, and many dancers report pain with *arabesque* (bending forward while standing on 1 straight leg with the other leg extended backward; Figure 5).

Radiographs should be taken in any athlete with low back pain and suspected spondylolysis. The radiographs should include standing anteroposterior, lateral, and possibly bilateral oblique lumbar imaging.[20,21] Nearly 90% of radiologically apparent defects are appreciated in the coned-down lateral view because it produces a clearer image of the posterior bone structures.[21] Acute pars injuries (first several months of pain/injury) may not routinely show up on radiographs but if apparent will include faint lucent lines in the pars region. Chronic pars injuries are more apt to be found with plain radiographs and may have wider fracture lines with or without increased bone deposition (sclerosis) adjacent to the fracture lines. Additional imaging with computed tomographic scan, single-photon emission computed tomography (SPECT) scan, or magnetic resonance imaging (MRI) should be pursued when a patient has negative plain films despite persistent symptoms. Single-photon emission computed tomography has high sensi-

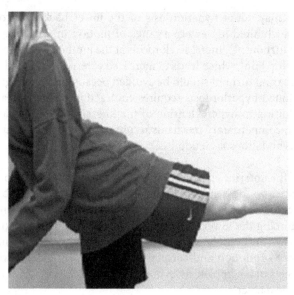

Fig 5. Arabesque dance position.

tivity but requires radiation exposure. Magnetic resonance imaging is associated with concerns about adequate visualization of stress injuries, but it does show soft tissue injuries and does not require radiation exposure. Treatment is aimed at pain resolution and bone healing (more apt to occur in the preadolescent than the older dancer), which requires rest from dancing until complete resolution of pain and dedicated physical therapy to correct the mechanical concerns that led to the injury. More than 80% of patients treated nonoperatively have resolution of symptoms.[20]

The sacroiliac joint is fundamentally involved in all actions of the spine and hip that are key to executing many dance elements. Movement of the sacroiliac joint helps decrease forward shearing at the L5/S1 junction during hip extension of gait.[22] Any restriction of sacroiliac joint mobility may disturb the mechanics of the spine and pelvis, leading to injury of the low back. Although opinions vary throughout the literature, many health professionals who specialize in dance medicine believe that sacroiliac dysfunction is the most common cause of low back pain in dancers.[22] Problems in either the lumbar spine or the hip may additionally manifest as pain in the sacroiliac joint, which can be viewed as a bridge between those 2 areas.

Examination should include palpating the posterior superior iliac spine while the patient bends forward with superior movement indicating decreased mobility of the joint on the side or using the Gilette or Stork test to assess sacroiliac mobility (Figure 6). Therapy should focus on mobilization on the lumbar spine and later attention to the sacroiliac joint.

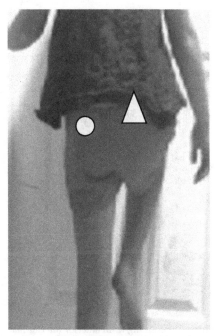

Fig 6. Normal Gilette or Stork test. With knee flexion, the ipsilateral posterior superior iliac spine (triangle) should be lower than the stance leg posterior superior iliac spine (circle). With restricted sacroiliac mobility, knee flexion leads to level or even raised ipsilateral posterior superior iliac spine.

TURNOUT IN CLASSICAL BALLET POSITIONS: EFFECT ON KNEES, ANKLES, AND FEET

All ballet movements start from 1 of 5 classical positions, each of which requires external rotation of the lower extremities for the orientation known as *turnout*. Ballet dancers devote immense time toward obtaining ideal turnout, which is defined as a 180-degree angle between the feet and knees of both legs.[23] Many dancers compensate for less than optimal external rotation by increasing lumbar lordosis, externally rotating the lower leg, everting the heels, and pronating the feet.[17,18] Increased stress of the knees, ankles, and feet by forcing turnout from the floor up instead of hips down can predispose the dancer to overuse injuries. The hyperflexible joints that enable dancers to achieve extreme range of motion may augment the risk for injury because the muscles are not strong enough in extremes of motion to bear the impact on the musculoskeletal system.[24]

Knee injuries account for 14% to 17% of injuries seen in dancers.[13] The patellofemoral joint is often a source of pain because of the multiple different forces on the joint. The joint consists of the patella and trochlear groove of the femur. It is evaluated by assessing the quadriceps angle (Q angle), which is formed by the lines connecting the anterior superior iliac spine and connecting the patella to the ante-

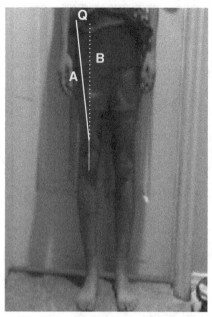

Fig 7. Q angle (Q) made from line running from anterior inferior iliac spine to patella (A) and extension of line running from patella to tibial tubercle (B).

rior tubercle (Figure 7). The Q angle tends to increase in females during the adolescent growth spurt because of widening of the pelvic region. Increased Q angles greater than 10 degrees in men and 15 degrees in skeletally mature women indicate laterally directed forces on the patella,[13] which can result in pain from abnormal contact forces and muscle traction forces between the patella and femur.

The quadriceps tendon places additional forces on the patella from its pull on the fixed patellar tendon insertion, which compresses the patella into the trochlea groove. Relative increased tightness of the lateral quadriceps, hamstrings, and iliotibial during the adolescent growth phase creates an even greater increased risk for patellofemoral disorders.

Additional forces leading to knee injury can be attributed to poor technique while dancer attempt to obtain ideal turnout. These forces can be assessed by having the dancer assume turnout in the second position (see Figure 2). A forced turnout from the knee creates a direction of force from the body, leg, and knee that is medial to foot rather than through the second metatarsal. This results in abnormal tensile forces directed across the medial aspect of the knee, leading to increased risk for patellofemoral pain or stress syndrome, patellar subluxation, and dislocation.[13,25,26]

Forcing turnout through excessive pronation of the foot also can lead to many ankle and foot injuries, including those of the flexor hallucis longus (FHL) and posterior tibialis tendons.

The FHL and posterior tibialis tendons can be placed under increased tension and compression when there is lack of appropriate alignment because of forced turnout. Dysfunction FHL tendon leads to pain in the tarsal tunnel as the tendon passes through the medial and lateral aspects of the posterior talus before entering the tarsal tunnel to exit under the flexor retinaculum.[27] Excessive pronation of the foot makes resupinating the foot to go en pointe more difficult, leading to potential entrapment and FLH tenosynovitis. Posterior tibialis tendinitis also can occur from forced turnout as a result of increased shear and tensile forces across the medial and lateral soft tissues of the foot and ankle secondary to malalignment.

EN POINTE: FOOT AND ANKLE CONCERNS

Advanced ballet dancers spend a great deal of time en pointe, which places them at risk for foot injuries while they are in full en pointe and ankle injuries while they are in slight dorsiflexion (known as demi-pointe) (Figure 8). While the dancer is in the full en pointe position, the ankle is relatively stable because the posterior lip of the tibia rests and locks on the calcaneus and the subtalar joint is locked with the heel in forefoot and varus.[27,28]

A dancer is more likely to acquire a midfoot than ankle sprain while en pointe.[22] Midfoot sprains result from a loss of balance while en pointe and performing spins leading to a hyperplantarflexion injury. Lisfranc injuries involve fractures or fracture-dislocations of the tarsometatarsal joint, usually between the lateral aspect of the medial cuneiform and medial base of second metatarsal with avulsion fractures of the Lisfranc ligament.[29] Less common midfoot injuries include

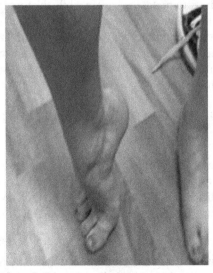

Fig 8. Demi-pointe position in ballet.

injuries to the dorsal ligaments between the talus and navicular or the calcaneus and cuboid.

The ankle is vulnerable to inversion injury when the dancer moves into slight dorsiflexion from the en pointe position. As the ankle progressively inverts, greater pressure is placed on the lateral ankle ligaments, particularly the anterior talofibular ligament. The talus is wider anteriorly and more narrow posteriorly. The inherent instability of the more narrow posterior talus combined with the vertical alignment of the anterior talofibular ligament place the ankle at risk for inversion while in plantarflexion but less so in the more stable en pointe position.

Underlying hypermobility and a history of ankle sprains are strong predictive factors for ankle sprains. Hypermobility of the ankle joint causes forces at the foot to be transferred proximally in suboptimal fashion, thus leading to injury.[30] The incidence of recurrent injury after initial acute ankle sprain has been reported to be as high as 70% in dancers.[28] Ankle sprains lead to reduced subtalar and ankle motion, which can result in increased compensatory stresses on muscle tendon units contributing to reinjures.[28] Impaired balance and proprioception can follow ankle sprains and last for several weeks after injury despite active rehabilitation.[28] Increased risk for injury can occur if neuromuscular coordination is not fully restored.

Dancers are susceptible to several unique fractures of the fifth metatarsal bone. Avulsion fracture of the styloid process of the fifth metatarsal, involving a fracture line perpendicular to the long axis of the bone, is associated with lateral ankle sprains because it usually is caused by sudden inversion of the foot. Acute metaphyseal-diaphyseal junction fractures, known as Jones fractures, occur with adduction of the fifth metatarsal, often while the foot is plantarflexed. They have a predilection for malunion because of the poor blood supply given that the metaphyseal-diaphyseal junction is a vascular watershed zone. Oblique spiral fracture through the mid to distal portion of the fifth metatarsal are known as dancer's fractures and usually occur with twisting or inversion of the foot while the dancer is on demi-pointe.

REPETITIVE LANDING AND JUMPING RESULTING IN FOOT AND SHIN INJURIES

The repetitive nature of dance training can lead to many overuse injuries involving the feet and shins, especially if dancers have any underlying limiting anatomy, poor form, or insufficient rest. The spectrum of repetitive overload injury ranges from soft tissue injury to bone stress reactions (increased bone resorption and production without frank fracture line) and eventually true stress fractures.

Hallux rigidus is caused by repetitive flexion and hyperextension of the metatarsophalangeal joint. It usually is the result of pronation of the great toe when the dancer attempts to force turnout. This movement restricts full dorsiflexion of the first metatarsophalangeal joint, with resultant prominent spur formation on the dorsal aspect of the first metatarsal head that prevents performing full relevé. Many dancers accommodate for this limitation by supinating the foot, which can lead to ankle sprains and fractures of the fifth metatarsal.[13]

A shin splint, or medial tibial stress syndrome, is a traction periostitis associated with diffuse anteromedial or posteromedial tibial pain that typically involves the distal third of the tibia. Medial tibial stress syndrome usually occurs at the beginning of the season after a long period of inactivity, whereas tibial stress fractures usually occur in the middle to late seasons. Lower-risk tibial stress fractures involve the proximal lateral or distal medial tibia. Dancers also are at risk for high-risk traction fractures of the anterior tibial cortex, which present as acute disability in male dancers after they land from a jump or more insidiously in female dancers who often have poor bone health because of components of the female athlete triad.

The sesamoid bones are at risk for stress injury given their vulnerable location beneath the base of the first metatarsal in the substance of the flexor hallucis brevis tendon. An exaggerated turned out position can lead to sesamoid overload because of rolling out, which increases medial loading of the first metatarsophalangeal joint.[27] The medial sesamoid bears more stress when dancers are in relevé and when they walk turned out because the line of progression exiting the foot is forced more medially under the first metatarsophalangeal joint rather than moving laterally between the first and second toes.

Another common site of stress fractures in dancers is the base of the second metatarsal, which is the longest metatarsal and therefore bears the bulk of weight while in the dancer is in the demi-pointe position. The distal aspect of the fibula, usually 10 cm above the lateral malleolus in the distal third of the shaft, also may be prone to stress fractures, which usually occur in the weight-bearing leg. Such fractures frequently occur when the dancer initiates a turn and are caused by poor balance and fatigue. Any medial midfoot pain, namely, in the dorsal aspect of the navicular bone, must be fully assessed for a navicular stress fracture, which is a high-risk traction injury that can result from repetitive jumping and landing on a plantarflexed foot.

In most stress fracture injuries, plain films typically are negative, so diagnosis requires MRI. Rest from loading activities for a minimum of 4 weeks usually is necessary for healing. During this time, a dancer can utilize yoga, Pilates, water-based exercise, and other nonimpact forms of rehabilitation to correct biomechanical issues that predisposed to the initial injury. Higher-risk stress fractures, such as the anterior tibial cortex and tarsal navicular, require initial nonweight-bearing on the injured limb, prolonged rest (several months), or surgical intervention and have a higher risk of adversely influencing the dancer's career.

INJURY PREVENTION RECOMMENDATIONS

Members of the dance medicine team should use the following guidelines to help educate and advocate for adolescent dancers and families.

- The American Academy of Pediatrics recommends rest periods from organized physical activity that include a minimum of 1 full day off per week and 2 to 3 months off per year.[31]
- Emerging evidence suggests that the risk of injury increases when the number of hours of organized sport/dance activity per week exceeds the age of the child in number of years (eg, a 14-year-old girl should not exceed 14 hours per week of organized dance activities).[32]
- Single sport or activity specialization at young ages can increase the risk of physical and emotional overuse, frequently leading to burnout and complete cessation of activity. Particular warning signs may include decreased interest in dance activities, lower school grades and attendance, less social interaction, changes in appetite or sleep, and mood alterations such as irritability, anger, or anhedonia. Incorporating recommended weekly and annual rest intervals along with varying the types of organized activities can reduce the potential for burnout.[2,31] (See *Overuse and Overtraining Injuries in Teenage Athletes*, pp. 79-99 in this issue.)
- Medical practitioners may be asked for their opinion on the readiness of young dancers to begin dancing en pointe, which is an advanced ballet skill that places extreme stress on the lower leg, ankle, and foot. Readiness recommendations focus not on chronologic age but on the presence of adequate whole body strength and balance (especially of the foot and ankle), lack of current restricting injuries, sufficient "pre-pointe" dance class exposure (minimum 3-4 years), and the future goals of the dancer.[33] Screening tests that can assess appropriate proximal strength, proprioception, and placement of extremities not only for pointe but for higher-level leaping are given in Table 1.

Table 1
Clinical screening tests for pointe readiness[33-35]

Screening test	Description
Airplane test	Dancer stands on 1 leg with the other leg in arabesque (hip extension; Figure 5. Dancer then must be able to perform 4 of 5 controlled pliés to touch hands to floor without the knee collapsing or losing balance.
Single-leg sauté test	Dancer performs 16 single-leg jumps (sautés), with at least 8 of 16 involving proper pelvic control and toe before heel landing. Test on both legs.
Topple test	From the 4th ballet position, dancer performs a series of outward turns (pirouettes) and must maintain balance without any lateral trunk movements.

- Medical professionals should maintain an open dialogue about adequate intake of calories and essential vitamins and minerals, and maintenance of healthy weight to best support ongoing dance activities.
- Physicians should respect the anatomic and emotional changes that occur during puberty without hesitating to modify or change focus to more basic skills to allow compensation for changes in movement patterns and coordination.

References

1. Russell JA. Preventing dance injuries: current perspectives. *Open Access J Sports Med.* 2013;4:199-210
2. DiFiori JP, Benjamin HJ, Brenner JS, et al. Overuse injuries and burnout in youth sports: a position statement from the American Medical Society for Sports Medicine. *Clin J Sports Med.* 2014;24(1):3-20
3. Burckhardt P, Wynn E, Krieg MA, Bagutti C, Faouzi M. The effects of nutrition, puberty and dancing on bone density in adolescent ballet dancers. *J Dance Med Sci.* 2011;15(2):51-60
4. Georgopoulos NA, Roupas ND, Theodoropoulou A, et al. The influence of intense physical training on growth and pubertal development in athletes. *Ann N Y Acad Sci.* 2010;1205:39-44
5. Steinberg N, Siev-Ner I, Peleg S, et al. Injuries in female dancers aged 8 to 16 years. *J Athl Train.* 2013;48:118-123
6. Mountjoy M, Sundgot-Borgen J, Burke L, et al. The IOC consensus statement: beyond the female athlete triad: relative energy deficiency in sport (RED-S). *Br J Sports Med.* 2014;48:491-497
7. De Souza MJ, Nattiv A, Joy E, et al. 2014 Female Athlete Triad Coalition consensus statement on treatment and return to play of the female athlete triad: 1st International Conference held in San Francisco, California, May 2012, and 2nd International Conference held in Indianapolis, Indiana, May 2013. *Clin J Sport Med.* 2014;24(2):96-119
8. Sousa M, Carvalho P, Moreira P, Teixeira VH. Nutrition and nutritional issues for dancers. *Med Probl Perform Art.* 2013;28:119-123
9. Golden NH, Carlson JL. The pathophysiology of amenorrhea in the adolescent. *Ann N Y Acad Sci.* 2008;1135:163-178
10. Loud KJ, Gordon CM. Adolescent bone health. *Arch Pediatr Adolesc Med.* 2006;160:1026-1032
11. Wyon M. Preparing to perform: periodization and dance. *J Dance Med Sci.* 2010;14:67-72
12. Schoene L. Biomechanical evaluation of dancers and assessment of their risk of injury. *J Am Podiatr Med Assoc.* 2007;97:75-80
13. Solomon R. The young dancer. *Clin Sports Med.* 2000;19:717-739
14. Shan G. Comparison of repetitive movements between dance and ballet dancers and martial artists: risk assessment of muscles overuse injuries and prevention strategies. *Res Sports Med.* 2005;13:63-76
15. d'Hemecort PA, Gerbino PG II, Micheli LJ. Back injuries in the young athlete. *Clin Sports Med.* 2000;19:663-679
16. Purcell L, Micheli L. Low back pain in young athletes. *Sports Health.* 2009;1:212-222
17. Steinberg N, Siev-Ner I, Peleg S, et al. Extrinsic and intrinsic risk factors associated with injuries in young dancers aged 8 to 16 years. *J Sports Sci.* 2012;30:485-495
18. Coplan JA. Ballet dancers' turnout and its relationship to self-reported injury. *J Orthop Sports Phys Ther.* 2002;32:579-584
19. Koutedakis Y, Jamurtas A. The dancer as a performing athlete: physiological consideration. *Sports Med.* 2004;24:651-661
20. Hu SS, Tribus CB, Diab M, Ghanayem AJ. Spondylolisthesis and spondylolysis. *J Bone Joint Surg.* 2008;90:656-671

21. Haidar R, Saad S, Khoury NJ, Musharrafieh U. Practical approach to the child presenting with back pain. *Eur J Pediatr.* 2011;170:149-156
22. DeMann LE. Sacroiliac dysfunction in dancers with low back pain. *Man Ther.* 1997;2:2-10
23. Toledo DT, Akuthota V, Drake DF, Nadler SF, Chou LH. Sports and performing arts medicine. 6. issues relating to dancers. *Arch Phys Med Rehabil.* 2004;85:75-78
24. Liederback M. General considerations for guiding dance injury rehabilitation. *J Dance Med Sci.* 2005;4:54-65
25. Steinberg N, Siev-Ner I, Peleg S, et al. Injury patterns in young, non-professional dancers. *J Sports Sci.* 2001;29:47-54
26. Motta-Valencia K. Dance related injury. *Phys Med Rehabil Clin N Am.* 2006;17:697-723
27. Macintyre J, Joy E. Foot and ankle injuries in dance. *Clin J Sports Med.* 2000;19:351-368
28. O'Laughlin PF, Hodgkins CW, Kennedy JG. Ankle sprains and instability in dancers. *Clin Sports Med.* 2008;27:247-262
29. Goulart M, O'Malley MJ, Hodgkins CW, Charlton TP. Foot and ankle fractures in dancers. *Clin Sports Med.* 2008;27:296-304
30. Foss KD, Ford KR, Myer GD, Hewet TE. Generalized joint laxity associated with increased medial foot loading in female athletes. *J Athl Train.* 2009;44:356-363
31. Brenner JS; American Academy of Pediatrics Council on Sports Medicine and Fitness. Overuse injuries, overtraining and burnout in child and adolescent athletes. *Pediatrics.* 2007;119:1242-1245
32. Jayanthi N. Intense, specialized training in young athletes linked to serious overuse injuries. April 22, 2013. Available at: www.loyolamedicine.org/newswire/news/intense-specialized-training-young-athletes-linked-serious-overuse-injuries. Accessed December 16, 2014
33. Shah S. Determining a young dancer's readiness for dancing on pointe. *Curr Sports Med Rep.* 2009;8:295-299
34. Elias E, Kruse D. Injury prevention guidelines. In: Koutures CG, Wong VYM, eds. *Pediatric Sports Medicine: Essentials for Office Evaluation.* Thorofare, NJ: SLACK; 2013:25
35. Walters E. Preparing for pointe work. CHKD Sports Medicine Blog. March 21, 2014. Available at: chkdsportsmed.com/2014/03/21/preparing-for-pointe-work. Accessed December 16, 2014

Adolesc Med 026 (2015) 163–173

Mental Health and Pressures in Teen Sports

Susannah M. Briskin, MD[a]*;
Kelsey Logan, MD, MPH[b]

[a]Assistant Professor of Pediatrics, Division of Pediatric Sports Medicine, Rainbow Babies
and Children's Hospital, Cleveland, Ohio; [b]Associate Professor of Pediatrics and Internal Medicine,
University of Cincinnati College of Medicine, Director, Division of Sports Medicine,
Cincinnati Children's Hospital Medical Center, Cincinnati, Ohio

INTRODUCTION

Within the United States, 60 million children between the ages of 6 and 18 years participate in some form of organized athletics.[1] Team sports participation accounts for approximately 27 million of these children, and individual sports account for the remainder.[1] Beyond the well-known physical benefits of sports are the multiple social and mental health benefits. For youth, these include the development of self-discipline, self-esteem, and valuable skills such as leadership, coping, and teamwork.[2] Participation in sports for 6- to 18-year-olds has a positive association with lower anxiety, fewer symptoms of depression, and improved academic performance.[3,4]

STRESS AND PRESSURES IN SPORTS

In general, physical activity is known to improve the psychological profile of adolescents and adults. Participation in sports can provide the benefit of reducing stress.[5,6] Exercise is a physical outlet for individuals of all ages, and it can help people develop important coping skills, especially related to stress. Sports provide a break from academics, can be fun, and can serve as a good opportunity for social interactions with peers. Whether this positive effect is the result of the social support experienced by many athletes, the cognitive benefits, or the biologic changes that occur with physical activity is largely unknown.

*Corresponding author
E-mail address: Susannah.briskin@uhhospitals.org

Some research has been done on the interaction of physical activity with positive body image and self-esteem. A study of college-aged women found that increased involvement with physical activity decreased symptoms of social phobia, generalized anxiety disorder, and obsessive-compulsive disorder.[7] Particularly important reductions were improvements in appearance, self-reported body fat, strength, and coordination.[7]

Sports can cause stress because of familial pressures to succeed, conflicts with coaches or teammates, and injuries.[8] Reeves et al[9] performed a longitudinal study on stress and youth soccer. They found that stressful experiences on the field include situations in which an athlete makes a mental or physical error, receives a bad call from an official, witnesses another athlete's cheating, or sees another athlete performing well. Sports-associated stress can cause loss of sleep or appetite, contribute to injury, affect the athlete's performance, and decrease enjoyment and satisfaction associated with playing sports.[10]

Parents can sometimes be the source of an athlete's stress. Negative parental behaviors include placing too much pressure on an athlete, being critical of an athlete's performance, placing an overemphasis on winning, being controlling or overinvolved, and engaging in a negative communication style.[11] An athlete's attitude, level of enjoyment, perception of achievement, his own expectation level, and his view of his own capabilities all are affected by the parent's behavior and attitude.[12,13] As parental pressure on the athlete increases, the child's reported enjoyment and satisfaction have been found to decrease.[14] In contrast, Sánchez-Miguel et al[15] found that as parents' support levels increased, the athlete's enjoyment level also increased. Therefore, parental behaviors have a direct effect on an athlete's enjoyment level.

Coaches also affect an athlete's self-perception and behavior.[16] Unfortunately, they often have minimal insight into the developmental issues, such as social pressures, that young athletes face. Adolescent athletes sometimes are subjected to demeaning behavior, including bullying, from their coaches.[17] Therefore, both parents and coaches may serve as sources of stress for youth athletes. A study of high-level athletes reported that 3% had been subjected to violence, with "verbal harassment or aggressions" being most common.[18]

Parents and coaches may directly influence how an athlete learns to cope.[19] Based on Lazarus' model of cognitive-motivational-relational theory, coping is defined as a "conscious effort of someone to manage demands that exceed one's resources or are considered taxing."[20] When an athlete is stressed, he may seek out social support, focus on improving technical skills, work harder, ignore the stressor, try to distance himself from the stressor, or use wishful thinking as tactics to reduce stress.[21] Because of the physical and psychological demands of their chosen sports, athletes often are unaware of abnormal negative consequences. For example, female athletes who overtrain (and undernourish) may experience amenorrhea and not realize that this is a red flag for more concerning medical problems. They may accept it as "normal" within certain sports since other athletes are also experiencing it. Also a gymnast may continue to practice with an arm or leg in a cast, just to avoid disapproval by coaches or teammates. This exemplifies how athletes are often not educated about how to manage stress within their athletic environment and how coping mechanisms vary by sport.

A large study of elite French adolescent and young adult athletes had several interesting psychological findings.[18] Athletes 17 years and younger were most likely to have at least 1 psychological disorder compared to those aged 22 years and older who were least likely. Generalized anxiety was the most prevalent issue across all ages. Depression, which is the largest mental health problem in the United States and many other countries, was much less likely in this group of French elite athletes.[22] Female athletes were 1.3 times more likely than male athletes to have at least 1 disorder, and the rate was even higher for anxiety disorders.[18] Generalized anxiety disorder had the highest prevalence in the so-called "aesthetic sports" (eg, figure skating, gymnastics, and synchronized swimming). The authors proposed that athletes participating in these sports are so dependent on judgment by others for their success that their perceived lack of power over this judgment negatively affects their self-esteem, which ultimately could lead to issues with anxiety or depression.

THE ELITE ATHLETE

Within recent decades, increased intensity of training that begins in early to middle childhood has become the trend within youth sports. Pressure from parents and coaches is common, and children often are encouraged to specialize in a single sport at a young age. This is referred to as *early sport specialization*. These youth exclude other sports and focus year-round on skill development and preparation at intense levels for a single sport.[23] Early sports specialization exposes young athletes to longer practice times, fewer days off, more intense competition, and tedious travel schedules. In return, they have less time to focus on their academic obligations and partake in other social activities. Early sports specialization has been linked to increased overuse injury rates, risk for quitting sports at a young age, and psychological stress.[24-26]

When an athlete competes at a high level, the culture around that athlete often changes. For many athletes who specialize in 1 sport and train extensively with the goal of select junior, college, or Olympic participation, the key relationships for the athlete become focused around those related to the sport. These relationships ultimately may replace those relationships considered typical for the adolescent, such as teachers and classmates. For example, an elite athlete who chooses alternative schooling (eg, online courses or homeschooling) can become isolated from school teachers and classmates. Coaches and teammates become increasingly important, and disruptions in those relationships can cause the athlete significant stress. Parents and other family members also can become stressed about the demands of the sport. It is essential for the physician to proactively discuss these issues with the high-level adolescent athlete and to recognize these relationships when dealing with the athlete's psychological stress. Internal and external sport pressures can be stressors and serve as catalysts for psychopathology. For example, the pattern of "obsessive attitudes towards exercising" can lead to negative psychological and physical conditions.[27]

SPORT TRANSITIONS

Athletes who give up a sport to which they were committed for a long time often also give up a significant part of their self-identify. Whenever athletes conclude their athletic "careers," the transition can be difficult and stressful. Athletes may undergo an adjustment-related depression as they lose their self-identity, struggle to find purpose, and have a difficult time finding new ways to cope and relieve stress.[28] Individuals may also feel a sense of failure if they couldn't make the team. This is common when athletes transition between middle and high school, a time when most youth already are struggling to find their identity.

Because the transition away from competitive sports is challenging, athletes may be tentative about expressing their desire to stop playing their sport. Frequent injuries or a hesitancy to return to sport after injury should be considered potential red flags that an individual may not want to return. Assessing an individual's desire to return to the sport, without the parent present, can be helpful in identifying individuals who may be ready to transition out of competitive sports. In these situations, the physician often has to help open lines of communication between the parent and the child, and sometimes with the coach.

As athletes transition from high school to college sports, they may face new and unique pressures. Some athletes may move from being 1 of the strongest members of a team to being among the weakest. They may have considerably less playing time, and they may have to deal with no longer being the focus of attention as they were in high school.[29] Balancing the demands of increased academic work with the greater time commitment of collegiate level sports is another adjustment for most athletes. Physicians can help athletes as they transition to college sports by discussing these areas of potential stress with them and helping them anticipate these challenges. Physicians also can aid athletes by identifying resources on their college campus should they require support services.

BURNOUT

Burnout occurs when an athlete decides to stop participating in sport as a direct result of the chronic stress associated with it. When an athlete feels that the demands being placed on him are excessive, his stress is increased. The athlete's stress level then can exceed his ability to cope, and he can develop exhaustion. This is the main symptom associated with burnout (see *Overuse and Overtraining Injuries in Teenage Athletes,* section on Overtraining Issues, pp. 79-99 in this issue).[30] Athletes with burnout also can develop changes in mood state, including depression, anger, and increased tension.[31] Athletes may experience a reduced sense of athletic accomplishment and may begin to devalue their sport participation.[32,33] Withdrawal is believed to occur when the athlete perceives he can no longer meet the physical and psychological demands of the sport.[10] When the exhaustion and mood symptoms are accompanied by an elevated heart rate, chronic muscle or joint pain, and impaired performance in sports or cognitive performance in school, the diagnosis of overtraining should be considered. This falls within the same spectrum as burnout but is characterized by the physiologic changes.[31,34]

Factors related to burnout can be categorized as personal characteristics and environmental factors. Personal characteristics that are related to burnout include nonassertive personality, an overfocus on one's athletic involvement, low self-esteem, high anxiety, a strong need to please others, and perfectionism. Several studies have demonstrated a negative relationship between optimism and both stress and burnout.[30,35,36] Environmental factors include extremely high training volumes and time demands, high performance expectations, frequent intense competition, inadequate social support, critically evaluated performance, little control over one's sports decision-making, and inconsistent coaching.[10,23,37,38] Females and athletes in individual sports who are participating at a very high level are thought to be at greatest risk for burnout.[38,39]

Not all withdrawals from sport are because of burnout. Athletes who discontinue sports do so for a variety of reasons. The most common reasons are time conflicts and interest in other activities. However, injury, low amount of playing time, lack of success or enjoyment, slow skill development, and boredom all may contribute to the decision to stop a sport.[40,41]

The diagnosis of burnout can be challenging. A thorough history should be completed with both the athlete and parent. Detailed information about frequency, duration, and intensity of practice sessions, competitions, and recovery time should be gathered. The physician should perform an in-depth assessment of sleep and nutrition habits because these factors can affect energy levels and mood. A complete physical examination to evaluate for physiologic changes associated with overtraining and other systemic conditions that can cause fatigue should be performed. Separating the athlete and parent for part of the history and physical examination will allow the athlete an opportunity to speak directly to the physician about his feelings and to be more forthcoming about his desire to withdraw from a sport.

DISORDERED EATING

Athletes with eating disorders have compromised physical and mental health and often have issues with athletic performance. Anorexia nervosa, bulimia nervosa, and eating disorder not otherwise specified are the conditions commonly considered when discussing eating disorders in athletes. The reported overall prevalence of eating disorders in athletes has not been consistent, ranging from as low as 5% up to 33%.[42] In addition, many athletes have disordered eating (DE) behaviors that do not fully meet the criteria for diagnosis (see *The Female Athlete Triad: Energy Deficiency, Physiologic Consequences, and Treatment,* section on Long-Term Bone Health and the Female Athlete Triad, pp. 126-127 in this issue) but still are at risk for psychological and physical harm.

Even without a diagnosable eating disorder, some traits of DE can be present and should be monitored for the athlete's health. Research has shown several recurring issues that should alert a physician that an athlete may be at risk for DE. Known risk factors for eating disorders are dissatisfaction with body image, perfectionism, an overachieving nature, lack of a support system or coping skills, and low self-esteem. When these risk factors are combined with the sport culture's increasing emphasis on low body weight, fitness, leanness, and speed, athletes may attempt to cope by exerting control over their body size and shape, leading to DE practices. Whether actual pressure to reach a particular weight or body composition is imposed by a sport or the athlete perceives it to be, it is the "preoccupation with dieting" that is seen as the most important trigger for DE.[43] In addition, evidence is emerging that underlying personal psychological issues, such as body uneasiness and anxiety traits, are associated with the risk for DE, independent of the level of competition.[44,45]

Pressure to control or lose weight, or to have a particular body shape (eg, among dancers), can lead to DE behaviors. Often these pressures are external. Franseen and McCann[46] studied US female Olympic athletes from 18 sports. In their study, athletes reported that coaches put the most pressure on them to lose weight. Parents, teammates, media, and magazines also were perceived sources of pressure. In a study of almost 1000 adolescent swimmers, external (societal) pressures caused more maladaptive weight control practices than did athlete concerns about swimming performance.[47] Although certain sports traditionally have been thought of as being higher risk for DE (eg, gymnastics, figure skating, long-distance running, and other endurance sports), the differentiation between sports and DE risk is less clear. One study found similar numbers of college female athletes to be at risk for DE, regardless of whether they were involved in a "lean-build" or "non–lean-build" sport.[48]

A study of 411 British young adult athletes explored the relationship between personal attachment style and risk for DE behaviors. Insecure (ie, anxious or avoidant) attachment styles had higher scores for eating psychopathology, with higher levels of depression and self-critical perfectionism and lower levels of self-esteem.[49] These attachment styles were independent of sport involvement and indicate that screening for relationship issues related to attachment style could help identify athletes at risk for DE. Counseling these athletes on these preexisting issues, similar to the risk factors identified earlier, could help prevent negative energy balance and its associated physical harms among athletes and improve psychological health in general.

Although it is common to think about female athletes when addressing DE, male athletes also can struggle with these issues. Sports that emphasize weight control and have weight classes, such as wrestling, often encourage DE (eg, fasting and dehydration before matches, large weight swings depending on season of competition) in their culture. Other sports associated with DE practices are distance running, bodybuilding, and horseracing (jockeys).

Anxiety and depression are common comorbid diagnoses in patients with anorexia nervosa, bulimia nervosa, and other eating disorders. Comorbid conditions must be addressed before DE behaviors can be changed. For athletes with bulimia nervosa, shame is common; they are distressed by their behavior. Patients with these diagnoses may not recognize their behavior as pathologic nor acknowledge the medical consequences of their behavior.

It is essential that the physician establish a good, trusting rapport with these patients. Pointing out performance issues rather than first focusing on the DE practices themselves may help the athlete initially discuss the problem.

Finally, the physician should realize that DE may not be intentional. Most adolescent athletes are not well educated about the nutritional needs for optimal growth, much less for their sport and performance. It is common for athletes to significantly increase the time or intensity of exercise without increasing caloric intake. Over time, this negative energy balance can lead to physical problems associated with eating disorders (eg, low bone mineral density, bony stress injuries, and amenorrhea) without the psychological aspects of DE. Simple education about the physical demands of a particular sport and the nutrition needed to support it can be sufficient to bring the athlete back to health. Physicians with adequate training may be a good position to address the requirements of a sport and counsel the athlete on potential issues (see *The Female Athlete Triad: Energy Deficiency, Physiologic Consequences, and Treatment*, section on Medical Nutritional Therapy, pp. 128-129 in this issue).

THE PHYSICIAN'S ROLE

It is beneficial to discuss sports opportunities with families early, when their child is still a toddler. It is at this young age that parents often initiate sports participation for their child.[50] Sports such as swimming, dance, gymnastics, and even soccer are offered for children in the toddler age range. These activities emphasize gross motor skills and often are an appropriate selection for the first sports experience. The physician can provide appropriate anticipatory guidance for readiness to a family who is considering starting their child in organized sports. By assessing a child's motor, cognitive, sensory, and social/emotional development, the physician may be able to offer an appropriate recommendation. Finding a sport with demands that match a child's growth and development is crucial for the child's enjoyment and success.[41,42] Providing this guidance to parents may help prevent unrealistic parent/coach expectations of a young child as well as help prevent the child's dropout from sports or loss of self-esteem.[51]

Physicians can play a crucial role in setting reasonable expectations and encouraging appropriate goals within sports. Coaches often are the greatest factor in encouraging an athlete to increase the intensity of training or to specialize in a single sport.[51,52] Physicians can help parents determine an athlete's developmental readiness to take this next step. As the child advances into more intense or specialized training, parents become more invested in their child's sports participation, making significant financial, emotional, and time commitments. The price that is often paid, both emotionally and psychologically, may not be considered as the adolescent advances through the competitive ranks and engages in increasingly more intense and complex sport schedules. The physician can help the adolescent and the family recognize the potential benefits, as well as the potential harms, of this level of participation. Families can invest thousands of dollars annually in sports participation fees, equipment, training time, travel, and coaching for an adolescent to participate in a year-round competitive sport.[53] However, many parents view this investment as necessary to put their child in the best possible position to obtain a college scholarship. Unfortunately, in reality very few youth athletes ever reach this level.

Depending on the sport, between 3.3% and 11.3% of all high school athletes continue to play sports at the NCAA level. Only 3 in 50 seniors on high school soccer teams ever play in college.[54] Unfortunately, most of these athletes play at a Division II and III level and are not eligible for an athletic scholarship. In fact, only about 2% of high school athletes are granted an athletic scholarship to an NCAA school. At the Division I level, not all athletes earn scholarships, and those who do may receive partial tuition scholarships, which cover only a portion of the total cost to attend a 4-year university.[55] Explaining these statistics to families may help them appreciate the challenge of earning an athletic scholarship. Therefore, physicians should emphasize the emotional and physical benefits of sports participation, rather than the potential for financial gain.

Physicians can provide guidance for healthy sports participation. They can educate families about the risks associated with early sports specialization and encourage appropriate limitations in training workload based on current recommendations from groups such as the American Academy of Pediatrics and the American Medical Society for Sports Medicine.[52] Because the parents' behavior can directly affect how an athlete views sports participation, physicians can review with parents the importance of serving as good role models and educate them on how to provide positive support for the young athlete.

References

1. National Council of Youth Sports. Report on Trends and Participation in Organized Youth Sports 2008. Available at: www.ncys.org/pdfs/2008/2008-ncys-market-research-report.pdf. Accessed September 3, 2014
2. Malina R. The young athlete: biological growth and maturation in a biosocial context. In: Smoll F, Smith R, eds. *Children in Youth Sports: A Biosocial Perspective*. Dubuque, IA: Brown and Benchmark; 1996:161-186
3. Strong W, Malina R, Blimkie C, et al. Evidence based physical activity for school-age youth. *J Pediatr*. 2005;146:732-737
4. Biddle S, Asare M. Physical activity and mental health in children and adolescents: a review of reviews. *Br J Sports Med*. 2011;45:88-95
5. Scully D, Kremer J, Meade M, Graham R, Dudgeon K. Physical exercise and psychological well-being: a critical review. *Br J Sports Med*. 1998;32:111-120
6. Hudd S. Stress at college: effects on health habits, health status, and self-esteem. *Coll Student J*. 2000;34:217-227
7. Herring M, O'Connor P, Dishman R. Self-esteem mediates associations of physical activity with anxiety in college women. *Med Sci Sports Exerc*. 2014;46:1990-1998
8. Kimball A, Freysinger V. Leisure, stress, and coping: the sport participation of collegiate student-athletes. *Leisure Sci*. 2003;25:115-141
9. Reeves C, Nicholls A, McKenna J. Longitudinal analyses of stressors, perceived control, and coping effectiveness among early and middle adolescent soccer players. *Int J Sport Psychol*. 2011;42:186-203
10. Matos N, Winsley R, Williams C. Prevalence of nonfunctional overreaching/overtraining in young English athletes. *Med Sci Sports Exerc*. 2011;43:1287-1294
11. Lauer L, Gould D, Roman N, Pierce M. Parental behaviors that affect junior tennis player development. *Psychol Sport Exerc*. 2010;11:487-496
12. Fredericks J, Eccles J. Parental influences on youth involvement in sports. In: Weiss M, ed. *Developmental Sport and Exercise Psychology: A Life-Span Perspective*. Morgantown, WV: Fitness Information Technology; 2004:145-164
13. Tofler I, Knapp P, Drell M. The achievement by proxy spectrum: historical perspective and clinical approach to pressured and high-achieving children and adolescents. *Child Adolesc Psychiatr Clin N Am*. 1998;7:803-820
14. Anderson J, Funk J, Elliot R, Smith P. Parental support and pressure and children's extracurricular activities: relationships with amount of involvement and affective experience of participation. *Appl Dev Psychol*. 2003;24:241-257
15. Sánchez-Miguel P, Leo F, Sánchez-Oliva D, Amado D, García-Calvo T. The importance of parents' behavior in their children's enjoyment and motivation in sports. *J Human Kinet*. 2013;36:169-177
16. Weiss M, Bredemeier B. Moral development in sport. *Exerc Sport Sci Rev*. 1990;18:331-377
17. Alexander K. Stafford A, Lewis R. *The Experiences of Children Participating in Organised Sport in the UK*. Edinburgh, Scotland: The University of Edinburgh/NSPCC Child Protection Research Centre; 2011
18. Schaal G, Tafflet M, Nassif H, et al. Psychological balance in high level athletes: gender-based differences and sport-specific patterns. *PLoS One*. 2011;6:e19007
19. Tamminen K, Holt N. Adolescent athletes' learning about coping and the roles of parents and coaches. *Psychol Sport Exerc*. 2012;13:69-79
20. Lazarus R. *Stress and Emotion: A New Synthesis*. New York: Springer; 1999
21. Holt N, Hoar S, Fraser S. How does coping change with development? A review of childhood and adolescent sport coping research. *Eur J Sport Sci*. 2005;5:24-39
22. US Burden of Disease Collaborators. The state of US health, 1990-2010: burden of diseases, injuries, and risk factors. *JAMA*. 2013;310:591-608
23. Malina R. Early sports specialization: roots, effectiveness, and risks. *Curr Sports Med Rep*. 2010;9:364-371

24. Gould D, Udry E, Tuffey S, Loehr J. Burnout in competitive junior tennis players: 1. A quantitative psychological assessment. *Sport Psychol.* 1996;10:322-340
25. Jayanthi N, Pinkham C, Dugas L, Patrick B, Labella C. Sports specialization in young athletes: evidence-based recommendations. *Sports Health.* 2013;5:251-257
26. Wall M, Cote J. Developmental activities that lead to dropout and investment in sport. *Phys Educ Sport Pedagog.* 2007;12:77-87
27. Silva L, Gomes A, Martins C. Psychological factors related to eating disordered behaviors: a study with Portugese athletes. *Spanish J Psychol.* 2011;14:323-335
28. Tofler I, Butterbaugh G. Developmental overview of child and youth sports for the twenty-first century. *Clin Sports Med.* 2005;23:783-804
29. Pritchard M, Wilson G, Yamnitz B. What predicts adjustment among college athletes? *J Am Coll Health.* 2007;56:15-21
30. Gustafsson H, Kenttä G, Hassmén P. Athlete burnout: an integrated model and future research directions. *Int Rev Sport Exerc Psychol.* 2011;4:3-24
31. Smith A, Link A. Sport psychology and the adolescent athlete. *Pediatr Ann.* 2010;29:310-316
32. Gustafsson H, Hassmén P, Kenttä G, Johansson M. A qualitative analysis of burnout in elite Swedish athletes. *Psychol Sport Exerc.* 2008;9:800-816
33. Raedeke T, Smith A. Development and preliminary validation of an athlete burnout measure. *J Sport Exerc Psychol.* 2001;23:281-306
34. Brenner JS; American Academy of Pediatrics Council on Sports Medicine and Fitness. Burnout in child and adolescent athletes. *Pediatrics.* 2007;119:1242-1245
35. Crosno J, Rinaldo S, Black H, Kelley S. Half full or half empty: the role of optimism in boundary-spanning positions. *J Serv Res.* 2009;11:295-309
36. Hayes C, Weathington B. Optimism, stress, life satisfaction, and job burnout in restaurant managers. *J Psychol.* 2007;141:565-579
37. Faigenbaum A, Kraemer W, Blimkie C, et al. Youth resistance training: updated position statement paper from the National Strength and Conditioning Association. *J Strength Cond Res.* 2009;23(Suppl 5):S60-S79
38. Cresswell S. Possible early signs of athlete burnout: a prospective study. *J Sci Med Sport.* 2009:12:393-398
39. Raglin J, Sawamura S, Alexiou S, Hassman P, Kentta G. Training practices and staleness in 13-18-year-old swimmers: a cross-cultural study. *Pediatr Exerc Sci.* 2000;12:61-70
40. Gould D. Understanding attrition in children's sport. In: Gould D, Weiss M, eds. *Advances in Pediatric Sport Sciences.* Champaign, IL: Human Kinetics; 1987:61-86
41. Malina R. Readiness for competitive youth sport. In: Weiss M, Gould D, eds. *Sport for Children and Youths.* Champaign, IL: Human Kinetics; 1986:45-50
42. Patel D, Greydanus D, Pratt H, Phillips E. Eating disorders in adolescent athletes. *J Adolesc Res.* 2003;18:280-296
43. Bonci C, Bonci L, Granger L, et al. National Athletic Trainers' Association position statement: preventing, detecting, and managing disordered eating in athletes. *J Athl Train.* 2008;43:80-108
44. Ravaldi C, Vannacci A, Zucchi T, et al. Eating disorders and body image disturbances among ballet dancers, gymnasium users and body builders. *Psychopathology.* 2003;36:247-254
45. Vardar E, Vardar S, Kurt C. Anxiety of young female athletes with disordered eating behaviors. *Eat Behav.* 2007;8:143-147
46. Franseen L, McCann S. Causes of eating disorders in elite female athletes: the United States Olympic Committee Study. *Olymp Coach.* 1996;6:13-14
47. Drummer G, Rosen L, Heusner W, et al. Pathogenic weight–control behaviors of young competitive swimmers. *Phys Sportsmed.* 1987;15;75-83
48. Beals K, Manore M. Disorders of the Female Athlete Triad among collegiate athletes. *Int J Sport Nutr Exerc Metab.* 2002;12:281-293
49. Shanmugam V, Jowett S, Meyer C. Eating psychopathology amongst athletes: links to current attachment style. *Eat Behav.* 2011;13:5-12

50. Baxter-Jones A, Maffulli N; TOYA Study Group. Parental influence on sport participation in elite young athletes. *J Sports Med Phys Fitness*. 2003;43:250-255

51. DiFiori J, Benjamin H, Brenner J, et al. Overuse injuries and burnout in youth sports: a position stand from the American Medical Society for Sports Medicine. *Br J Sports Med*. 2014;48:287-288

52. Hill G, Simons J. A study of the sport specialization on high school athletics. *J Sport Soc Issues*. 1989;13:1-13

53. King M, Rothlisberger K. Family financial investment in organized youth sport. January 1, 2014. Research On Capitol Hill 2014. *Research on the Hill (Salt Lake City)*. Paper 17. Available at: digitalcommons.usu.edu/poth_slc/17. Accessed February 17, 2015

54. National Collegiate Athletic Association. Estimated probability of competing in athletics beyond the high school interscholastic level. September 24, 2013. Available at: www.ncaa.org/sites/default/files/Probability-of-going-pro-methodology_Update2013.pdf. Accessed September 27, 2014

55. National Center for Education Statistics. Who reports participation in varsity intercollegiate sports at 4-year colleges? December 1996. Available at: nces.ed.gov/pubs/web/97911.asp. Accessed September 27, 2014

Adolesc Med 026 (2015) 174–188

Performance-Enhancing Substances

Joseph N. Chorley, MD*;
Roberta H. Anding, MS, RD/LD, CDE, CSSD

*Baylor College of Medicine, Texas Children's Hospital, Department of Pediatrics,
Section of Adolescent Medicine and Sports Medicine, Houston, Texas*

PERFORMANCE-ENHANCING SUPPLEMENTS

Every 2 years, the world watches as elite athletes compete in the Olympics. Their hard work and dedication may be rewarded with a gold medal that signifies that they are the best in the world in their sport. The Olympic motto of "Citius, Altius, Fortius" (faster, higher, stronger) motivates athletes and many young people to continually strive to improve and pursue their dreams of excellence. The reality of this level of competition is much less idyllic. In the classic *Sports Illustrated* interview of elite Olympic athletes in 1997, 98% of athletes would take a performance-enhancing substance if they would win and not be caught for doping. More disturbing, if they could take a substance that would be undetectable and they would win all their competitions for the next 5 years and then die, 50% still would take the supplements.[1] The rewards for success have become so alluring that common sense arguments will not change risky behavior. Physicians who treat children and adolescents must understand the reasons for the use of performance-enhancing substances, the risks and purported benefits, and the safe, effective alternatives.

DEFINITIONS AND CATEGORIZATION OF SUPPLEMENTS

The 1994 Dietary Supplement Health and Education Act (DSHEA) significantly liberalized the definition of dietary supplements (DS) and markedly increased their availability in the United States. It also significantly limits the ability of the US Food and Drug Administration (FDA) to regulate DS, does not ensure the

---

*Corresponding author
E-mail address:* jchorley@bcm.edu

quality of products, and does not require research for the recommended dosage. A DS is a product that is intended to supplement the diet and contains 1 or more of the following: a vitamin, a mineral, an herb or other botanic, or an amino acid.[2] A subgroup of DS are *performance-enhancing supplements,* which improve sports performance by increasing strength, power, speed, or endurance or by altering body weight or body composition. Substances that improve performance by causing changes in behavior, arousal level, or perception of pain should be considered performance enhancing.[3] The World Anti-Doping Agency (WADA) defines a performance-enhancing drug (PED) as any substance or method that meets any 2 of the following 3 criteria: (1) it has the potential to enhance or enhances sports performance; (2) it represents an actual or potential health risks to the athlete; and (3) it violates the spirit of sport.

These drugs include anabolic steroids and their precursors, erythropoietin, hormone manipulation, metabolic modulators (eg, insulins), blood manipulators, gene doping, stimulants, and narcotics. In order to ensure safe use of all these substances by athletes, they have been categorized into 4 groups according to scientific merit.[4]

1. Group A (approved DS): There is evidence that they "provide true performance benefit when used according to a specific protocol in specific situation"
2. Group B (DS under consideration): They have insufficient evidence of efficacy
3. Group C (DS with no clear proof of beneficial effects)
4. Group D (banned DS): "directly banned by the WADA Code or provide a high risk of producing positive doping outcome"

This categorization has been adopted recently by the American College of Sports Medicine (ACSM), the American Dietetic Association (ADA), and the Dietitians of Canada.[5]

EPIDEMIOLOGY: NATIONAL POPULATION SURVEYS IN THE UNITED STATES

In the United States, sales of DS grew from $27 billion in 2009 to $37.6 billion in 2014.[6] Adolescents are a significant driving market for this industry. In 2012, a study showed that 1.2 million athletes younger than 18 years in the United States reported using a DS specifically to enhance sport performance in the past 30 days.[7] Multivitamin/mineral supplements accounted for 90% of the DS used, and creatine for 2%.[7] In surveys of older children, creatine use is higher, especially in males. Annual use increases by age (males: middle school 3%-4%, high school 11%-17%; females: middle school 1%-2%, high school 6%-9%) and was relatively stable from 2005 to 2013.[8,9] A higher proportion of creatine users also use androstenedione and anabolic androgenic steroids (AAS) compared to non-creatine users.[8] The use of androstenedione (4%) and AAS (2%) in high school males peaked in 2001 (the same year that Barry Bonds set the single-season Major League Baseball home run record). The prevalence of steroid use in males is approximately twice that of age-matched females. Most studies have shown that overall use has decreased by 40% to 50% in the past 10 years (androstenedione 0.7%, AAS 1.3%).[8,10] Use of human growth hormone (hGH) has been considered low (5%) and stable until a recent study showed a marked increase in the annual prevalence to 11% of high school students.[11] This increase may be related to more 1-time users (experimenters), but with the high cost of hGH, studies are needed to clarify this trend.[7-11]

HIGH SCHOOL USE OF DS

The National Federation of High School Associations reports that in 2013, high school sports participation was at an all-time high with 7.7 million participants (58% male, 42% female). Football has nearly twice the number of participants (1,086,627) than other sports (male: track/field 580,672, basketball 538,676; female: track/field 472,939, basketball 433,120).[12] Adolescent athletes, especially males, are more likely to use protein or other muscle-enhancing substances compared to females (Table 1). The same trend exists when comparing high school to middle school male students (use of protein odds ratio 1.70, other muscle-enhancing substances odds ratio 1.73). Those participating on sports teams were significantly more likely to report more "muscle-enhancing behaviors," specifically, to change their diet and be more likely to exercise and use protein supplements than those not involved in sports. Steroid use is similar among athletes and non-athletes.[13] Rates of DS use have been reported as high as 58% among high school athletes.[14] In the transition from adolescence to adulthood, young adult males who played a sport in high school were 15.6% more likely to use legal performance-enhancing DS and were 2.7% more likely to use steroids than their non-athletic peers. This effect was less significant in former female high school athletes compared to female non-athletes.[15] Adolescents who strength train at a non-school-based workout facility may be exposed to increased availability of PEDs. A survey at workout facilities found that 18% of

Table 1
Muscle-enhancing behavior among adolescents < 18 years within the past year

	Percentage of males	Percentage of females
Exercise more	80	63.8
Protein powder	18.7	8.2
Steroid use	3.1	1.2
Other substance use	6.4	2.3

From Eisenberg ME, Wall M, Neumark-Sztainer D. Muscle enhancing behaviors among adolescent girls and boys. *Pediatrics.* 2012;130:1019-1026.

males reported use of androstenedione or other adrenal hormones, 25% reported ephedrine use, and 5% reported anabolic steroid use.[16]

COLLEGE USE OF DS

The National Collegiate Athletic Association (NCAA) reported that from 2012 to 2013, 265,645 male and 203,565 female athletes competed in collegiate sports (Divisions I, II, and III).[17] College athletes demonstrate a higher use of DS (as high as 88%) than high school athletes. The most commonly used DS were vitamins (73%), herbs (21%), calorie replacement drinks (47%), protein (40%), and creatine (31%).[18] Three percent of male NCAA student athletes admitted to using at least 1 of the 11 illegal PEDs.[19] The NCAA uses the National Center for Drug-Free Sport to provide information on medications and DS to their athletes. From 2009 to 2010, 89% of inquiries were for DS. Most inquiries coincided with the beginning of the school year, and football accounted for a disproportionately higher number of inquiries (24%). The most common DS inquiries were for amino acids (20%), vitamins (19%), herbs (13%), creatine (10%), stimulants (9%), and nitric oxide (7%).[20]

REASONS FOR USING DS

Health care professionals providing care for an athlete who admits to using or has questions about performance-enhancing DS should explore the athlete's motivations.[3] Motivation for DS use is different for each individual, but there are some patterns of use. In high school athletes, males are more concerned about gaining muscle and increasing energy, while females are more interested in preventing illness and increasing energy.[14] Pursuit of muscularity and low body fat has become important for athletes and non-athletes, especially related to their body image.[21] Male adolescents (aged 11-21 years) who were more dissatisfied with their bodies or were attempting to lose or gain weight were more likely to support doping in sport.[22] In the general population, overweight and obese males and females were more likely to report protein powder and steroid use than those with an average body mass index.[13,23-25]

The reasons for use of performance-enhancing supplements in college have been studied primarily in athletes. Athletes who perceive their competition is gaining a performance edge by using DS or PED may be more likely to use.[26,27] Male athletes reported a higher use for increasing size, speed, and power, and for general performance enhancement.[28] Female athletes were more concerned with body fat and health benefits (weight loss and multivitamin DS) compared to male athletes.[29,30] Male and female athletes in the non-lean sports (eg, basketball, football, lacrosse, softball) were more likely to use DS that purported to increase muscle mass than did those in the lean sports (eg, swimming, wrestling, track and field, gymnastics).[31] In collegiate non-athletes, the highest likelihood of using illicit PEDs, such as AAS, was in those who used supplements advertised to burn fat and build muscle. Independent of gender, the strongest predictor of positive belief about AAS was body image disturbance, compulsive exercise, illicit drug use, and perfectionism.[32]

RISK FOR OTHER HIGH-RISK BEHAVIORS

While assessing for motivation for DS use, health care professionals should evaluate for other substance use. Twenty-nine percent of adolescents report lifetime use of herbal or other natural products to feel better or to perform better in sports or school. Adolescents using these products were more likely to have used cigarettes or marijuana (2.2 times), alcohol (3.5 times), inhalants (4.4 times), cocaine (5.9 times), methamphetamines (6.8 times), intravenous drugs (8.1 times), heroin (8.8 times), and AAS (14.5 times).[33]

Although a comprehensive review of DS and PEDs is beyond the scope of this article, specific information about the most often used DS will allow health care professionals to provide accurate information to adolescents. Creatine is one of the most popular performance-enhancing supplements. Elite and non-elite athletes are increasingly using hGH. Nitrates are the newest DS to gain the attention of athletes, especially at the collegiate level.

Creatine

The performance-enhancing ability of creatine is based on the anaerobic phosphate system, which supplies energy for short-burst, high-intensity exercise for 5 to 8 seconds. Creatine phosphate is able to rapidly rephosphorylate adenosine diphosphate (ADP) to adenosine triphosphate (ATP) in working muscles. Creatine is produced endogenously but requires 1 g/day from the diet to maintain homeostasis. Creatine stores are located in skeletal muscle (95%), and intracellular creatine concentration is regulated by the creatine transporter proteins, which are located in the plasma and mitochondrial membranes.[34] Higher extracellular creatine concentration will facilitate intracellular transport. Carbohydrate (CHO) ingestion increases total muscle creatine related to insulin's stimulation of the creatine transporter system.[35] A common creatine use protocol starts with a 5-day loading phase of 20 g/day, then a maintenance dose of 3 to 5 g/day until discontinuing use of the supplement.

In the adult male population of athletes, creatine demonstrates improvement in anaerobic performance, especially in activities with repeated short-burst exercise to exhaustion, such as football and soccer. Increased lean muscle mass also has been demonstrated, but some of this effect is related to fluid retention required with creatine storage. Performance outcomes indicate there are individual differences in response to creatine use. "Responders" have a greater proportion of type II (fast twitch) muscle fibers and lower muscular creatine and phosphocreatine concentrations than "nonresponders."[36] Because muscle biopsy is required to obtain this information, it is not feasible to screen an individual's potential to respond to creatine supplementation. The ACSM states that the evidence on potential and real side effects of creatine supplementation in the population younger than 18 years is inadequate to formulate valid conclusions as to the risk-to-benefit ratio of creatine supplementation. Thus, creatine supplementation is not advised for the pediatric population (ie, <18 years of age).[37] Although the American Academy of Pediatrics agrees with this recommendation,[3] the International Society of Sports Nutrition states that younger athletes could consider taking creatine if they are postpubertal, are involved in training that may benefit from creatine supplementation, and are eating an appropriate diet. Furthermore, the athletes and their parents should understand the effects of creatine and approve of its use. A "quality" creatine should be used (those certified by NSF International), should not exceed the "recommended dosage" (mentioned above), and should be supervised by the athlete's parents, trainers, coaches, and physician.[38]

Human Growth Hormone

Human growth hormone (hGH) is released under the control of gonadotropin hormone-releasing factor in a pulsatile manner at all ages, but the amplitude of the pulses is 3 times higher during the adolescent physiologic growth spurt than in the prepubertal period.[39] Endogenous hGH release can be stimulated by deep sleep, exercise, heat stress, hypoglycemia, and some amino acids. It is inhibited by obesity, a CHO-rich diet, and medications (eg, beta-2 agonists, clonidine, L-DOPA, estrogens).[40] Supplements advertised as growth hormone stimulators under DSHEA (not the FDA) often use this information to entice sales with little evidence of efficacy. Prescribing hGH is tightly regulated by federal legislation, and hGH use for athletic performance is a felony punishable by 5 to 10 years in prison.[41]

The benefits of hGH for athletes have been described in the nonmedical literature for 30 years. As with AAS, the doses of hGH in years past were well above physiologic replacement requirements, and its efficacy in the gym and field of competition was recognized much earlier than in the scientific community. The effects of hGH in individuals with growth hormone deficiency include improved aerobic fitness (VO_{2max}) as a result of increased erythropoiesis and cardiac output, and increased lean mass as a result of lipolysis of adipose tissue and increased protein synthesis.[42] Scientific studies have found these effects to not be statistically significant in normal subjects and athletes.[43] Athletes probably use higher dosing regimens than those used in scientific studies, which may be sufficient for a performance effect that could provide a competitive advantage. The Mitchell report in 2007 described growth hormone abuse in Major League Baseball as widespread,[44] and the 1996 Atlantic Olympic Games have been called the "Growth Hormone Games."[45] Drug testing for hGH is based on the measurement in blood samples of the ratio of isoforms of hGH, and the test result will be positive for only 10 to 20 hours after administration. Given this brief detection period, no positive tests have been reported in the Olympics, but some Olympians have admitted use as part of drug investigations. Research to improve hGH drug testing is ongoing and will help identify its abuse. The side effects of hGH in a non–growth hormone-deficient individual may include carpal tunnel syndrome, fluid retention, and acromegaly. We do not endorse hGH use in non–growth hormone-deficient individuals.

Nitrates

Dietary nitrates have been linked with cardiovascular health and improvement in athletic performance.[46] Nitrates are converted to nitrites and then to nitric oxide, which is an effective and powerful vasodilator. Most dietary nitrate (80%–95%) comes from fruits and vegetables (eg, spinach, celery, beet root, lettuce, leeks, parsley), and a diet with high fruit and vegetable content (at least 5-7 servings) will lower the risk of heart disease and high blood pressure. The higher nitrate content of the Mediterranean diet may be responsible for its blood pressure-lowering effect.[47] The average consumption of dietary nitrate from food in European countries is 31 to 185 mg/day and is 40 to 100 mg/day in the United States. Most dietary nitrite comes from nitrite food additives and added nitrite in processed cured meats and baked goods and cereal.[48]

The VO_2 at a given exercise intensity was significantly reduced with the use of beet root juice, which allowed athletes to perform at higher intensity at a lower percentage of their maximum (5% reduction of VO_{2max} with moderate intensity, 1%-2% reduction of VO_{2max} in high-intensity endurance training).[49-51] Given that the daily amount of beet root juice (500 mL) needed to affect exercise performance is not practical, most athletes use a nutritional product. Long-term studies on the safety and adverse reactions of beet root juice products have not been performed. We recommended including beets and other high nitrate foods in the athlete's diet.

THE ATHLETE'S PLATE

The most effective and healthy ways to improve performance is to optimally meet each athlete's unique needs. The concept of the "athlete's plate" emphasizes that the nutritional requirements for sports are specific to the type, intensity, and duration of activity. In adolescence, the energy demands for growth and development must be added. The science for the nutrient requirement in sports is strong. The challenge is providing these recommendations in a way that are understandable and practical.

Carbohydrate

Carbohydrate (CHO) is the primary fuel of exercising muscle and the central nervous system. Although keto-adaptation from fat and gluconeogenesis from protein can meet some of the body's energy needs, CHO remains the primary fuel for the young exercising athlete. Carbohydrate needs are based on the intensity and duration of activity and can be quantified as grams per kilogram

Table 2
Carbohydrate needs based on intensity and duration of sport

Training type		Recommended grams carbohydrate per kilogram body weight
Light-weight management	Low-intensity skill based	3-5
Moderate	1 h/day	5-7
High	Endurance 1-3 h/day of moderate-to high-intensity practices	6-10
Intense	Extreme commitment 4-5 h/day, with 2 practices per day	8-12

(Table 2).[52] For many high school athletes, it is not game day or the event that drives CHO need but rather practice. For example, a 100 m-sprinter runs 10 to 13 seconds during a race and thus requires minimal total energy, whereas training involves interval work and core work for an hour per day. The quality of CHO is a key component of an athlete's plate. The focus should be on minimally processed whole grains (oatmeal, 100% whole wheat bread, 100% whole grain cereals) and moderation of the portion size and the amount of dietary fat consumed along with the CHO. Defining quality CHO includes the glycemic index, glycemic load, fiber, and nutrients in these foods.

Glycemic index (GI) quantifies CHO-containing foods according to their ability to elevate plasma glucose rapidly or slowly. Glycemic index is the ratio of the area under the blood response curve of glucose for a portion of food that contains 50 g of available CHO divided by 50 g of reference food (glucose or white bread).The GI is classified as low (<55), moderate (55-70), or high (>70).[53] In athletic performance, both low and high glycemic foods have a role in performance and recovery from sport. Whereas GI illustrates the glycemic response to a defined portion of CHO, the amount of food eaten is the major determinant of postprandial hyperglycemia. Atkinson et al[53] compiled data on the GI and glycemic load (GL) for nearly 2500 foods.

Glycemic load is defined as GI times the amount of food eaten (in grams). For a single serving, GL is considered high (>20), medium (11-19), or low (<10). Foods that have a high GI may have a low GL if the amount eaten is a standard serving. For example, watermelon has a GI of 72, yet given the serving size of watermelon, the GL is only 4. Because meals consist of more than CHO, other dietary components may affect the postprandial rise in blood sugar. Ice cream is one such example. Given the high fat content of the food, the postprandial rise in blood sugar is blunted, but this does not make this food an everyday choice. Mixed food, or foods with a substantial amount of low glycemic sugars such as fructose or undesirable amounts of fats, can contribute to energy density, a low GI, and undesirable health outcomes. However, when the focus is on patterns of food intake and not just the contribution of the GI and GL of a single food, some trends exist.

An ad lib, low GI diet may be more effective in reducing obesity than a traditional calorie-controlled diet in which energy is controlled but the quality of CHO is not.[54] Low GI diets can promote weight loss and improved glycemic control in persons at risk for diabetes. Recommending higher CHO availability for athletes undergoing intense training should focus on those food sources that promote long-term health and improved athletic performance. When planning diets for athletes, there may be some advantages to stressing the use of low glycemic CHOs in pre-competition meals. During exercise, this strategy will provide continued availability of CHO. In contrast, a high glycemic meal can be used in the postexercise period to promote rapid restoration of the glycogen used during sustained aerobic exercise. For postexercise recovery, 1 g CHO per kilogram body weight per hour within the first hour after exercise and an additional meal within 2 hours can promote glycogen restoration.[55] If CHO stores are exhausted (eg, after marathon, tournament), the athlete should consume 7 to 12 g/kg over the next 24 hours.[56] The addition of protein to the postexercise meal is controversial, and not all studies indicate that protein is needed in the recovery meal if CHO is adequate.

In addition to the GI, minimally processed CHO are good sources of fiber and magnesium, which are considered at-risk nutrients for children and teens. Currently, 90% of children and adolescents do not meet the Institute of Medicine recommendations for fiber.[57] Higher-fiber diets should be introduced gradually to reduce gastrointestinal stress, especially in athletes.

Busy practicing physicians need a method to recommend the appropriate amount of CHO to their athletic patients. Some CHO-containing foods and an estimate of the grams of CHO per serving are listed in Table 3. When recommending diets with high CHO availability, dairy products, grains, and fruits have the highest content per serving. The dietitians at the United States Olympic Committee developed a plate method for athletes based on the intensity and duration of physical activity to visually illustrate the amount of CHO needed

Table 3
Carbohydrate content of foods

Food	Serving size estimate	Grams carbohydrate
Milk, yogurt (plain)	8 ounces	12
Fruit	4 ounces juice, 1 medium piece	15
Vegetables	½ cup cooked, 1 cup raw	5
Breads, cereal, pasta, rice, potatoes	1 slice bread; ½-¾ cup cereal; ½ cup pasta, rice, potatoes	15
Meat		0
Fats, oils		0

Adapted from *The exchange list system for diabetic meal planning*. The American Diabetes Association and the American Dietetic Association, 1995. Available at: www.uaex.edu/publications/pdf/FSHED-86.pdf. Accessed March 13, 2015.

for easy, moderate, and hard training (www.teamusa.org/About-the-USOC/Athlete-Development/Sport-Performance/Nutrition/Resources-and-Fact-Sheets). This tool is now in the validation stage and represents an excellent graphic and teaching tool for patients (Figure 1).

Protein

Protein needs for adolescents are higher than those for adults: 1 g/kg vs 0.8 g/kg, respectively.[58-60] Although protein requirements increase during growth and development, national data suggest that adolescents overconsume protein, and 31% of adolescent boys aged 14 to 18 years consume more than twice the recommended daily allowance for protein.[61]

However, adolescents may be at risk for marginal or low protein intakes if they severely restrict calories, are vegans, or live in food-insecure households. Vegetarian and vegan diets can meet protein needs if they are well planned, requiring guidance from a registered dietitian nutritionist.[62] The primary role of protein is to build and repair tissue; however, just eating extra protein does not translate into more lean mass. Sex hormones are essential for accrual of lean weight, along with a quality strength program.[3] Protein needs can be estimated based on the type of exercise performed. Aerobically driven athletes require 1.2 to 1. 4 g/kg, and strength trained athletes need 1.2 to 1.7 g/kg.[62] Intakes of more than 2 g/kg per day do not confer any additional benefit, with few exceptions, such as during weight loss. Adolescents are better served meeting protein needs with food rather than protein supplements. As with CHO, the type of protein matters for muscle protein synthesis and optimal health. Whey and milk proteins have a

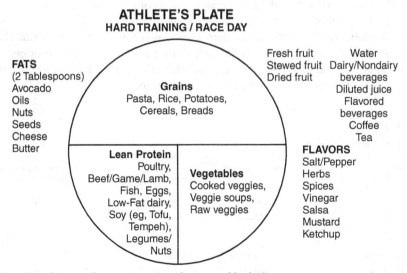

Fig 1. United States Olympic Committee dietitians athlete's plate.

unique role in the synthesis of mitochondrial and myofibrillar proteins. The benefit of diary protein may be linked to the rich content of branch chain amino acids, particularly leucine.[63] Lactose intolerance can be addressed by using lactose-reduced milks or lactase enzyme. The amount of protein needed at a meal to promote muscle protein is estimated to be between 20 to 40 g. Table 4 lists the protein content in some foods. For example, 2 scrambled eggs, 2 slices of toast, and an 8-ounce glass of milk provide 28 g of protein and the needed essential amino acids for muscular growth and development.

Dietary Fat

The diets of traditional athletes often focus on increased amounts of dietary fat to increase calories for weight gain. National surveys indicate that adolescents overconsume saturated fat and cholesterol.[62] Other athletes who wish to lose weight may significantly restrict dietary fat. All athletes benefit by choosing healthier monounsaturated fats such as olive or canola oil, regardless of their weight status. Higher-fat foods such as avocado, nut butters, and trail mix can increase the caloric density of a meal without a significant increase in volume. For athletes who have exceptionally high CHO needs, such as elite distance runners, choosing lower-fat foods and meats allows for the needed CHO and moderation of fat intake. Omega-3 fatty acids from coldwater fish, flax, and almonds are beneficial for athletes in promoting cardiovascular health and reducing inflammation and muscle soreness after exercise.[64] The American Heart Association recommends adolescents consume 2 coldwater fish meals per week.

Fruits and Vegetables

Children and adolescents do not consume the recommended daily amounts of fruit and vegetables.[65] A greater percentage of children aged 2 to 5 years consumed adequate fruits vegetables than did adolescents aged 12 to 19 in the United States.[65] As calorie needs increase during adolescence, the amounts of fruits and vegetables should increase. Lean athletes can drink 100% fruit juice as a valuable source of CHO, vitamin C, and potassium.

Table 4
Protein content of foods

Food	Serving size	Grams of protein
Milk, soymilk, yogurt	8 ounces	8
Fruit	4 ounces juices, 1 medium piece	0
Vegetables	½ cup cooked, 1 cup raw	2
Meat, beans, nut butters, eggs	1 ounce meat, ½ cup beans, 2 tbsp nut butter, 1 egg	7
Breads, grains, pasta, rice	1 slice bread; ½ cup cooked	3
Fats and oils	1 teaspoon	0

The role of fruits and vegetables in the athlete's diet is multifactorial. Fruits and vegetables are approximately 90% fluid, and as such they contribute a small amount of fluid to the diet. Given their high fluid volume, fiber, and low caloric density, fruits and vegetables contribute to increased satiety and are valuable in promoting calorie control and weight management. Fruits and vegetables are a rich source of vitamins and minerals, including vitamin B, vitamin C, beta-carotene, folic acid, potassium, magnesium, and others. Foods and teas rich in flavonoids have shown beneficial effects for the central nervous system.[66] Anthocyanins, a subset of flavonoids, are abundant in dark-colored fruit such as blueberries, Concord grapes, and acai fruits, and have been shown to possess potent antioxidant and anti-inflammatory activities. Tart cherries contain compounds associated with reduction of muscle soreness. Given the potential benefits of these fruits and vegetables, their consumption is recommended.

Polyphenolic compounds and their phytochemicals (concentrated in the pigments of fruits, vegetables, and spices) are being recognized for their nutritional importance and health benefits.[67] A common-sense approach is to choose a variety of fruits and vegetables with different colors on the plate to maximize the variety of these compounds. A good example is curcumin, found in turmeric, which reduces pro-inflammatory cytokines. In most studies, 150 to 500 mg of curcumin was sufficient to reduce the inflammatory response.[67] Curry spices combined with vegetables can provide a synergistic effect and benefit.

It is essential for physicians to understand the importance of body image and sports performance of adolescents. Physicians who discuss supplement use during health maintenance visits can provide adolescent athletes with effective, proven strategies of nutrition while they look for other health risk behaviors associated with DS use. The athlete's plate is an easy and effective strategy for planning diets and meal plan strategies that can assist young athletes to improve performance. When the diet is properly selected, nutrition status can be improved, with a resulting improvement in performance. More than just discussing optimal performance, it is important to emphasize the benefits of sports and competition. As the Olympic creed states: "The most important thing in the Olympic Games is not to win but to take part, just as the most important thing in life is not the triumph but the struggle. The essential thing is not to have conquered but to have fought well."

References

1. Bamberger M, Yaeger, D. Over the edge. *Sports Illustrated.* 1997:62-70
2. Public Law 103-417. Dietary supplement health and education act of 1994. 103rd Congress. October 25, 1994
3. Gomez JM, American Academy of Pediatrics Committee on Sports Fitness. Use of performance-enhancing substances. *Pediatrics.* 2005;115:1103-11064
4. Burke LM, Cort M, Cox GR, et al. Supplements and sports food. In: Deakin V, Burke LM. eds. *Clinical Sports Nutrition.* 3rd ed. Sydney, Australia: McGraw-Hill; 2006: 485-579

5. Rodriguez NR, DiMarco NM, Langley S. Position of the American Dietetic Association, Dietitians of Canada, and the American College of Sports Medicine on Nutrition and athletic performance. *J Am Diet Assoc.* 2009;109:509-527

6. Nutrition Business Journal Supplement Business Report 2013. In *Nutrition Business Journal*, edited by Penton Media Inc. Boulder, CO, 2013. Available at: www.marketresearch.com/Nutrition-Business-Journal-v2520/Supplement-Business-8436979. Accessed November 21, 2014

7. Evans MW Jr, Ndetan H, Perko M, Williams R, Walker C. Dietary supplement use by children and adolescents in the United States to enhance sport performance: results of the National Health Interview Survey. *J Prim Prev.* 2012;33:3-12

8. Johnston LD, O'Malley PM, Bachman JG, Schulenberg JE, Miech RA. *Monitoring the Future National Survey Results on Drug Use.* Ann Arbor, MI: Institute for Social Research, University of Michigan; 2014

9. Field AE, Austin SB, Camargo CA Jr, et al. Exposure to the mass media, body shape concerns, and use of supplements to improve weight and shape among male and female adolescents. *Pediatrics.* 2005;116:e214-e220

10. Kann L, Kinchen S, Shanklin SL, et al. Youth risk behavior surveillance—United States. *MMWR Surveill Summ.* 2014:1-168

11. The Metlife Foundation. 2010 Partnership Attitude Tracking Study sponsored by the Metlife Foundation and The Partnership at Drugfree.org. Released April 6, 2011. Available at: www.drugfree.org/wp-content/uploads/2014/05/FULL-REPORT-FINAL-PATS-Teens-and-Parent-April-6-2011-1.pdf. Accessed November 21, 2014

12. The National Federation of State High School Associations. 2012-13 high school athletics participation survey. Available at: www.nfhs.org/ParticipationStatics/PDF/2013-14%20NFHS%20Handbook_pgs52-70.pdf. Accessed November 21, 2014

13. Eisenberg ME, Wall M, Neumark-Sztainer D. Muscle-enhancing behaviors among adolescent girls and boys. *Pediatrics.* 2012;130:1019-1026

14. Kayton S, Cullen RW, Memken JA, Rutter R. Supplement and ergogenic aid use by competitive male and female high school athletes. *Med Sci Sports Exerc.* 2002;5S:193S

15. Dodge TL, Jaccard JJ. The effect of high school sports participation on the use of performance-enhancing substances in young adulthood. *J Adolesc Health.* 2006;39:367-373

16. Kanayama G, Gruber AJ, Pope HG Jr, Borowiecki JJ, Hudson JI. Over-the-counter drug use in gymnasiums: an underrecognized substance abuse problem? *Psychother Psychosom.* 2001;70:137-140

17. Irick E. NCAA sports sponsorship and participation rates report, 1981-2 to 2012-3. Available at www.ncaapublications.com/p-4334-1981-82-2012-13-ncaa-sports-sponsorship-and-participation-rates-report.aspx. Accessed November 21, 2014

18. Burns RD, Schiller MR, Merrick MA, Wolf KN. Intercollegiate student athlete use of nutritional supplements and the role of athletic trainers and dietitians in nutrition counseling. *J Am Diet Assoc.* 2004;104:246-249

19. Buckman JF, Farris SG, Yusko DA. A national study of substance use behaviors among NCAA male athletes who use banned performance enhancing substances. *Drug Alcohol Depend.* 2013;131:50-55

20. Ambrose PJ, Tsourounis C, Uryasz FD, Patterson E. Characteristics and trends of drug and dietary supplement inquiries by college athletes. *J Am Pharm Assoc.* 2013;53:297-303

21. Cafri G, van den Berg P, Thompson JK. Pursuit of muscularity in adolescent boys: relations among biopsychosocial variables and clinical outcomes. *J Clin Child Adolesc Psychol.* 2006;35:283-291

22. Yager Z, O'Dea JA. Relationships between body image, nutritional supplement use, and attitudes towards doping in sport among adolescent boys: implications for prevention programs. *J Int Soc Sports Nutr.* 2014;11:13

23. Cafri G, Thompson JK, Ricciardelli L, et al. Pursuit of the muscular ideal: physical and psychological consequences and putative risk factors. *Clin Psychol Rev.* 2005;25:215-239

24. Boutelle K, Neumark-Sztainer D, Story M, Resnick M. Weight control behaviors among obese, overweight, and nonoverweight adolescents. *J Pediatr Psychol.* 2002;27:531-540

25. Neumark-Sztainer D, Story M, Hannan PJ, Perry CL, Irving LM. Weight-related concerns and behaviors among overweight and nonoverweight adolescents: implications for preventing weight-related disorders. *Arch Pediatr Adolesc Med.* 2002;156:171-178

26. Papadopoulos FC, Skalkidis I, Parkkari J, Petridou E. Doping use among tertiary education students in six developed countries. *Eur J Epidemiol.* 2006;21:307-313

27. Mazanov J, Petroczi A, Bingham J, Holloway A. Towards an empirical model of performance enhancing supplement use: a pilot study among high performance UK athletes. *J Sci Med Sport Sports Med Austr.* 2008;11:185-190

28. Muller SM, Gorrow TR, Schneider SR. Enhancing appearance and sports performance: are female collegiate athletes behaving more like males? *J Am Coll Health.* 2009;57:513-520

29. Nieper A. Nutritional supplement practices in UK junior national track and field athletes. *Br J Sports Med.* 2005;39:645-649

30. Ziegler PJ, Nelson JA, Jonnalagadda SS. Use of dietary supplements by elite figure skaters. *Int J Sport Nutr Exerc Metab.* 2003;13:266-276

31. Rudd NA, Carter J. Building positive body image among college athletes: a socially responsible approach. *Clothing Textiles Res J.* 2006;49-64

32. Hildebrandt T, Harty S, Langenbucher JW. Fitness supplements as a gateway substance for anabolic-androgenic steroid use. *Psychol Addict Behav.* 2012;26:955-962

33. Yussman SM, Wilson KM, Klein JD. Herbal products and their association with substance use in adolescents. *J Adolesc Health.* 2006;38:395-400

34. Greenhaff PL, Bodin K, Soderlund K, Hultman E. Effect of oral creatine supplementation on skeletal muscle phosphocreatine resynthesis. *Am J Physiol.* 1994;266:E725-E7230

35. Green AL, Hultman E, Macdonald IA, Sewell DA, Greenhaff PL. Carbohydrate ingestion augments skeletal muscle creatine accumulation during creatine supplementation in humans. *Am J Physiol.* 1996;271:E821-E826

36. Snow RJ, Murphy RM. Factors influencing creatine loading into human skeletal muscle. *Exerc Sport Sci Rev.* 2003;31:154-158

37. Terjung RL, Clarkson P, Eichner ER, et al. American College of Sports Medicine Roundtable. The physiological and health effects of oral creatine supplementation. *Med Sci Sports Exerc.* 2000;32:706-717

38. Buford TW, Kreider RB, Stout JR, et al. International Society of Sports Nutrition position stand: creatine supplementation and exercise. *J Int Soc Sports Nutr.* 2007;4:6

39. Martha PM Jr, Rogol AD, Veldhuis JD, et al. Alterations in the pulsatile properties of circulating growth hormone concentrations during puberty in boys. *J Clin Endocrinol Metab.* 1989;69:563-570

40. Yilmaz D, Ersoy B, Bilgin E, et al. Bone mineral density in girls and boys at different pubertal stages: relation with gonadal steroids, bone formation markers, and growth parameters. *J Bone Miner Metab.* 2005;23:476-482

41. Rogol AD. Growth hormone and the adolescent athlete: what are the data for its safety and efficacy as an ergogenic agent? *Growth Hormone IGF Res.* 2009;19:294-299

42. Widdowson WM, Healy ML, Sonksen PH, Gibney J. The physiology of growth hormone and sport. *Growth Hormone IGF Res.* 2009;19:308-319

43. Birniece V, Nelson A, Ho K. Growth hormone administration: Is it safe and effective for athletic performance. *Endo Metab Clin North Am.* 2010;39(1):11-23

44. Mitchell GJ. Report to the commissioner of baseball of an independent investigation into the illegal use of steroids and other performance enhancing substances by players in major league baseball. Reported by Major League Baseball. 2007

45. Yesalis CE, Bahrke MS. Anabolic-androgenic steroids and related substances. *Curr Sports Med Rep.* 2002;1:246-252

46. Bryan NS. Pharmacological therapies, lifestyle choices and nitric oxide deficiency: a perfect storm. *Pharmacol Res.* 2012;66:448-456

47. Appel LJ, Obarzanek E, Vollmer WM, et al. A clinical trial of the effects of dietary patterns on blood pressure. *N Engl J Med.* 1997;336(16):1117–1124

48. Hord NG, Tang Y, Bryan NS. Food sources of nitrates and nitrites: the physiologic context for potential health benefits. *Am J Clin Nutr.* 2009;90:1-10
49. Larsen FJ, Weitzberg E, Lundberg JO, Ekblom B. Effects of dietary nitrate on oxygen cost during exercise. *Acta Physiol.* 2007;191:59-66
50. Cermak NM, Gibala MJ, van Loon LJ. Nitrate supplementation's improvement of 10-km time-trial performance in trained cyclists. *Int J Sport Nutr Exerc Metab.* 2012;22:64-71
51. Wylie LJ, Mohr M, Krustrup P, et al. Dietary nitrate supplementation improves team sport-specific intense intermittent exercise performance. *Eur J Appl Physiol.* 2013;113:1673-1684
52. Nutrition Working Group of the International Olympic Committee. Nutrition for Athletes. Athletes' Medical Information (Guide prepared by the Nutrition Working Group of the International Olympic Committee). 2012;1-66
53. Atkinson FS, Foster-Powell K, Brand-Miller JC. International tables of glycemic index and glycemic load values: 2008. *Diabetes Care.* 2008;31:2281-2283
54. Ebbeling CB, Leidig MM, Sinclair KB, Hangen JP, Ludwig DS. A reduced-glycemic load diet in the treatment of adolescent obesity. *Arch Pediatr Adolesc Med.* 2003;157:773-779
55. McLellan TM PS, Lieberman HR. Effects of protein in combination with carbohydrate supplements on acute or repeat endurance exercise performance: a systematic review. *Sports Med.* 2014;44(4):535-550
56. Tarnopolsky MA, Zawada C, Richmond LB, et al. Gender differences in carbohydrate loading are related to energy intake. *J Appl Physiol.* 2001;91:225-230
57. American Academy of Pediatrics Council on Sports Medicine and Fitness; McCambridge TM, Stricker PR. Strength training by children and adolescents. *Pediatrics.* 2008;121:835-840
58. Gong E, Heald F. *Diet, Nutrition and Adolescence: Modern Nutrition in Health and Disease.* Philadelphia: Lea & Febiger; 1994:759-769
59. Shils ME. National Dairy Council Award for Excellence in Medical and Dental Nutrition Education Lecture, 1994. Nutrition education in medical schools—the prospect before us. *Am J Clin Nutr.* 1994;60:631-638
60. Subcommittee on the Tenth Edition of the RDAs Food and Nutrition Board, Commission on Life Sciences, National Research Council. *Recommended dietary allowances.* Washington, DC: National Academy Press; 1989
61. Gleason PM, Suitor CW. Children's diets in the mid-1990s: dietary intake and its relationship with school meal participation. US Department of Agriculture, Food and Nutrition Service, Office of Analysis and Evaluation, Alexandria, VA; 2001, report no. CN-01-CD1. Available at: www.fns.usda.gov/childrens-diet-mid-1990s-dietary-intake-and-its-relationship-school-meal-participation. Accessed October 21, 2014
62. Ogata BN, Hayes D. Position of the Academy of Nutrition and Dietetics: nutrition guidance for healthy children ages 2 to 11 years. *J Acad Nutr Diet.* 2014;114:1257-1276
63. Phillips SM, Van Loon LJ. Dietary protein for athletes: from requirements to optimum adaptation. *J Sports Sci.* 2011;29(Suppl 1):S29-S38
64. Jouris KB, McDaniel JL, Weiss EP. The effect of omega-3 fatty acid supplementation on the inflammatory response to eccentric strength exercise. *J Sports Sci Med.* 2011;10:432-438
65. Nielsen SJ, Rossen LM, Harris DM, Odgen CL. Fruit and vegetable consumption of U.S. Youth, 2009-2010. NCHS Data Brief. 2014; No. 156;1-8
66. Meeusen R. Exercise, nutrition and the brain. *Sports Med.* 2014;44(Suppl 1):S47-S56
67. Prasad S, Gupta SC, Tyagi AK, Aggarwal BB. Curcumin, a component of golden spice: from bedside to bench and back. *Biotechnol Adv.* 2014;32:1053-64

Adolesc Med 026 (2015) 189–207

The Traveling Athlete

Holly J. Benjamin, MD, FAAP, FACSM[a]*;
Nicole T. Boniquit, MD[b];
Elisabeth S. Hastings, MPH, RD, CSSD, LD[c]

[a]Associate Professor of Pediatrics and Orthopedic Surgery, Director of Primary Care Sports Medicine, University of Chicago, Chicago, Illinois; [b]Resident Physician, Department of Pediatrics, University of Chicago, Chicago, Illinois; [c]Instructor, Baylor College of Medicine, Department of Pediatrics, Section of Adolescent Medicine and Sports Medicine, Houston, Texas

PREPARATION FOR TRAVEL

Adolescent athletes need to prepare mentally, physically, and logistically well in advance of traveling to a competitive event in order to increase their chances for success.[1] The basic components of any travel plan include making sure identification and passports are up-to-date, visas are in order (if needed), travel arrangements are finalized, housing and transportation are available upon arrival, and confirming that cash, checks, and credit cards are packed. Review of venue rules and regulations includes confirming all necessary paperwork, considering updated physical and dental examinations, checking immunization status, and determining whether any prophylactic medications are needed. Athletes with a chronic disease or who have a potentially life-threatening allergy should wear a medical identification bracelet and should always travel with up-to-date medical records, including documentation of prescription medications and proof of health insurance.[2,3] Use of the current US universal preparticipation screening evaluation form is recommended whenever possible for all athletes needing clearance to participate in sports at home or abroad.[4,5] All athletes younger than 18 years of age who are not traveling with a parent or guardian should have appropriate contact information in case consent for treatment is needed.

Further preparation includes verifying meeting places and times, especially if traveling in a group. Traveling in team uniforms allows for easy identification.

---

*Corresponding author
E-mail address: hbenjamin@peds.bsd.uchicago.edu

Equipment regulations should be verified ahead of time if traveling with sports equipment. Make sure adequate baggage allowance is available, and consider insurance for expensive equipment. Carry on important items for competition, such as shoes, uniforms, and small equipment whenever possible. Include a warm, comfortable change of clothes, which often is needed on long flights. Allow sufficient travel time to spare in case weather or other unforeseen circumstances result in delays, and consider a backup plan.[1]

Immunizations

Athletes should be up-to-date on immunization requirements, including tetanus, diphtheria, pertussis, measles, mumps, rubella, hepatitis B, hemophilus influenza B, varicella, and polio.[6] Immunizations that are optional for adolescents but are strongly encouraged include the human papilloma virus vaccine (HPV), meningococcal vaccine, pneumococcal vaccine, hepatitis A vaccine, and an annual flu shot. General immunization indications include (1) routine health maintenance; (2) catch-up immunizations; (3) high-risk groups; (4) close contact with a known infected individual; (5) recent exposure to an infectious agent; and (6) travel planned to an endemic area. Athletes who will be traveling internationally to endemic countries must allow for a minimum of 4 months to properly receive additional immunizations, such as yellow fever, typhoid, malaria, or cholera.[7] The Centers for Disease Control and Prevention (CDC) travel Web site (www.cdc.gov/travel/destinations/list) is an excellent resource for recommended immunizations as well as up-to-date information on current infectious disease outbreaks in countries of destination. All athletes should travel with proof of immunization status.[2,6]

Infectious Disease and Athletes

Mass sporting events have been associated with outbreaks of a variety of infectious diseases; therefore, athletes constitute a high-risk population.[8] Many unanticipated illnesses can occur during the course of traveling. Decisions to train or compete are based on general guidelines that pertain primarily to the illness or injury itself, with consideration of the venue setting. For example, several evidence-based guidelines are available to aid in determining sport participation for athletes with common conditions, including concussions, febrile illnesses (eg, influenza, infectious mononucleosis), chronic diseases, skin infections, and various orthopedic injuries.[3,4,9-15] Whether a physician is functioning as a team physician or is simply tasked with evaluating an athlete's health and readiness to participate in the activity, several important guidelines must be consistently followed to ensure safety (Table 1).[16-19] The physician must obtain a medical history and evaluate the illness or injury (including causality and natural history) and the known risks of participation during or immediately after diagnosis. Assessment of psychological factors, readiness, and coping mechanisms as well as performance of any diagnostic or functional testing necessary to determine

Table 1
Factors necessary to evaluate clearance for return to play

Health status (past medical history, family medical history, signs and symptoms of acute illness/injury)
Nature of illness/injury (mechanism of injury, natural history, participation risks)
Psychological factors (readiness, coping mechanisms)
Diagnostic and functional testing (may be sport specific, eg, gait assessment)
Participation risk of specific sport, position, and competitive level of play
Role of taping, bracing, or orthoses
Role of medical therapies (analgesics, injections, inhalers, fluids, topical agents)
Risk to other athletes (from contact with bracing or casting, disease transmission)

---

readiness to return to play are essential. An important part of evaluating the athlete's participation risk includes understanding the demands of the sport; the role of taping, bracing, or orthoses; and the role of medical therapies such as analgesics, topical agents, injections, inhalers, and fluids. With each athlete, a comprehensive treatment plan that includes short- and long-term treatment components and an appropriate timeline for restoration of musculoskeletal, cardiopulmonary, psychological, and neurologic function is needed. A brief assessment of the risks that clearance to play may pose to other athletes (eg, injury from contact with the brace or disease transmission) is required.[3,16-19] Once the evaluation is complete, the physician needs a system to ensure the appropriate medical documentation is completed and the return to play plan is communicated to the player, the family, coaches, athletic trainers, or any other personnel involved in the athlete's care.[20] Any requests for release of information should follow pre-established Health Insurance Portability and Accountability Act (HIPAA) compliance protocols.[4,16] The final steps in determining clearance are compliance with the rules and regulations of the governing bodies of certain sports as well as identification of applicable local, state, federal, or international regulations relevant to traveling to compete.[1,10,16,18-20]

Practical advice that is used frequently by physicians who communicate with parents and athletes is as follows: (1) Utilize a buddy system whenever there is a suspected injury, such as a concussion, so that the athlete is never alone in a locker room or a hotel room; (2) Do not treat potentially severe illnesses with excessive pain or anti-inflammatory medication in an attempt to let the athlete play; (3) Do not let the athlete drive if injured, particularly if there is a suspected head injury because slowed reaction times are common; (4) If a coach or physician at the venue contacts the parents to inform them that their child has been injured, the coach or physician then should attempt to monitor the child for signs of severe or worsening injury-related symptoms and be prepared to provide additional information or consent emergent treatment is needed.[3,4,8-11] If a musculoskeletal injury occurs, guidelines to withhold clearance include joint swelling, instability, and an inability to perform sport-specific activities with minimal to no pain, such as running, jumping, or throwing.[4,16] Clearance to train or compete with bacterial skin infections such as impetigo, cellulitis, furuncles, carbuncles, erysipelas, or abscesses should follow the National Federation of High Schools Guidelines, which state that an athlete must be on oral antibiotics for 48 hours with no draining, oozing, or moist lesions, and all wounds must be completely and securely covered with an occlusive dressing.[21] Athletes who become ill while traveling or at a competition should follow general guidelines nicknamed "the neck check." If above-the-neck symptoms such as cough and congestion are present, then the athlete may play as tolerated. However, if below-the-neck or systemic symptoms such as fever, malaise, dehydration, or gastrointestinal symptoms are present, then no exercise is recommended, and the athlete should refrain from competition and training.[8,11-13,17] Risks associated with systemic symptoms (eg, fever) are increased caloric and fluid requirements, and decreased muscle strength, pulmonary perfusion, and cognitive function.[11-13]

Traveler's diarrhea (TD) warrants special mention with regard to athletes who travel to train or compete. Acute infectious diarrhea is the most common travel illness. Traveler's diarrhea is benign and self-limiting but is particularly detrimental to athletes because of dehydration and impaired performance. Other common causes of diarrhea in athletes include viral gastroenteritis and physiologic diarrhea ("runner's trots").[22,23] Travel from a developed country to a developing country puts athletes at highest risk for TD. Highest-risk areas include Central and South America, Africa, the Middle East, and parts of Asia, although TD can occur during domestic travel as well.[24]

Traveler's diarrhea is caused by ingestion of food or water that is contaminated with pathogenic containing fecal material. Easily contaminated foods and beverages include raw or unpeeled fruits and vegetables, tap water or ice, unpasteurized dairy products, and raw or inadequately cooked meats and seafood. Unsafe foods include unrefrigerated street vendor food, reheated foods, and condiments, sauces, salsas, and dressings. Understanding hygiene standards and safety of fluids and foods while traveling in foreign or unfamiliar places is important. Wash hands regularly or use hand sanitizer before meals and when handling fluids and foods. Following food safety tips (Table 2) can help athletes prevent unwanted gastrointestinal discomfort while traveling and competing.[22-24]

Traveler's diarrhea presents with nausea, malaise, vomiting, abdominal cramping, anorexia, fever, and at least 3 diarrheal stools within 24 hours. The onset of symptoms usually occurs within the first 4 to 14 days of travel. In contrast, food poisoning characteristically has an acute onset of symptoms 1 to 6 hours after ingestion of the toxin and typically has complete resolution within 48 hours. TD is generally self-limited, with symptoms lasting 1 to 5 days. In the absence of severe symptoms or complications of infection, supportive management with oral rehydration or intravenous rehydration, rest, and dietary modification is adequate. Avoidance of caffeine, nonsteroidal anti-inflammatory drugs, and high carbohydrate-containing beverages or foods may speed up recovery and

Table 2
Dietary tips to prevent acute diarrheal illnesses during travel

Avoid salads and raw vegetables that are often washed with contaminated water	Do not drink tap water and check the seal on all bottles
Peel all fruits	Keep all tap water out of the mouth during bathing and washing
Avoid seafood, particularly raw or undercooked	Avoid ice in drinks
Avoid raw or undercooked meats	Avoid ice cream and foods requiring strict refrigeration
Avoid unpasteurized foods	
Avoid reheated food	Avoid spicy foods, salsas, condiments, and dressings
Avoid food served by street vendors or street markets	Avoid trying new foods
	Eat in well-known restaurants

minimize symptoms. Antidiarrheal medications are not generally recommended because of depressive central nervous system effects and alterations in the body's thermoregulatory system.[22,23] Antibiotics may be indicated to treat moderate to severe diarrhea (>4 stools per day) associated with prolonged symptoms over 1 week or systemic symptoms including fever, severe dehydration, and blood, pus, or mucus in the stool. Routine stool cultures for bacteria, viruses, and ova and parasites are indicated for athletes who are systemically ill or have prolonged symptoms and are helpful in guiding appropriate use of antibiotics.[24,25] The CDC does not recommend routine antibiotic prophylaxis, although it may be effective in some cases. Bismuth subsalicylate and probiotics may decrease the incidence of TD and can be considered for use.[25]

The Medical Team

It is important to know what medical support will be available at the event or venue that the athlete will be attending. Will a physician, a medical tent, and medical supplies or care be available on site?[16,26] Some teams are fortunate to travel with medical personnel, such as a certified athletic trainer or physician, who is familiar with the athletes and who will have a variety of accessible medical supplies. A head team physician should be well trained in sports medicine and be able to provide basic emergency care for almost any illness or injury suffered by an athlete. The type of competition, the location, the number of athletes, the level of medical care, and the availability of medical facilities at the destination site all influence the selection and preparation of the medical team. Venue medical staff members typically include a head team physician and at least 1 certified athletic trainer. Adjunctive medical staff members often include paramedics, nurses, physical therapists, massage therapists, and chiropractors.[26] The duties and expectations for each medical team members are always clearly defined before travel and athletic teams are introduced to their medical team.[16,27] Proper licensure, malpractice insurance coverage, and transportation of medical equipment and supplies, such as syringes, scalpels, sutures, medications, and automatic external defibrillators, need to be verified before travel. Medical information pertaining to the team should be kept by the head team physician in carry-on luggage in a secure but accessible location. Even if the medical team is not traveling with an athlete, it is reasonable to carry a small portable medical kit that should include first aid items, hand sanitizer, a thermometer, and over-the-counter medications such as fever or pain relievers and antidiarrheal medications.[16]

Jet Lag versus Travel Fatigue

The travel component of an athlete's schedule plays a critical role in his well-being and general performance. Athletes must learn how to minimize the negative effects of travel and adjust relatively quickly.[1,28] Jet lag is the result of circadian desynchronization and resolves with resynchronization at an average rate of 1 day per time zone. Jet lag tends to occur in episodes and can be characterized by gastrointestinal complaints, including heartburn, indigestion, and diarrhea. Sleep disturbance, fatigue, and impaired concentration are other key manifestations.[28,29] In contrast, travel fatigue is the consequence of chronic fatigue accumulating over the course of a season and requires ongoing monitoring of the athlete to detect and address the fatigue. It is characterized by long-term persistent fatigue, recurrent illness, changes in behavior and mood, and loss of motivation.[30] Chronic fatigue is often a sign of overtraining syndrome, and care must be taken to identify and address these issues promptly in adolescent athletes to decrease the risk of experiencing health issues or impaired performance.[1,31-33]

A travel management program is a comprehensive approach to the management of jet lag and travel fatigue, incorporating the time before, during, and after travel. Taking a brief sleep history during the medical visit and obtaining a month-long sleep log will help to identify athletes with sleep disturbances and individuals who are prone to jet lag and travel fatigue. Adaptation before travel may be difficult because of busy schedules but ideally would include the 7 days before travel. Teams may adopt modified training schedules that focus on reducing training volume and intensity. Promoting time for rest before competition is important. If possible, it would be advantageous to adjust training to the destination time zone a few days before departure and arrive in the new time zone days before competition. One-day adjustment for each time zone shift is recommended.[1,28,29,34,35] Readjustment is slightly quicker with westward travel. It is of paramount importance that athletes get enough sleep before travel to reduce sleep debt by sleeping at night and avoiding prolonged daytime naps.[1,28]

During travel, athletes should adjust their watches to the destination time zone as soon as they board the plane. This helps prepare them mentally for the time adjustment. A comfortable environment should be created using a personal pillow, blanket, or lumbar support. Distractions such as electronic devices should be minimized. Eye masks, earplugs, and noise-canceling devices should be used to encourage relaxation and rest, rather than overstimulation or poorly timed sleep.[29] For those wearing contact lenses, keeping contact solution and a lens case in a carry-on is helpful. Eyes may become irritated on long flights if lenses are not removed. Getting up to stretch in order to prevent stiffness, leg swelling, or deep venous thrombosis is critical, especially on longer trips. In-flight meals should be eaten on the destination schedule, which may be easier to do if athletes bring their own meals. Staying hydrated should remain a priority. Onboard sleep should coincide with the destination schedule. Using hypnotics or melatonin is controversial; downsides include unpredictable effects, prolonged drowsiness, and slowing adjustment to new time zones.[1] The body will need alternating periods of light and dark to adapt to a new sleep-wake cycle if the athlete is traveling through several time zones. This means staying awake during the "day" using artificial light or sunlight and sleeping at night while avoiding prolonged or frequent daytime naps.[35,36]

After travel, the activities of the athlete, including meals, sleeping, rest, and recovery, should be strategically planned by the support team to promote rapid circadian adjustment. Avoidance of large meals and caffeine late at night helps to minimize disrupted sleep patterns, but maintenance of hydration is vital.[29,35]

ENVIRONMENTAL CONSIDERATIONS

Altitude

Acclimatization to the destination environment is a gradual process. One of the most difficult adjustments that cause physiologic stress to the athlete's body is an abrupt change in altitude.[37] When competing in a destination of high altitude, the transition can be made easier by initially reducing training intensity. It is important to have longer rest and recovery periods. Increased volume or intensity of training may contribute to symptoms of overtraining, including overall body aches, general fatigue, headache, inability to sleep, or loss of appetite. It is critical to get plenty of rest and eat plenty of carbohydrates and iron-rich foods.[37,38] Because the sun is more intense at high altitudes than at sea level, sun protection is important. Athletes may also become more dehydrated at higher altitudes, so ensuring adequate fluid intake is paramount. In the setting of prolonged stays at altitude, the ideal situation is to "live high and train low." This allows for adaptation to high altitude with low oxygen levels while still training at sea level. The optimal height for sleeping at high altitude is around 2200 to 3100 meters for approximately 4 weeks in order to see physiologic adaptations.[39] Unfortunately, most well-controlled scientific studies to date have failed to show a consistent positive systematic effect on endurance performance, mostly likely because of the wide variability in adaptive responses of athletes.[37-39]

Cold Climates

Performing in cold climates can be particularly challenging, especially if the athlete is not accustomed to the environment. The maximum rate at which the body can use oxygen is often reduced in cold climates. Lactic acid will accumulate at lower levels of activity, which can lead to a reduction in performance.[40,41] In order to optimize performance in cold climates, it is recommended that the athlete wear several layers of clothing as opposed to 1 thick layer to promote comfort and facilitate regulation of individual body temperature. Avoid moisture directly against the skin because damp clothing will increase the rate at which heat is lost from the body. Bring ample amounts of extra clothing (layers) to change into when necessary. If athletes will be exposed to snow, be sure hands, feet, and any other portions of skin that are exposed are well protected. In addition, it is critical to protect eyes from wind using goggles.[42] As with any environmental change or stressor, athletes must adapt their hydration and nutrition to meet energy needs. Energy expenditure is higher in colder temperatures. Plan a snack every 2 hours when training or competing in cold weather to maintain energy levels. Dehydration must be avoided even in cold environments, so maintaining adequate hydration is important.[40,41]

HYDRATION IN SPORTS

Hydration is among the most important concerns for athletes. Optimal hydration plays a critical role in allowing peak athletic performance. As athletes move muscles during exercise, they produce heat. Sweat is the body's way of dissipating this heat. If athletes do not replace the water and electrolytes lost in sweat, then dehydration and, in severe cases, heat illness or injury can ensue. As little as 2% of body weight lost via sweat can impair athletic performance.[43,44] Often, athletes do not realize they are dehydrated or that suboptimal hydration can negatively influence their performance.[43-47]

Proper daily hydration is important whether athletes are in practice or competition. Attention to hydration should be a focus during the preseason when athletes are less acclimatized, when they are traveling to new climates for, competition and during summer and early fall sports because of heat issues. Factors that contribute to the development of heat-related stress and injury (listed Table 3) should be avoided.[43,45,48,49]

Table 3
Factors that contribute to the development of heat-related stress and injury

Poor hydration and nutritional status
Fatigue
Prolonged heat exposure
Wearing clothing that impedes sweat evaporation or bulky protective equipment
Recent acute illness
Rapid increase in training
Low fitness level
Sleep deprivation
Sickle cell trait or other chronic medical illness that may alter hydration or thermoregulation
Medications that alter hydration or thermoregulation

Acclimatization

Coping with the heat can be very challenging, especially if the athlete is not accustomed to the environment. Common heat intolerance symptoms include headache, nausea, dizziness, disorientation, extreme thirst, lack of coordination, and poor performance. Symptoms may indicate dehydration or early stages of heat illness. If the athlete has concurrent symptoms of fever, upper respiratory infection, or diarrhea, then medical evaluation is necessary.[8,11,12] If an athlete has a chronic disease, illness, or other medical condition that can be exacerbated by acute climatic changes and sports participation (eg, sickle cell trait), then it is vital for the athlete to allow adequate time for acclimatization or consider refraining from participation.[3,49-51] Recommendations for acclimatization include training for 60 to 100 minutes per day for at least 2 to 3 days. Increased fluid intake to maintain hydration status and a shaded environment before the event are critical. Sunscreen should be worn to prevent sunburn even on cloudy days. Mild skin erythema can be uncomfortable and lead to impaired temperature regulation for several days. Sun protection for the eyes in the form of sunglasses or goggles with UV protection is recommended. Sunscreen should be used liberally and reapplied frequently during periods of prolonged sun exposure. The risk of sunburn is sometimes increased around water because of sun reflection as well as loss of protection if the sunscreen washes off. Shade or air conditioning after activity will help to reduce body temperature after exercise. Various acclimatization guidelines (ksi.uconn.edu/prevention-strategies/high-school-state-policies/heat-acclimatization-state-policies/) for preseason practices and conditionings in warm or hot environments are available to help high school staff support the athlete's gradual exposure to duration and intensity of exercise and prevent dehydration.

Fluid Recommendations

It is challenging to make global recommendations for fluid intake that apply to all adolescent athletes; however, familiarity with general guidelines is helpful and important for the athlete to follow. Ideally, an athlete will learn to make adjustments to meet his or her individual needs. Total body water (about 60%) is a large proportion of body weight. Sweat rates can vary greatly between individuals. A common base range between 0.5 and 2 L/h is often significantly higher in very hot and humid conditions.[43,46,50] Sweat loss rate depends on many factors, including genetics, gender, age, exercise intensity and duration, presence of equipment or clothing, environmental temperature and humidity, fitness level, acclimatization, indoor versus outdoor exercise, travel, altitude, illness, and injury or surgery.[43,44,46,47] Generally, males and genetically determined "heavy sweaters" have higher sweat rates than females.[45] Heavy sweaters are often recognized by the significant salty residue left on their face, body, and clothing after exercise. Also, despite previous literature that reported thermoregulation and performance capacity were inferior in children compared to adults, recent studies have disproved these results by showing that thermoregulation in acclimatized children, particularly postpubertal adolescents, is not impaired in hot weather conditions as previous speculated.[51,52] When correcting for body size, pubertal and postpubertal adolescents are similar to adults with regard to body sweat losses. However, prepubertal adolescents (males only) demonstrate significantly lower sweat water losses than their adult counterparts, likely because of their lack of androgenic hormonal stimulation.[51] General fluid guidelines have been adopted and supported by multiple accredited organizations (Table 4).[43-46]

Barriers to Optimal Hydration

There are many barriers to hydration, including inexperience with importance of optimal hydration, lack of awareness of thirst, limited opportunities to consume fluids, and frequent opportunities for multiple games or tournament play. Adolescent athletes should practice their game-day hydration strategies during team or individual practices to identify their optimal fluid intake needs. Although athletes should always drink when they are thirsty and recognize signs of thirst, thirst is a not an ideal mechanism to rely on for prevention of dehydration. An exception is seen in runners, who tend to drink more adequately than athletes in other sports.[43,46] Furthermore, adolescent athletes involved in weight class sports may purposefully ignore thirst to dehydrate themselves intentionally in order to make weight.[44,45,47,51] Athletes should be aware of and try to prevent the signs and symptoms of dehydration, which include flushed skin, headache, weakness, poor concentration, light-headedness, increased core temperature and heart rate, nausea, vomiting, loss of coordination, and muscle cramps.[43-45]

Table 4
General fluid guidelines

Time	Amount	Practical translation
2-3 hours before workout or event	Drink 16 oz fluid	1 standard water bottle
15-30 minutes before workout or event	Drink 8-16 oz fluid	½-1 water bottle
During workout or event	Drink 3-6 oz of fluid every 15-20 minutes (about 16-24 oz per hour)	2-5 gulps every 15-20 minutes or 1 water bottle per hour Make sure to drink when thirsty Consider mouth rinses if fluids are not tolerated during sports
After workout or event	Drink 16-24 oz per pound of weight lost (150% body weight lost) or at least 2 mL per pound of body weight[6]	1+ water bottles depending on sweat rate or weight lost and how often the athlete consumed fluid during practice

Many adolescents are not motivated to adequately hydrate. Ad libitum drinking volumes, estimated at 6 mL per pound of body weight per hour, are comparable in pubertal adolescent athletes and adults. This hydration rate is not considered adequate to prevent postevent dehydration.[51] In a study by Arnaoutis et al,[53] more than 89% of adolescents were found to be hypohydrated (urine specific gravity [USG] ≥1.02 mg/dL) based on first morning urine sample and more than 76% remained hypohydrated after training. This finding emphasizes the need for athletes to be euhydrated at the start of practice and games. Parents, coaches, and physicians need to promote this early hydration strategy because educational interventions can lead to better ad libitum fluid consumption in adolescents, thus improving hydration status.[52,54] When developing policies and event schedules, it is important to allow enough time both for recovery between contests and for frequent fluid drinking opportunities. This can minimize a carryover effect of fatigue, dehydration, or heat exposure so that the athlete is competing sufficiently replenished and recovered.[50,55-57] The amount of time needed depends on several factors, including the climate, the age and level of conditioning of the athlete, and the sport type and intensity level.[50] Bergeron[50] demonstrated that elite junior tennis players who competed in a hot, humid environment had difficulties maintaining adequate hydration with short rest periods between same-day matches. He noted that prior same-day exercise increased cardiovascular and thermal strain as well as the effort perception in subsequent activity bouts. He further showed that the extent of earlier exercise-heat exposure could affect performance and competition outcome.[50] Governing bodies of youth sports need to address this issue and provide more specific, appropriate, evidence-based guidelines for minimum rest periods between same-day contests for all levels of tournament play in the heat.[33,50,55] Strategies to promote optimal hydration in adolescent athletes are listed in Table 5.[43-45,47,58,59]

Assessing Hydration Status

Teaching athletes how to properly monitor hydration and encouraging mandatory hydration breaks during practices and competitions are key prevention methods.[43,45,55] Although there is no universal measure, several practical parameters for assessing hydration status can be used. Urine color, volume, and fre-

Table 5
Strategies to promote optimal hydration

Assess availability of fluid intake before and during school hours (be aware of rules and regulations on water bottles and consumption at school)

Ensure and promote access to fluids throughout the day

Take advantage of all drinking opportunities during sport (not all sports have convenient fluid breaks, so requiring them often is essential)

Use fluid drinking challenges among team members or staff and peers to promote better hydration

Encourage consumption of foods with high fluid content (eg, fruits, vegetables, smoothies, soups)

---

quency along with daily morning measurements of body weight and sweat rate determination are common field measures of hydration.

Athletes should urinate at least every 3 hours with adequate volume. Straw- or lemonade-colored urine is indicative of good hydration status. Dark-colored urine indicates dehydration. Changes in body weight during practice may be the optimal way to observe changes in an athlete's hydration status[52] (USG ≤1.020 g/mL is indicative of euhydration).[43] Genetically heavy sweaters may benefit from learning how to calculate a sweat rate during exercise in order to help gauge the appropriate amount of postexercise fluid to consume.[43-45] Table 6 details how athletes can check individual sweat rates, which can help them determine fluid needs before, during, and after exercise.[43-45] Online urine color charts can help assess hydration (www.ncaa.org/sites/default/files/Assess%2BYour%2BHydration%2BStatus.pdf). Dipping urine for USG measure, using a refractometer, and checking blood osmolality levels are more sophisticated techniques that require supplies and investment and produce precise measurements of hydration.[43-48]

Types of Fluid Replacement

For low-to-moderate intensity workouts or events lasting less than 60 minutes, water is the ideal fluid replacement for most adolescent athletes. For intense training (>30 minutes) or long workouts (>60 minutes), added carbohydrates or fluid replacement drinks containing 4% to 8% carbohydrate (ie, sports drinks) are preferred.[43-45,52-57] These drinks are rapidly available glucose sources for muscles during sport that are well tolerated.[43,44,46,53] Varying the source of carbohydrate (glucose, sucrose, and fructose) helps to maximize carbohydrate transport and may be optimal for athletes with frequent gastrointestinal distress.[45] Athletes should begin hydrating with palatable fluids as early as tolerated during a workout or event.

Adolescent athletes should avoid carbonated and highly caffeinated beverages at all times, including during sport participation. Energy drinks contain substances that are not found in sports drinks and act as stimulants, such as caffeine, guarana, and taurine. Caffeine has been linked to a number of harmful health effects

Table 6
Calculating sweat rate

A. Record body weight before moderate-to-intense exercise.
B. Record body weight after moderate-to-intense exercise.
C. Determine the change in body weight (A − B).
D. Record any drink volume consumed during exercise (oz × 30 = mL).
E. Record any urine volume excreted before postexercise weight (oz × 30 = mL).
F. Determine sweat loss: C + D − E.
G. Record exercise time (in minutes or hours).
H. Calculate sweat rate: F/G in mL/min or mL/h.

in children, including effects on the developing neurologic and cardiovascular systems. The American Academy of Pediatrics states that energy drinks are never appropriate for children or adolescents. In contrast, sports drinks, which contain carbohydrates, minerals, electrolytes, and flavoring, are intended to replace water and electrolytes lost through sweating during exercise. However, sports drinks have no place in the routine diet of adolescents and are not an appropriate source of dietary calories or healthy nutrition in a nonathletic setting.[57,58] For athletes who participate in high-intensity or endurance sports that result in a need to use sports drinks, there are alternatives to commercially available beverages. Homemade sports drink recipes are budget friendly and easy to make (combinations of water, sugar or fruit juice, salt, and flavoring agent as needed). For those who are prone to cramps or those with genetically high sweat rates, a higher-sodium specialty sports drinks or adding extra salt to fluids and foods may be advantageous.[43-48] Table 7 lists common fluid replacement options and their respective carbohydrate and electrolyte compositions.

Athletes who drink early and often are better at remaining hydrated. Preventing fluid losses more than 2% of body weight during exercise and promoting daily euhydration are crucial.[48,50] Table 8 outlines an ideal sample daily hydration plan for an adolescent male athlete training in an afternoon school sport.

Hyponatremia

Hyponatremia as a result of overhydration is decreased sodium levels relative to total body water. Hyponatremia is a serious and sometimes deadly condition. Although it occurs less frequently than dehydration, hyponatremia can be difficult to differentiate from dehydration because the symptoms are similar. Symptoms of hyponatremia include fatigue, bloating, nausea, headache, swollen hands and feet, confusion, and disorientation.[43-45]

Table 7
Comparison of popular rehydration fluids

Beverage (8oz)	CHO %	CHO (g)	Calories	Sodium (g)	Potassium (g)
Water	0	0	0	0	0
Propel Sport Water	1	3	12	78	38
Pedialyte	2.5	6	25	252	192
G2	3	7	20	110	30
Coconut water	4	10	44	64	404
Vitamin water	5.5	13	52	0	0
Gatorade	6	14	50	110	30
Powerade	8	19	72	102	44

From USDA National Nutrient Database for Standard Reference, Release 27. Available at: ndb.nal. usda.gov/ndb.

Table 8
Sample daily hydration plan for a student athlete

Time	Meal/event	Fluid intake
7 a.m.	Breakfast	1-2 cups water or other healthy fluid
Mid morning	Classes	Take regular sips of water or other healthy fluid (about 2 cups)
Mid day	Lunch	2-3 cups water or other healthy fluid
3 p.m.	Pretraining session	1-2 cups water; can top off again 15-30 minutes before workout as tolerated
4-5 p.m.	Training session	2-5 gulps every 20 minutes
6 p.m.	Post-training	Consume fluid to replace 150% of body weight lost during training; drink recovery milk or other nonwater beverage
7-8 p.m.	Evening/recovery meal	2 cups water or other healthy fluid
9-10 p.m.	Bedtime	1 cup water or other healthy fluid

Hyponatremia risk increases during long durations of exercise (4+ hours).[43] Risk factors include drinking fluids with low sodium content, high sodium sweat losses, less-trained athletes, smaller athletes or females, and those with low sodium intake in their diet.[1] Hyponatremia prevention includes avoiding excessive water loading before events and excessive water consumption during exercise (>1 L/h for several hours) as well as consuming salty foods and fluids before and during exercise.[43,46,59] Sodium helps the body retain water and stimulates thirst. Decreased urine output and weight gain after exercise are signs of possible overhydration and hyponatremia.[43] Not all athletes are at risk for hyponatremia because many underhydrate and consume high dietary salt content.[43]

Travel Hydration

Pressurized plane cabins and air-conditioned environments increase risk for dehydration because of increased fluid losses from skin and lungs, especially when travel times are long.[58,59] Although fluids are provided during commercial travel, the portions often are small and not readily available. Athletes should bring their own fluids while traveling and drink a minimum of 1 cup per hour to maintain adequate hydration.[58] Water and sports drinks are ideal fluid replacements during travel.[57,58] Unfamiliar or caffeinated fluids are not recommended.[45,46,58] Table 9 lists selected resources for athlete hydration replacement.

TRAVEL AND PORTABLE NUTRITION

Consuming proper nutrition can be difficult when traveling for sport. Stress, poor decision-making, special diets or food allergies, irregular meal times, unfamiliar foods and food culture, overconsumption of convenience or tempting foods, inactivity or boredom eating, increased fluid loss during travel, and

Table 9
Online hydration resources

Gatorade Sports Science Institute:
www.gssiweb.org/en/publications/sports-nutrition
NCAA Nutrition:
www.ncaa.org/health-and-safety/nutrition-and-performance/nutrition
Sports, Cardiovascular, and Wellness Nutrition (SCAN) Sports Nutrition Fact Sheets:
www.scandpg.org/sports-nutrition/sports-nutrition-fact-sheets/
US Olympic Committee "Team USA" Sports Nutrition Resources and Fact Sheets:
www.teamusa.org/About-the-USOC/Athlete-Development/Sport-Performance/Nutrition/
Resources-and-Fact-Sheets.aspx
American College of Sports Medicine Public Information Factsheets:
www.acsm.org/access-public-information/brochures-fact-sheets/fact-sheets
Australian Sports Commission Factsheets:
www.ausport.gov.au/ais/nutrition/factsheets

consumption of unsafe foods are obstacles athletes face while traveling.[58,59] Exercising sound nutritional judgment at restaurants, fast food outlets, and "all you can eat" or buffet-style dining halls can be difficult for athletes. Pre-trip food planning with adult supervision (parents, coaches) and recognition of these obstacles are keys to healthy travel nutrition. Adaptations include timing meals to destination time zones and packing extra, familiar snacks in case of delays, which can help prevent skipping meals or consumption of excessive non-nutritional "convenience" foods. Snacks to restore glycogen stores during travel are important but should not be abused or overconsumed.[59] Table 10 offers some nutritious restaurant fast food meal suggestions for athletes who are traveling.

Table 10
Sample restaurant fast food meal suggestions and recovery snacks during travel

Restaurant meals

2 slices of cheese or vegetable pizza with added grilled chicken, green salad, 100% juice
Turkey and cheese sandwich, baked chips, fruit, low-fat milk
2 grilled chicken soft tacos, rice, beans, tomatoes, corn
Spaghetti with marinara or meat sauce, bread, green salad, low-fat milk or juice
Baked potato with chili and broccoli
2 single burgers with extra veggies, no fries, water

Restaurant recovery snacks

Fruit smoothie made with yogurt or milk
Half turkey sandwich with piece of fruit
Peanut butter and banana sandwich
Yogurt with berries and granola
Bowl of broth-based soup with crackers and low-fat cheese
Oatmeal made with milk, raisins, and almonds
Vegetable omelet with toast
Liquid fluid replacement or meal bar

Same Day Competitions and Tournament Eating

Time can be a limiting factor during travel and tournament play when athletes have multiple events per day or consecutive days of play. Adolescent athletes often struggle with food tolerance and limited time to replenish energy between bouts of activity, which leads to subsequent decreased performance.[50,53] Longer rest and recovery periods are beneficial to athlete performance and safety.[55] Consuming easily tolerated and frequent recovery snacks and fluids during rest time is paramount. Organized team portable food supplies can help provide healthy nutrition for game day. Table 11 lists useful foods and supplies for traveling athletes and teams.

CONCLUSION

Athletes aspire for maximal performance and physical health while competing at competitive events away from home, yet traveling to these events triggers unique stressors and inevitable challenges. Careful planning and preparation across many factors, from medical to nutritional to psychological and beyond, are required for the optimal performance and safety of athletes as they travel. Adolescent athletes should be educated on travel recommendations and develop subsequent strategies to prevent undue illness, injury, and stress while on the

Table 11
Useful foods and supplies for traveling

Beans
Lean lunch meats
Breads/cereals
Spreads (nut butters, honey)
Crackers or other carbohydrate snack of choice
Long-life cheeses
Granola/cereal bars
Dried fruit
Fresh fruits and vegetables if washed with known safe water source
Nut mix or trail mix
100% juice or ultrapasteurized, shelf-stable milk (can be frozen ahead of time to retain temperature)
Quick-cook rice or noodles
Sports drinks
Liquid meal supplements or recovery shakes
Powdered drinks
Sports bars
Sports gels, tablets, goos
Snap-lock bags or plastic containers
Bowl or plate and cutlery
Single cup heater to boil water
Bottled water
Hot pot or other travel friendly cooking device

move. Because adolescent athletes are less experienced with travel, parents, coaches, athletic trainers, and all those who work with athletes should appreciate their distinct travel challenges, advocate for necessary equipment and food, and assist athletes with travel preparations.

References

1. Samuels, CH. Jet lag and travel fatigue: a comprehensive management plan for sport medicine physicians and high-performance support teams. *Clin J Sport Med.* 2012;22:268-273
2. Hagmann S, Neugebauer R, Schwartz E, et al; GeoSentinel Surveillance Network. Illness in children after international travel: analysis from the GeoSentinel Surveillance Network. *Pediatrics.* 2010;125:e1072-e1080
3. American Academy of Pediatrics Committee on Nutrition and the Council on Sports Medicine and Fitness; Rice SG. Medical conditions affecting sports participation. *Pediatrics.* 2008;121:4 841-848
4. Caswell SV, Cortes N, Chabolla M, et al. State-specific differences in school sports preparticipation physical evaluation policies. *Pediatrics.* 2015;135:26-32
5. Bernhardt DT, Roberts WO, eds. *PPE: Preparticipation Physical Evaluation.* 4th ed. Elk Grove Village, IL: American Academy of Pediatrics; 2010
6. American Academy of Pediatrics Committee on Infectious Diseases. Recommended Childhood and Adolescent Immunization Schedule—United States, 2014. *Pediatrics.* 2014;133:357-363
7. Gärtner BC, Meyer T. Vaccination in elite athletes. *Sports Med.* 2014;44:1361-1376
8. Jaworski CA, Donohue B, Kleutz J. Infectious disease. *Clin Sports Med.* 2011;30:575-590
9. American Academy of Pediatrics Council on Sports Medicine and Fitness; Halsted ME, Walter KD. Clinical report: sports-related concussion in children and adolescents. *Pediatrics.* 2010;126:3 597-615
10. American Academy of Pediatrics Council on Sports Medicine and Fitness and the Council on School Health; Halsted ME, McAvoy K, Devore CD, et al. Clinical report: returning to learning following a concussion. *Pediatrics.* 2013;132:948-957
11. Metz JP. Upper respiratory tract infections: who plays, who sits? *Curr Sports Med Rep.* 2003;2:84-90
12. Glezen WP. Clinical practice: prevention and treatment of seasonal influenza. *N Engl J Med.* 2008;359:2579-2585
13. Putukian M, O'Connor FG, Stricker PR, et al. Mononucleosis and athletic participation: an evidence-based subject review. *Clin J Sport Med.* 2008;18:309-315
14. Benjamin HJ, Nikore V, Takagishi J. Practical management: community-associated methicillin-resistant Staphylococcus aureus (CA-MRSA): the latest sports epidemic. *Clin J Sport Med.* 2007;17:393-397
15. Sedgwick PE, Dexter WW, Smith CT. Bacterial dermatoses in sports. *Clin Sports Med.* 2007;26:383-396
16. Herring SA, Kibler WB, Putukian M. Team physician consensus statement: 2013 update. *Med Sci Sports Exerc.* 2013;45:1618-1622
17. Creighton DW, Shrier I, Shultz R, Meeuwisse WH, Matheson GO. Return-to-play in sport: a decision based model. *Clin J Sport Med.* 2010;20:379-385
18. Matheson GO, Shultz R, Bido J, et al. Return-to-play decisions: are they the team physician's responsibility? *Clin J Sport Med.* 2011;21:25
19. Shrier I, Charland L, Mohtadi NG, Meeuwisse WH, Matheson GO. The sociology of return-to-play decision-making: a clinical perspective. *Clin J Sport Med.* 2010;20:333-335
20. Roberts WO, Löllgen H, Matheson GO, et al. Advancing the preparticipation physical evaluation: an ACSM and FIMS joint consensus statement. *Clin J Sport Med.* 2014;24:442-447
21. Lindenmayer JM, Schoenfeld S, O'Grady R, et al. Methicillin-resistant *Staphylococcus aureus* in a high school wrestling team and the surrounding community. *Arch Intern Med.* 1998;158:895-899

22. Casey E, Mistry DJ, MacKnight JM. Training room management of medical conditions: sports gastroenterology. *Clin Sport Med.* 2005;24:525-540
23. Rendi-Wagner P, Kollaritsch H. Drug prophylaxis for travelers' diarrhea. *Clin Infect Dis.* 2002;34:628-33
24. Dupont HL, Ericsson CD. Prevention and treatment of travelers' diarrhea. *N Engl J Med.* 1993;328:1821-1827
25. Boggess BR. Gastrointestinal infections in the traveling athlete. *Curr Sports Med Rep.* 2007;6:125-129
26. McCloskey B, Endericks T, Catchpole M, et al. London 2012 Olympic and Paralympic games: public health surveillance and epidemiology. *Lancet.* 2014;282:2083-2089
27. Olympia RP, Brady J. Emergency preparedness in high school-based athletics: a review of the literature and recommendations for sport health professionals. *Phys Sportsmed.* 2013;41:15-25
28. Lee A, Galvez JC. Jet lag in athletes. *Sports Health.* 2012;4:211-216
29. Schoebersberger W, Schobersberger B. The traveling athlete: from jet leg to jet lag. *Curr Sports Med Rep.* 2012;11:222-223
30. Leatherwood WE, Dragoo JL. Effect of airline travel on performance: a review of the literature. *Br J Sports Med.* 2013;47:561-567
31. American Academy of Pediatrics Council on Sports Medicine and Fitness; Brenner, JA. Overuse injuries, overtraining and burnout in child and adolescent athletes. *Pediatrics.* 2007;119:1242-1245
32. DiFiori JP, Benjamin HJ, Brenner JS, et al. A position statement from the American Medical Society for Sports Medicine. Overuse injuries and burnout in youth sports: a position statement. *Br J Sports Med.* 2014;48:287-288
33. Luke A, Lazaro RM, Bergeron MF, et al. Sports-related injuries in youth athletes: is overscheduling a risk factor? *Clin J Sports Med.* 2011;21:307-314
34. Schwellnus MP, Derman WE, Jordaan E, et al. Elite athletes traveling to international destinations > 5 time zone differences from their home country have a 2-3-fold increased risk of illness. *Br J Sports Med.* 2012;46:816-821
35. Forbes-Robertson S, Dudley E, Vadgama P, et al. Circadian disruption and remedial interventions: effects and interventions for jet lag for athletic peak performance. *Sports Med.* 2012;42:183-208
36. Fowler PM, Duffield R, Morrow I, Roach G, Vaile J. Effects of sleep hygiene and artificial bright light interventions on recovery from simulated international air travel. *Eur J Appl Physiol.* 2015;115:541-545
37. Schommer K, Menold E, Subudhi AW, Bartsch P. Health risk for athletes at moderate altitude and normobaric hypoxia. *Br J Sports Med.* 2012;46:828-832
38. Zafren K, Prevention of high altitudes illness. *Travel Med Infect Dis.* 2014;12:29-30
39. Roach GD, Schmidt WF, Aughey RJ, et al. The sleep of elite athletes at sea level and high altitude: a comparison of sea-level natives and high altitude natives (ISA3600). *Br J Sports Med.* 2013;47(Suppl 1):i114-i120
40. Jett DM, Adams KJ, Stamford BA. Cold exposure and exercise metabolism. *Sports Med.* 2006;36:643-656
41. Yamane M, Oida Y, Ohnishi N, Matsumoto T, Kitagawa K. Effects of wind and rain on thermal responses of humans in a mildly cold environment. *Eur J Appl Physiol.* 2010;109:117-123
42. Burtscher M, Kofler P, Gatterer H, et al. Effects of lightweight outdoor clothing on the prevention of hypothermia during low-intensity exercise in the cold. *Clin J Sport Med.* 2012;22:505-507
43. Sawka MN, Burke LM, Eichner ER, et al. American College of Sports Medicine position stand: exercise and fluid replacement. *MSSE.* 2007;377-390
44. Clark N. *Sports Nutrition Guidebook.* 5th ed. Champaign, IL: Human Kinetics; 2014
45. Iammartino C, Rosenbloom C. *The Sports Nutrition Care Manual.* Chicago, IL: Academy of Nutrition & Dietetics; 2014
46. International Olympic Committee (IOC); Maughan R, Burke LM. Nutrition for athletes: a practical guide to eating for health and performance. Available at: www.olympic.org/documents/reports/en/en_report_833.pdf. Accessed August 27, 2014

47. Burke L. *Practical Sports Nutrition.* Champaign, IL: Human Kinetics; 2007
48. American Academy of Pediatrics Council on Sports Medicine and Fitness and Council on School Health; Bergeron MF, Devore C, Rice SG. Policy statement: climatic heat stress and exercising children and adolescents. *Pediatrics.* 2011;128:e741-e747
49. Casa DJ, Csillan D; Inter-Association Task Force for Preseason Secondary School Athletics Participants, et al. Preseason heat-acclimatization for secondary school athletics. *J Athl Train.* 2009;44:332-333
50. Bergeron MF. Youth sports in the heat. *Sports Med.* 2009;39:513-522
51. Rowland T. Fluid replacement requirements for child athletes. *Sports Med.* 2011;41:279-288
52. Kavouras SA, Arnaoutis G, Makrillos M, et al. Educational intervention on water intake improves hydration status and enhances exercise performance in athletic youth. *Scand J Med Sci Sports.* 2012;22:684-689
53. Arnaoutis G, Kavouras SA, Angelopoulou A, et al. Fluid balance during training in elite young athletes of different sports. *J Strength Cond Res.* 2014;[Epub ahead of print]
54. Armstrong LE, Johnson EC, Kunces LJ, et al. Drinking to thirst versus drinking ad libitum during road cycling. *J Athl Train.* 2014;49:624-631
55. Bergeron MF. Youth sports in the heat: recovery and scheduling considerations for tournament play. *Sports Med.* 2009;39:513-522
56. Holway F, Spriet L. Sport-specific nutrition: practical strategies for team sports. *J Sports Sciences.* 2011;29(SI):S115-S125
57. American Academy of Pediatrics Committee on Nutrition and the Council on Sports Medicine and Fitness. Sports drinks and energy drinks for children and adolescents: are they appropriate? *Pediatrics.* 2011;127:1182-1189
58. Reilly T, Waterhouse J, Burke LM, Alonso JM. Nutrition for travel. *J Sports Sci.* 2007;25(Suppl 1):S125-S134
59. US Anti-Doping Agency (USADA); Berning JR, Kendig A. *TrueSport Nutrition Guide: Nutritional Requirements of Athletes.* Colorado Springs, CO: USADA; 2013

Adolesc Med 026 (2015) 208–220

Extreme Sports and the Adolescent Athlete

Andrew R. Peterson, MD, MSPH, FAAP[a]*;
Andrew J. Gregory, MD, FAAP, FACSM[b]

[a]Assistant Professor, University of Iowa Carver College of Medicine,
Stead Family Department of Pediatrics, Iowa City, Iowa; [b]Associate Professor of Orthopedics,
Pediatrics and Neurosurgery, Vanderbilt University School of Medicine, Nashville, Tennessee

The benefits of sport participation by children and adolescents are well described.[1-4] However, these benefits do not come without risk. Rates of severe musculoskeletal injury and concussion are well reported in organized high school sports,[5,6] and many steps have been taken to improve the safety of adolescent athletes competing in school-sanctioned athletics. However, many adolescents participate or compete in alternative activities such as extreme sports, mixed martial arts (MMA), parkour, and outdoor sports, and these alternative sports may be much riskier than the contact and collision sports in which their classmates commonly compete in school. Some of the alternative activities are quite dangerous, such as BASE (Building, Antenna, Span, Earth) jumping, which carries a high risk of both injury and death.[7] Other sports, such as boxing, seem dangerous but have lower rates of injury than many high school sports.[8-11] This review aims to identify some of the risks associated with extreme sports and to help the medical practitioner better understand the demands placed on the athletes who compete in them.

X GAMES

The X Games is an annual festival of extreme sports. It is owned and operated by ESPN Inc., a joint venture between the Walt Disney Company and the Hearst Corporation. ESPN is best known as a subscription television sports broadcasting service based in Connecticut in the United States. The X Games is a made-for-television event tailored to attract viewers who may not otherwise watch ESPN for more traditional sports coverage.

---

*Corresponding author
E-mail address: Andrew-r-peterson@uiowa.edu

The fact that the events in the X Games are designed for television cannot be overemphasized. The growth and popularity of the X Games can be directly attributed to how television-friendly the events are. ESPN frequently changes the sports that are included in the festival in an effort to maximize the television audience. This makes it very difficult for most medical practitioners to keep up with the sports included in the games and the risks and demands facing the athletes. There are multiple other extreme sports competitions and tours (eg, Red Bull Rampage, Dew Action Sports Tour, Fuel TV, Gravity Games), but X Games is the largest and most popular. This section focuses primarily on X Games sports, but be aware that athlete patients may be competing in similar events in other venues.

The types of demands, and even the basic rules of many of the X Games sports, are difficult to determine. Unlike traditional athletic events, X Games sports are not generally overseen by any national governing body (NGB). Most X Games sports are not World Anti-Doping Agency (WADA) signatories and do not fall under the jurisdiction of any national federations or the Court of Arbitration for Sport. Little has been written about them in the medical literature, and popular media accounts of the risks of X Games sports tend to focus on catastrophic injuries. With few exceptions, there are no useful epidemiologic data on extreme sports and very little descriptive analysis of the risks of such sports.[12] Some data on injuries that occurred while athletes were surfing, bicycle motocross (BMX) cycling, or competing in motocross events have been reported,[13-19] but they are not specific to the types of competitions and demands seen in X Games sports.

A list of current and past X Games sports is given in Table 1. The types of sports, the physical demands, and the level of risk are quite diverse. For this reason, we encourage the medical practitioner who is evaluating X Games athletes to ask them more about the specifics of their sport and to search the Internet to learn more about it in order to better partner with them in making meaningful shared medical decisions.

It is particularly difficult for the medical practitioner who is not familiar with the X Games to distinguish between the demands of sound-alike sports. For example, within the BMX category, there are multiple types of BMX competition. Epidemiologic studies of BMX have traditionally lumped these remarkably different disciplines together and measured injuries sustained on BMX-style bicycles.[16] BMX Street is a relatively safe, slower-paced event requiring lower amplitude skills. Athletes are judged on skills that are performed on mostly flat ground with a few small rails, steps, and ramps. There are no large ramps, and most injuries occur from falls of only a few feet. In contrast, BMX Big Air uses a mega ramp, which consists of a roll-in section that drops from a height of at least 40 feet to allow the athlete to gain speed.[20] It then transitions to a long gap of 25 to 75 feet over which the athlete jumps while performing a judged skill. Finally, the athlete rolls into a large quarter-pipe jump in which the he launches himself

Table 1
X Game sports

Current Summer Sports	Previous Summer Sports
Current Summer Sports	Snowmobile Speed and Style
	Snocross
Moto X Speed and Style	Snocross Adaptive
Moto X Best Whip	Real Video Snow
Moto X Freestyle	Real Video Ski Backcountry
Men's Moto X Endurocross	
Women's Moto X Endurocross	**Previous Summer Sports**
Moto X Step Up	
Moto X Adaptive Racing	Vert Skating
Men's Moto X Racing	Vert Skating Triples
Women's Moto X Racing	Vert Skating Best Trick
Mountain Bike Slopestyle	Street Skating
Rallycross Lites	Park Skating
Rallycross SuperCar	BMX Flatland
Gymkhana Grid	BMX Downhill
Stadium Super Trucks	BMX Vert Doubles
Skateboard Vert	BMX Vert Best Trick
Men's Skateboard Park	Skateboard Big Air Rail Jam
Women's Skateboard Park	Downhill Skateboarding
Street League Skateboarding	Skateboard Vert Doubles
SLS Select Series	Women's Skateboard Vert
Women's Skateboard Street	Skateboard Vert Best Trick
Skateboard Big Air	Skateboard Game of SK8
BMX Vert	Climbing
BMX Park	Street Luge
BMX Street	X-Venture Race
BMX Big Air	Motocross Supercross
BMX Dirt	Wakeboarding
Real Video Surf	Skysurfing
Real Video Women	Bungee Jumping
Real Video Street	Barefoot Jumping
Red Bull Phenom Mountain Bike Slopestyle	Barefoot Waterski Jumping
Red Bull Phenom Skateboard Street	Motocross Best Trick
Red Bull Phenom BMX Street	Mountain Bike Trials
	Mountain Bike Slalom
Current Winter Sports	Mountain Bike Giant Slalom
Ski Big Air	**Previous Winter Sports**
Men's Ski Slopestyle	
Women's Ski Slopestyle	Super Modified Snow Shovel Racing
Men's Ski Superpipe	Snow Mountain Bike Racing
Women's Ski Superpipe	Skiboarding
Snowboard Big Air	Ice Climbing
Women's Snowboard Slopestyle	Ultracross
Men's Snowboard Slopestyle	Snowskating
Men's Snowboard Superpipe	Hillcross
Women's Snowboard Superpipe	Snowmobile Best Trick
Men's Snowboard X	Men's Skier X
Women's Snowboard X	Women's Skier X
Snowmobile Freestyle	Mono Skier X

directly into the air in an attempt to attain the highest possible height off the lip and return safely to the quarter-pipe transition. The total score for the run is a combination of the judged score and the height of the jump. This is obviously a much more dangerous event than slower-paced BMX events such as BMX Street, which tends to have very few high-energy crashes. BMX Big Air has fairly frequent high-energy crashes and potential for catastrophic injuries. Both of these sports stand in stark contrast to BMX Racing, which is a head-to-head timed racing sport included in the summer Olympic Games. It is important for medical practitioners to understand the demands of specific sports so that they can better counsel the athlete about the risks of returning to sport, prepare the athlete for the specific challenges an injury may pose, or assist in problem-solving and adaptation so that the athlete can return to sport despite the injury.

Catastrophic injuries and deaths are remarkably rare in the X Games. Only 1 death has occurred during X Games competition. Caleb Moore was killed in a snowmobile freestyle competition in 2013.[21] In contrast to the highly visible injuries and single death that have occurred on camera, it is impossible to know how many athletes have been injured training for, or mimicking, the events that are seen by the viewing public. Usually only training injuries that occur to high-profile athletes are reported in the media. For example, popular Canadian freestyle skier Sarah Burke was killed during training in 2012.[22] This incident was widely reported in the popular media because, in addition to her competitive success, Ms Burke was instrumental in the successful campaign to have half-pipe freestyle skiing added to the Winter Olympics.[23] The sport made its Olympic debut at the 2014 Games in Sochi, Russia, and many of the athletes dedicated their performances to Ms Burke.

In response to these deaths, the X Games removed 5 sports that were perceived to be the most dangerous.[24] These Best Trick sports rewarded high-amplitude, very risky skills by allowing competitors multiple attempts to successfully complete a skill and charging no penalty for failed attempts. Best Trick events took place within the Moto-X, skate, BMX, snow, and vertical skate competitions. These events were targeted for removal because of their perceived danger rather than any catastrophic injuries or deaths that had occurred during training or competition.

In addition to traditional sporting venues, the X Games includes 2 categories of video-based competition. The Real Video Series competitions pit athlete-submitted videos against each other in an online tournament in the areas of surfing, street, and backcountry snow, as well as in a separate women's category. Large cash prizes are awarded to the winners of these competitions, and the most competitive entrants tend to be professional athletes. The Red Bull Phenom competition is of similar format but is only open to 14- to 19-year-old athletes in the areas of mountain bike slope style, skateboard street, and BMX Street.

The X Games festival and ESPN are large structured organizations, but there is little infrastructure surrounding the individual X Games sports. No coaching certifications or credentials are necessary for most of the X Games sports. Former athletes and coaches from other disciplines occasionally are employed as coaches by athletes. Some high-profile athletes with copious resources may hire multiple coaches to help them with different aspects of their sport. However, many X Games athletes do not have the resources to hire a coach or do not feel they need a coach. Many X Games athletes leverage modern video recording and display technologies to rapidly evaluate their skill development during training instead of relying on the watchful eye of a coach.

X Games sports do not have NGBs. No mechanisms are in place for punishing or penalizing athletes who do not follow the rules of their sport. In fact, most X Games sports do not have rules governing conduct outside of the competitive arena. As X Games sports have become more popular, several athletes have experienced difficulty transitioning into more mainstream sporting structures. The most prominent example occurred in the pre-X Games era of downhill snowboarding. Before 1998, snowboarding was perceived as an extreme fringe sport, much like the current X Games sports. Men's snowboarding was included in the 1998 Olympic Games in Nagano, Japan. Ross Rebagliati was the first gold medalist in the Giant Slalom event. However, he tested positive for marijuana and was temporarily stripped of his medal (it was later reinstated). This transition from the unregulated world of extreme sports to the rigid infrastructure of Olympic competition and NGBs can be difficult for some athletes.

MIXED MARTIAL ARTS

Mixed martial arts is a combat sport that combines striking and grappling techniques. Fighters from diverse backgrounds compete to submit, knock out, or outscore their opponents using techniques borrowed from other combat sports such as Jiu-Jitsu, boxing, wrestling, karate, and Muay Thai. Successful MMA fighters rarely are specialists, although many have a background in a single combat sport. Fighters need to be able to fight and defend themselves in many styles and in any position.

Mixed martial arts is a descendent of the ancient Greek sport of pankration, which was a hybrid sport of boxing and wrestling. Pankration had few rules other than prohibition of biting and eye gouging. The term *pankration* is still commonly used to describe youth MMA leagues. Modern MMA began with the development of several leagues in Brazil, Japan, and the United States in the late 20th century. Each of these leagues began with minimal rules and regulations and had a reputation of being bloody and lawless. However, as the popularity of the sport spread, it became clear that some rules and equipment were necessary to protect the health of the athletes and to help the development of MMA into a legitimate sport.

The first rules involved the development of weight classes. In early MMA, it was common for fighters of very different sizes to compete against one another. As technique improved, larger fighters clearly had an advantage, especially when using and escaping from submission holds. Now, most leagues classify athletes into at least 9 different weights.

Small, open-fingered striking gloves were introduced early in the development of modern MMA. This development likely did little to contribute to athlete safety. Striking gloves actually increase the amount of striking in a fight. The gloves usually do more to protect the hands of the striker than the target of the strike. Gloves also help to decrease the number of facial cuts, which in turn decreases the number of stoppages.

Most leagues require use of a mouthguard to prevent dental injuries and a protective cup to prevent testicular injuries in males. Rarely, a league requires the use of boxing headgear or foot protectors such as those used in Taekwondo. No other protective equipment is commonly used or required.

In most leagues, fighters younger than 18 years are not allowed to strike or kick above the collarbone. Otherwise, youth MMA is very similar to the adult sport. Likewise, amateur MMA is essentially the same sport as professional MMA, unlike boxing. In boxing, rule and equipment differences between amateur and professional bouts lead to much lower injury risk at the amateur level.[9] MMA has no such protections. Much like boxing injuries, which likely occur at a higher rate in unsanctioned or informal events,[25] "backyard" MMA is likely to be quite dangerous; however, useful epidemiologic data are lacking.

Male participants commonly fight in baggy "fight shorts" or tight-fitting spandex shorts. The torso is rarely covered by a compression shirt, tank top, or fighting robe (such as the Karate "gi" or Taekwondo "dobok"). Women wear similar attire with the addition of a sports bra or compression top.

Injury epidemiology in MMA is poorly described in the literature. Most data are focused on sanctioned professional matches, and no data on the number of injuries sustained during training or in unsanctioned "backyard" bouts are available. Ngai et al[26] reviewed injuries from 635 professional bouts over 5 years and found 300 total injuries, for an injury rate of 26 per 100 exposures. They also reported a concussion rate of 15.4 per 1000 exposures. Scoggin et al[27] reported similar rates of 55 injuries and 11 concussions in 116 professional bouts.

PARKOUR

Parkour is a discipline of obstacle course training in which participants, or traceurs, attempt to traverse a course or environment in the most efficient way possible using only their bodies and their surroundings. Parkour is not traditionally a competitive sport but rather a holistic training discipline. However, a growing number of parkour competitions focus on either the aesthetic aspects of the discipline or timed trials through set courses, or both.

Traceurs aim to move through their environment using the most efficient movement for the given situation. This can include running, climbing, swinging, jumping, rolling, vaulting, and specialized landing techniques. Traceurs train to improve their efficiency with each of these movements so that they can be used on new obstacles and environments as needed. Some traceurs can land on solid ground without injury after jumping from remarkable heights. There is some evidence that parkour precision landing techniques produce less maximal vertical landing force and landing loading rates than traditional landing techniques.[28] Although the physical training of parkour is an important aspect of the discipline, visualization of the environment and creativity in movement also play major roles. There is some evidence that this type of spatial awareness causes traceurs to perceive their environment differently than non-practitioners. For example, trained traceurs estimate the height of a scalable wall as lower than do untrained novices.[29]

Despite a long history of similar disciplines and the widely used practice of classic obstacle course methods in military training, modern parkour did not develop until the 1980s. The sport grew in popularity throughout the 1990s and 2000s as a result of documentaries and exhibitions. As the Internet became more widely available, videos of traceurs completing amazing feats of athleticism drove rapid growth in the mid- to late-2000s. The James Bond film *Casino Royale* opened with a chase scene involving very technical parkour techniques and is largely credited with the current popularity of the discipline.

Around the time *Casino Royale* was released, case reports of parkour-related injuries began to appear in the medical literature.[30] By 2008 there were case reports of severe injuries and warnings that growth of the discipline would lead to a higher number of injured traceurs presenting to emergency departments.[31]

The first epidemiologic study of parkour-related injuries was not published until 2013.[32] This retrospective cross-sectional study of 266 German traceurs used an online survey to query subjects about injuries sustained in the previous year. Traceurs reported 1.9 injuries per subject per year and 5.5 injuries per 1000 hours of training. Upper extremity injuries accounted for 58% of all injuries and lower extremity injuries for 27%. Head and back injuries were relatively rare. Most injuries were minor, with 70% of all reported injuries being simple abrasions. Muscle injuries accounted for 13% of injuries, and 6% were dislocations. Sixty-one percent of injuries occurred during landing. Overestimating (23%) and misjudging (20%) were the most common reasons given for injury. Only 12% of traceurs used any type of precautionary equipment or measure.

Although the current evidence suggests that most parkour-related injuries are minor, there are case reports of catastrophic injuries[33] and popular media accounts of deaths. In 2012, a 24-year-old Russian woman fell to her death after she attempted a very difficult jump between 2 rooftops in what was reported to be her first parkour lesson.[34] In 2013, popular Russian traceur Pavel Kashin fell to his death when he lost his balance doing a back flip on the edge of a 16-story building in St. Petersburg.[35] Unfortunately, both of these accounts illustrate a common misconception about parkour. The popular media commonly equates daredevil acts with the practice of parkour. Although there may be an element of danger in some aspects of parkour, most traceurs would not attempt such risky maneuvers, and parkour purists are quick to point out that such death-defying feats have nothing to do with the deliberate progressive physical training that is central to parkour practice.

WILDERNESS SPORTS

Access to activities in the wilderness seems almost unlimited now that air travel is frequent to remote locations. People often enter the wilderness with little knowledge, preparation, or planning. Mort and Godden[36] performed a systematic review of 50 articles on injuries that occurred in individuals participating in mountain and wilderness sports from 1987 to 2010. Most mountain and wilderness sports injuries are minor to moderate, and occur in young adults (20-39 years of age) and in males (70%-90%). The percentage of severe injuries ranged from 5% to 10%, with less than 10% of participants admitted to the hospital. Deaths related to wilderness activities are relatively uncommon. Newman et al[37] reviewed all deaths of children between 1 and 20 years of age involving a wilderness recreational activity in 5 western Washington counties over 10 years (from 1987 to 1996) based on medical examiners' logs. Of the 40 cases that were found, 90% were male, and 83% were 13 to 19 years old. Hiking (33%), swimming (20%), and river rafting (10%) were the most common activities resulting in death. Death most often was the result of drowning (55%) or closed head injury (26%). All children younger than 10 years were accompanied by an adult compared to only 26% of children 10 years or older. No victim wore a personal flotation device (PFD) or helmet, and only 5% had foul weather gear. Parental accompaniment, preparation, planning, and use of safety equipment should be encouraged for any wilderness trip even if the activity is considered to be low risk, such as hiking.

Whitewater Rafting

Whitewater rafting is a common pastime for families in the mountains of eastern and western United States. In general, guided rafting trips are thought to be fairly safe; however, individual rivers are very different, and conditions may vary significantly based on recent rainfall and current weather conditions. Attarian and Siderelis[38] reviewed commercial whitewater rafting injuries that occurred on the New and Gauley rivers in West Virginia from 2005 to 2010. They found that musculoskeletal injuries (sprains/strains 21%, dislocations 14%, fractures 12%) comprised the majority (47%) of incidents, followed by soft tissue injuries (lacerations 29%, abrasions 13%, contusions 2%). Almost half of all injuries (44%) occurred to the head, neck, and shoulders, followed by the lower extremity (foot/ankle/leg/knee/hip 34%) and the upper extremity (hand/wrist/arm 14%). Over one-third of injuries occurred when the occupant was ejected from the raft. This finding emphasizes the importance of wearing PFDs and helmets while rafting.

Kayaking

Like other outdoor sports, kayaking in rivers, lakes, and oceans is becoming more popular. Little is known about kayaking injuries in children, although they frequently participate with their adult counterparts. Different types of kayaks include whitewater, expedition, fishing, and inflatable versions. In 2000, Schoen and Stano[39] surveyed 319 whitewater canoe and kayak paddlers of all ages and found 388 acute and 285 chronic injuries. The joints of the upper extremity were the most common sites of injury. The most common acute injuries were sprains/strains (26%), followed by lacerations (17%) and contusions (17%). The most common chronic injury was tendinitis (44%), followed by sprain/strain (27%). Only 47% of acute and 36% of chronically injured paddlers sought medical attention. Injuries as a result of portage or carrying the boat on land were common. Giardia infection is not unusual in whitewater paddlers, so bottled water or water purification systems are recommended.

Sea kayakers face their own unique risks when tides, currents, and wind come into play. Bailey[40] reviewed 50 sea kayaking incident reports from 1992 to 2005 collected by Kiwi Association of Sea Kayakers (KASK) in New Zealand. Of the incidents, 56% occurred in groups, with 20% of those injuries sustained by overseas tourists and 72% in recreational private trips. Most injuries (85%) occurred in men 24 to 39 years old, and 48% were inexperienced. Severity of injury was greater when the capsized kayaker became separated from the kayak, when a PFD was not worn, or when fishing was involved. Hypothermia and sprains were common. Collision with a powered vessel often was fatal. When sea kayaking, the kayaker should take particular care to be aware of weather conditions, tides, and the presence of powered vessels. All kayakers should wear a PFD.

Surfing

Surfing was invented in Hawaii and involves being carried along the face of a breaking wave as it approaches shore, usually on a surfboard. The 2 main types of surfboards are longboards and shortboards, but people may also use knee-boards, boogie boards, kayaks, surf skis, or just their bodies. Various maneuvers that are performed while riding the wave include turning, carving, and banking off the top of the wave. A surfer who is "riding the tube" maneuvers into a position where the wave curls over the top of the surfer before the wave crashes down. Although the incidence is unclear, drownings and near-drownings are significant threats to the surfer. The surfboard may assist a surfer in staying buoyant, but it cannot be relied upon for flotation. An athlete who cannot handle the water conditions without a board should not go into the water to surf. Undertow can cause leashes (a safety device) to become caught on reefs, holding the surfer underwater. Collisions can be caused by impact with either the surfboard nose or fin, causing lacerations and contusions, or with objects under the surface of the water. Impact with sand, coral, or rocks may cause loss of consciousness or even death. Surfers must also be aware of exposure to sea life, including sharks, stingrays, and jellyfish.

Nathanson et al[41] surveyed 1348 surfers of all ages from 1998 to 1999 and found 1237 acute injuries and 477 chronic injuries. Of the acute injuries, lacerations were most common (42%), followed by contusions (13%), sprains/strains (12%), and fractures (8%). Acute injuries were evenly distributed between the lower extremity (37%) and the head and neck (37%). Most occurred from contact with the surfer's own board (55%), from another surfer's board (12%), or from the sea floor (17%). Older surfers, expert surfers, and those surfing large waves have a higher relative risk for significant injury. Surfers should take steps to decrease the risk for injury. Just like with swimming, surfers should always surf in pairs. Beginners should take lessons and use soft foam or rubber surfboards. Rubber-soled water shoes will protect feet from kicking the reef or stepping on sea life. Lycra shirts (rash guards) can protect surfers from friction rash and sunburn. Surfers should wear leashes to keep them tethered to their boards.

River Rope Swings

River rope swings are popular outdoor activities for teenagers. The person uses a rope tied to a tree to swing out over and then drop into the water. Injuries can occur from drowning, hitting unseen objects in the water (shallow water), hitting the bank, or getting tangled in the rope. Sorey et al[42] reviewed cases of injuries associated with falls from river rope swings from 2002 to 2006 from the National Electronic Injury Surveillance System (NEISS). Finger fractures were the most commonly reported injury. The risks of severe injuries, such as lower extremity fractures, concussions, and spinal cord injuries, are similar to those for traditional rope swings. Drowning, finger avulsions, and genital lacerations are more common with river rope swings. Cervical spine injuries may occur with dives from ropes. Drowning is the most common cause of death related to river rope swings. Hazardous features of river rope swings are shallow water, extreme fall height, presence of a small-diameter retrieval line, and use of the rope by a nonswimmer. Before using a river rope swing, the participant should always check the water for proper depth and unseen obstacles.

Rock Climbing

The popularity of rock climbing continues to rise, with people of all ages regularly participating in the sport. This activity can be practiced in indoor climbing gyms or outside on various elements. Bouldering involves free climbing without a rope, usually at lower heights. A safety rope using a belay system is recommended for climbing at any height greater than the person's own height. Using a belay system involves 2 climbers wearing harnesses that attach to the waist (chest can be included for younger climbers), a length of rope, and a belay device that can stop the rope. The rope can be attached at the top of the wall or rock (top roping) or brought up by a climber from the bottom and attached to the wall or rock on the way up (lead climbing). Using a belay requires instruction and practice to be performed correctly and safely.

Schöffl et al[43] prospectively evaluated all attendees of an indoor climbing gym in Stuttgart, Germany, over 5 years from 2007 to 2011. Thirty climbing injuries were recorded (22 in males and 8 in females; mean age 28 ± 11 years). Acute injuries occurred in 6 cases while bouldering, in 16 while lead climbing, and in 7 while top roping. Bouldering injuries were mostly the result of falls onto the mat. The overall injury rate was 0.02 injuries per 1000 hours of climbing activities. Few injuries were sustained, suggesting that indoor climbing has a low risk of acute injury. The injuries were of minor to moderate severity, and no fatalities occurred. Indoor climbing seems to be a fairly safe activity because it is practiced in a relatively controlled and monitored environment.

Outdoor rock climbing seems to be inherently more dangerous than indoor rock climbing because many more variables are at play, including weather, rock conditions, and lack of familiarity with the climb. Lack et al[44] reviewed the Rocky Mountain Rescue Group rock climbing incident reports from 1998 to 2011 in Boulder County, Colorado. Rock climbing rescues accounted for 428 of a total of 2198 (20%) mountain and wilderness rescues. Most rock climbing victims were male (78%) and were between the ages of 20 and 29 years (46%). Roped climbers accounted for 58% of climbing victims, and unroped climbers accounted for 34%. Belay incidents accounted for 12% of climbing victims, and rock falls accounted for 5% of victims. Most victims were uninjured (43% stranded or lost), but the most common injury occurred to the lower extremity (30%). A total of 6% of climbing victims were fatally injured (23 victims: 9 from unroped falls, 5 from lead falls, 3 during lower off, 2 from anchor failure, 2 rock falls and 2 during mountaineering). A large fraction of incidents and fatalities resulted from unroped climbing. Incidents of lost or uninjured stranded climbers and belay incidents accounted for more than half of victims. These incidents likely can be prevented by climbers gaining appropriate experience, seeking local information, and applying some simple safety measures for control of rope belays.

CONCLUSION

The term *extreme sports* encompasses a wide range of activities, from competitive events (such as X Games sports) to training disciplines (such as parkour) to recreational activities (eg, whitewater rafting). Although each of these sports has relatively few participants, the collective rate of participation across the multitude of extreme sports is high. It is unlikely that the medical practitioner who does not participate in any of these sports will truly understand the demands placed on the sport's participants. For this reason, it is important for the physician to discuss the specific requirements, demands, risks and challenges of the sport with the patient. Partnering with the patient to solve challenges of risk mitigation, adaptive exercise, and return to sport can be a rewarding experience for patient and physician alike.

References

1. Taliaferro LA, Rienzo BA, Miller MD, Pigg RM Jr, Dodd VJ. High school youth and suicide risk: exploring protection afforded through physical activity and sport participation. *J School Health*. 2008;78:545-553
2. Yang X, Telama R, Hirvensalo M, Viikari JS, Raitakari OT. Sustained participation in youth sport decreases metabolic syndrome in adulthood. *Int J Obes*. 2009;33:1219-1226
3. Brown DR, Galuska DA, Zhang J, et al. Psychobiology and behavioral strategies. Physical activity, sport participation, and suicidal behavior: U.S. high school students. *Med Sci Sports Exerc*. 2007;39:2248-2257
4. Babiss LA, Gangwisch JE. Sports participation as a protective factor against depression and suicidal ideation in adolescents as mediated by self-esteem and social support. *J Dev Behav Pediatr*. 2009;30:376-384
5. Marar M, McIlvain NM, Fields SK, Comstock RD. Epidemiology of concussions among United States high school athletes in 20 sports. *Am J Sports Med*. 2012;40:747-755
6. Darrow CJ, Collins CL, Yard EE, Comstock RD. Epidemiology of severe injuries among United States high school athletes: 2005 to 2007. *Am J Sports Med*. 2009;37:1798-1805
7. Soreide K, Ellingsen CL, Knutson V. How dangerous is BASE jumping? An analysis of adverse events in 20,850 jumps from the Kjerag Massif, Norway. *J Trauma*. 2007;62:1113-1117
8. Bianco M, Pannozzo A, Fabbricatore C, et al. Medical survey of female boxing in Italy in 2002 to 2003. *Br J Sports Med*. 2005;39:532-536
9. Zazryn T, Cameron P, McCrory P. A prospective cohort study of injury in amateur and professional boxing. *Br J Sports Med*. 2006;40:670-674
10. Butler RJ, Forsythe WI, Beverly DW, Adams LM. A prospective controlled investigation of the cognitive effects of amateur boxing. *J Neurol Neurosurg Psychiatry*. 1993;56:1055-1061
11. Porter MD. A 9-year controlled prospective neuropsychologic assessment of amateur boxing. *Clin J Sport Med*. 2003;13:339-352
12. Caine DJ. The epidemiology of injury in adventure and extreme sports. *Med Sport Sci*. 2012;58:1-16
13. American Academy of Pediatrics Committee on Injury and Poison Prevention. Snowmobiling hazards. *Pediatrics*. 2000;106:1142-1144
14. Rice MR, Alvanos L, Kenney B. Snowmobile injuries and deaths in children: a review of national injury data and state legislation. *Pediatrics*. 2000;105(3 Pt 1):615-619
15. Decou JM, Fagerman LE, Ropele D, et al. Snowmobile injuries and fatalities in children. *J Pediatr Surg*. 2003;38:784-787
16. Illingworth CM. Injuries to children riding BMX bikes. *Br Med J*. 1984;289:956-957

17. Gobbi A, Tuy B, Panuncialman I. The incidence of motocross injuries: a 12-year investigation. *Knee Surgery Sports Traumatol Arthrosc.* 2004;12:574-580

18. Gorski TF, Gorski YC, McLeod G, et al. Patterns of injury and outcomes associated with motocross accidents. *Am Surg.* 2003;69:895-898

19. Nathanson A, Haynes P, Galanis D. Surfing injuries. *Am J Emerg Med.* 2002;20:155-160

20. Higgins M. A Skateboarding ramp reaches for the sky. November 1, 2006. Available at: www.nytimes.com/2006/11/01/sports/othersports/01ramp.html. Accessed September 1, 2014

21. Caleb Moore dies after crash. January 31, 2013. Available at: xgames.espn.go.com/article/8901435/caleb-moore-died-snowmobile-accident-x-games-aspen. Accessed September 1, 2014

22. Sarah Burke Dies from injuries. January 15, 2012. Available at: xgames.espn.go.com/skiing/article/7466421/sarah-burke-dies-injuries-suffered-utah. Accessed September 1, 2014

23. Keh A. Sarah Burke, freestyle skier, dies from injuries in training. January 20, 2012. Available at: www.nytimes.com/2012/01/20/sports/skiing/sarah-burke-canadian-freestyle-skier-dies-from-injuries.html. Accessed September 1, 2014

24. Associated Press. In wake of Caleb Moore death, X Games drops best tricks events for snowmobile, Moto X competitions. March 13, 2013. Available at: www.nydailynews.com/sports/more-sports/x-games-drops-events-wake-athlete-death-article-1.1287897. Accessed September 1, 2014

25. Potter MR, Snyder AJ, Smith GA. Boxing injuries presenting to U.S. emergency departments, 1990 to 2008. *Am J Prev Med.* 2011;40:462-467

26. Ngai KM, Levy F, Hsu EB. Injury trends in sanctioned mixed martial arts competition: a 5-year review from 2002 to 2007. *Br J Sports Med.* 2008;42:686-689

27. Scoggin JF 3rd, Brusovanik G, Pi M, et al. Assessment of injuries sustained in mixed martial arts competition. *Am J Orthop.* 2010;39:247-251

28. Puddle DL, Maulder PS. Ground reaction forces and loading rates associated with parkour and traditional drop landing techniques. *J Sports Sci Med.* 2013;12:122-129

29. Taylor JE, Witt JK, Sugovic M. When walls are no longer barriers: perception of wall height in parkour. *Perception.* 2011;40:757-760

30. McLean CR, Houshian S, Pike J. Pediatric fractures sustained in Parkour (free running). *Injury.* 2006;37:795-797

31. Miller JR, Demoiny SG. Parkour: a new extreme sport and a case study. *J Foot Ankle Surg.* 2008;47:63-65

32. Wanke EM, Thiel N, Groneberg DA, Fischer A. [Parkour—"art of movement": and its injury risk]. *Sportverletz Sportschaden.* 2013;27:169-176

33. Derakhshan N, Zarei MR, Malekmohammady Z, Rahimi-Movaghar V. Spinal cord injury in Parkour sport (free running): a rare case report. *Chin J Traumatol.* 2014;17:178-179

34. Reilly J. Russian "parkour" girl, 24, falls 17 storeys to her death after building jump goes horribly wrong. June 4, 2012. Available at: www.dailymail.co.uk/news/article-2154373/Russian-parkour-girl-24-falls-17-storeys-death-building-jump-goes-horribly wrong.html. Accessed September 1, 2014

35. Pavel Kashin falls to death. July 7, 2013. www.farang-mag.com/?P=4378. Accessed September 1, 2014

36. Mort A, Godden D. Injuries to individuals participating in mountain and wilderness sports: a review. *Clin J Sport Med.* 2011;21:530-536

37. Newman LM, Diekema DS, Shubkin CD, Klein EJ, Quan L. Pediatric wilderness recreational deaths in western Washington State. *Ann Emerg Med.* 1998;32:687-692

38. Attarian A, Siderelis C. Injuries in commercial whitewater rafting on the New and Gauley rivers of West Virginia. *Wilderness Environ Med.* 2013;24:309-314

39. Schoen RG, Stano MJ. Year 2000 whitewater injury survey. *Wilderness Environ Med.* 2002;13:119-124

40. Bailey I. An analysis of sea kayaking incidents in New Zealand 1992 to 2005. *Wilderness Environ Med.* 2010;21:208-218

41. Nathanson A, Haynes P, Galanis D. Surfing Injuries. *Am J Emerg Med.* 2002;20:155-160

42. Sorey WH, Cassidy LD, Crout J, Blount P. River tree rope swing injuries. *South Med J.* 2008;101:699-702

43. Schöffl VR, Hoffmann G, Küpper T. Acute injury risk and severity in indoor climbing: a prospective analysis of 515,337 indoor climbing wall visits in 5 years. *Wilderness Environ Med.* 2013;24:187-194

44. Lack DA, Sheets AL, Entin JM, Christenson DC. Rock climbing rescues: causes, injuries, and trends in Boulder County, Colorado. *Wilderness Environ Med.* 2012;23:223-230

Note: Page numbers of articles are in **boldface** type. Page references followed by "*f*" and "*t*" denote figures and tables, respectively.

metabolic adjustments, 119
nutritional therapy, 128–129
orthorexia, 129
osteoporosis, 121, 127
physiology, 118–120
protein needs, 131
race and ethnicity, 124–125
repartitioning of energy away from growth
    and reproduction, 119
simple 500-calorie nutritional additions, 132
Tanner stage, 130
treatment, 127–134
vegetarians/vegans, 129, 131
Female Athlete Triad Coalition Consensus
    Paper (2014), 124, 127, 132–134
FERPA. *See* Federal Educational Rights and
    Privacy Act (FERPA)
FFM. *See* Fat-free mass (FFM)
FHL tenosynovitis. *See* Flexor hallucis longus
    (FHL) tenosynovitis
Fifth position (ballet), 145*f*
Finger fracture, 54, 56, 57
First position (ballet), 145*f*
Flexor hallucis longus (FHL) tenosynovitis,
    156–157
Fluid replacement, 200–201, 201*t*
FMS. *See* Functional Movement Screen (FMS)
Focal peripheral nerve injury, 60
Folliculitis, 27*t*
Foot injuries (dance), 156–159
Football helmet, 47*t*, 48
Fourth position (ballet), 145*f*
Fracture
    avulsion fracture of the pelvis, 64–65, 65*f*
    dancer's, 158
    Jones, 158
    Maisonneuve, 68
    on-the-field emergency, 7, 8*t*
    physeal, 73–75
    scaphoid, 55–56, 55*f*
    Seymour, 54–55, 54*f*
    skull, 44
    stress, 24, 71–73, 125, 159
Fracture splinting, 7, 8*t*
Fructose, 181
Fruits and vegetables, 184–185
Functional knee valgus, 101, 102*f*
Functional Movement Screen (FMS), 101–104,
    104*f*, 105*f*, 112
Functional outcomes questionnaire, 112
Functional reserve, 28
Functional screening, 13

G

G2 (rehydration fluid), 201*t*
Gamekeeper's thumb, 57
Gastrointestinal examination, 25–26
Gatorade, 201*t*

Gatorade Sports Science Institute, 203*t*
GCS. *See* Glasgow coma score (GCS)
Gene doping, 175
General musculoskeletal screening
    examination, 24
Generalized anxiety disorder, 165
Genitourinary examination, 26
Ghent criteria, 23
GI. *See* Glycemic index (GI)
Giardia infection, 216
Gilette test, 155*f*. *See also* Stork test
GL. *See* Glycemic load (GL)
Glasgow coma score (GCS), 42, 45
Gluten restriction, 128
Glycemic index (GI), 181
Glycemic load (GL), 181
Good Samaritan laws, 1
Grade I spondylolisthesis, 92, 92*f*
Greater trochanter, 64
Growth and development, 148–149
Growth hormone abuse, 176, 179–180
Gymnast
    back pain, 91–93
    bone accumulation and loss, 123–124
    stress management, 165
    wrist pain, 85–86
Gymnast wrist, 85–86

H

Hallux rigidus, 158
Hamstring, 88, 89*t*
Hamstring injuries, 110–111
Hamwi equation, 130
Hand injuries, 53–58
    central slip rupture, 56–57
    jersey finger, 57
    mallet finger, 56
    scaphoid fracture, 55–56, 55*f*
    Seymour fracture, 54–55, 54*f*
    skier's thumb, 57–58, 58*f*, 59*f*
    ulnar collateral ligament (UCL) injury,
        57–58, 58*f*, 59*f*
Harris-Benedict equation, 120
Head lice, 27*t*
Head injury. *See* Concussion
Heads Up Program, 47*t*
Health care team, 2–3
Health Insurance Portability and
    Accountability Act (HIPAA), 11
Heat acclimatization, 197. *See also* Hydration
    in sports
Heat exhaustion, 10–11
Heat illness, 10–11, 13, 196, 196*t*, 197
Heat stroke, 10
Heat tolerance symptoms, 197
Helmets, 47*t*, 48
Hematologic examination, 30
Herbal products, 178